Social Insurance and Social Justice

Social Security, Medicare, and the Campaign Against Entitlements

Leah Rogne, PhD, is associate professor of sociology at Minnesota State University, Mankato. She is the coordinator of Minnesota State, Mankato's Applied Sociology program and former interim director of its Gerontology Program/Center on Aging. She is a founding member of Concerned Scientists in Aging.

Carroll L. Estes, PhD, is professor of sociology at the University of California, San Francisco in the School of Nursing and founding and first director of the Institute for Health and Aging (1979–1998). Dr. Estes is a member of the Institute of Medicine of the National Academy of Sciences, and she is past president of the Gerontological Society of America, the American Society on Aging, and the Association for Gerontology in Higher Education. She has served as consultant to U.S. Commissioners of Social Security and Congressional Committees on Aging.

Brian R. Grossman, MSPH, is a doctoral candidate in sociology at the University of California, San Francisco. He is an instructor in the Health Science Department at San Jose State University and in the Department of Sociology and the Graduate Program in Gerontology at San Francisco State University. He is a project associate with Students for Social Security.

Brooke A. Hollister, PhD, is assistant professor of sociology at the University of California, San Francisco. Brooke is the national director and cofounder of Students for Social Security and Concerned Scientists in Aging. She is currently serving as vice chair of the Gray Panther's National Board of Directors.

Erica Solway, MSW, MPH, is a doctoral candidate in sociology in the Department of Social and Behavioral Sciences at the University of California, San Francisco. She is a project associate with Students for Social Security.

Social Insurance and Social Justice

Social Security, Medicare, and the Campaign Against Entitlements

LEAH ROGNE, CARROLL L. ESTES,
BRIAN R. GROSSMAN, BROOKE A. HOLLISTER
AND ERICA SOLWAY

EDITORS

SPRINGER PUBLISHING COMPANY
New York

Springer Publishing Company, LLC
11 West 42nd Street
New York, NY 10036–8002
www.springerpub.com

Acquisitions Editor: Jennifer Perillo
Project Manager: Cindy Fullerton
Cover design: Steve Pisano
Composition: Aptara Inc.

09 10 11 12/ 5 4 3 2 1

Ebook ISBN: 9780826116154

Library of Congress Cataloging-in-Publication Data

Social insurance and social justice : social security, medicare, and the campaign against entitlements / Carroll L. Estes . . . [et al.].
p. cm.
Includes index.
ISBN 978-0-8261-1614-7 (alk. paper)
1. Social security – United States. 2. Social justice – United States.
I. Estes, Carroll L.
HD7125.S585 2009
368.4′300973–dc22 2008054123

Printed in the United States of America by Bang Printing.

Contents

PART V: TEACHING SOCIAL INSURANCE: CRITICAL PEDAGOGY AND SOCIAL JUSTICE

Contributors

W. Andrew Achenbaum, PhD, is a professor of history and social work at the University of Houston.

Nancy J. Altman is the author of *The Battle for Social Security: From FDR's Vision to Bush's Gamble* (2005).

Robert M. Ball, who first went to work for the Social Security Administration in 1939, served as commissioner of the Social Security Administration under Presidents Kennedy, Johnson, and Nixon. He died January 30, 2008, at the age of 93.

Robert H. Binstock, PhD, is professor of Aging, Health, and Society at Case Western Reserve University.

Patricia K. Cianciolo, PhD, is a professor in the Sociology and Social Work Department at Northern Michigan University.

Fay Lomax Cook, PhD, is director of the Institute for Policy Research and professor of human development and social policy in the School of Education and Social Policy at Northwestern University.

John Cornman, a former executive director of the Gerontological Society of America, is a principal with Consultants on Purpose, LLC, formed in 1996 to help nonprofit organizations succeed in competitive, changing markets.

Meredith B. Czaplewski is a doctoral candidate in the department of political science and a graduate fellow at the Institute of Policy Research at Northwestern University.

G. William Domhoff, PhD, is a research professor of sociology at the University of California, Santa Cruz.

C. Joanne Grabinski, MA, ABD, is president/educator and consultant for AgeEd in Mt. Pleasant, Michigan; lecturer in the gerontology program, Eastern Michigan University; and visiting professor in human development: gerontology at Saint Joseph College in West Hartford, Connecticut.

Madonna Harrington Meyer, PhD, is director of the Syracuse University Gerontology Center.

Martha Holstein, PhD, teaches health care ethics at Loyola University; professional ethics at Northwestern University; and serves as codirector of the Center for Long-Term Care Reform at the Health and Medicine Policy Research Group in Chicago.

Malcolm Johnson, PhD, is professor of gerontology and end-of-life care at the University of Bath in England.

Barbara B. Kennelly, president and CEO of the National Committee to Preserve Social Security and Medicare, served 17 years as a member of the U.S. Congress. In 2006, she was appointed to the Social Security Advisory Board by Speaker of the House Nancy Pelosi.

Eric R. Kingson, PhD, professor of social work and public administration, is a member of the faculty of the Syracuse University School of Social Work.

Philip R. Lee, MD, PhD, is senior scholar in the Philip R. Lee Institute for Health Policy Studies and professor emeritus of social medicine, Department of Medicine, School of Medicine at the University of California, San Francisco.

Phoebe S. Liebig, PhD, is a professor emerita of gerontology and public administration at the University of Southern California.

Harry R. Moody, PhD, is director of academic affairs for AARP.

Thomas R. Oliver, PhD, is associate professor of population health sciences at the University of Wisconsin School of Medicine and Public Health. He also serves as associate director for health policy at the University of Wisconsin Population Health Institute.

Chris Phillipson, PhD, is professor of applied social studies and social gerontology at Keele University, UK.

Edgar E. Rivas, MS, MPP, is a portfolio manager for AARP's Office of Diversity and Inclusion in Washington, DC.

James H. Schulz, PhD, is professor emeritus of economics at the Florence Heller Graduate School, Brandeis University.

E. Percil Stanford, PhD, is the chief diversity officer of AARP and professor emeritus at San Diego State University.

Bernard A. Steinman, MS, is a researcher at the Andrus Gerontology Center and a doctoral candidate at the Davis School of Gerontology at the University of Southern California in Los Angeles.

Debra Street, PhD, is an associate professor and director of graduate studies in the Department of Sociology at SUNY-Buffalo and faculty fellow of the University at Buffalo Regional Institute.

Judie Svihula, PhD, is a research scientist at the Institute on Aging, University of North Carolina at Chapel Hill. She is a fellow of the NIH-NIA funded Carolina Program for Health and Aging Research at the Institute.

Amanda Torre-Norton currently serves as the research associate for the evaluation of Project Home, conducted by the Cornell Institute for Translational Research on Aging (CITRA).

Valentine M. Villa, PhD, is a professor of social work at California State University, Los Angeles, and adjunct associate professor at the UCLA School of Public Health, Department of Community Health Sciences, and senior researcher with the UCLA Center for Health Policy Research.

Alan Walker, PhD, is professor of social policy and social gerontology at the University of Sheffield, UK.

Steven P. Wallace, PhD, is professor at the UCLA School of Public Health, vice-chair of the Department of Community Health Sciences, and associate director of the UCLA Center for Health Policy Research.

Donna L. Yee, PhD, is CEO of the Asian Community Center (ACC) in Sacramento, California, a nonprofit organization that serves older adults.

Foreword

We can never insure one hundred percent of the population against one hundred percent of the hazards and vicissitudes of life, but we have tried to frame a law which will give some measure of protection to the average citizen and to his family against the loss of a job and against poverty-ridden old age.

—President Franklin D. Roosevelt upon signing the Social Security Act, 1935

Poverty-ridden old age. It is hard to imagine our not-so-distant past when many Americans faced old age without income, assets, or even the basic necessities of life. In 1935, more half of the nation's elderly were poverty stricken. Today, this sad part of our history is gone. Far fewer American seniors live in poverty or are denied access to medical care thanks to social insurance programs like Social Security and Medicare. Though benefits are modest, the programs are a lifeline for millions of families. Like other risk pools designed to insure individuals against physical and material losses, social insurance continues to provide income protection for workers and their families, retirees, and the disabled.

Unfortunately, many conservatives and private market advocates ridicule social insurance as an archaic system of government handouts. Over the years, opponents of social insurance have fomented intergenerational warfare, pitting the young against the old in an effort to erode support for Social Security and Medicare among those unfamiliar with the programs' many virtues. In fact, the Social Security system reflects the ways in which the generations are interdependent. The system contributes to the well being of Americans by providing a foundation of retirement income that permits seniors to live in dignity and independence. In addition to retired worker and spousal benefits, wage earners receive insurance protection for themselves and their families if they should become disabled or die.

Through economic crises, natural disasters, and wartime, America's social insurance programs have remained reliable constants in a changing world. These are *not* the antiquated and archaic programs portrayed by those opposed to any government social insurance role. In fact, quite the contrary is true. Social insurance programs showcase the best of what government *can* do for its citizens and create a lasting compact between our citizens and their government.

In January 2007, Kathleen Casey-Kirschling applied for Social Security retirement benefits. Although thousands of people apply for benefits every day, this one single act is notable because Casey-Kirschling is the Nation's unofficial "first baby boomer." Her retirement begins a new era in American history—one in which our government's ability to support generations of retirees will be tested as never before.

The fact is, baby boomers are no different from anyone else; there are simply more of them than the age cohorts before and behind them. And it will take them at least 2 decades before they have all left the workforce. This will create a long-term funding gap for Social Security, but it does not create an insurmountable crisis. Baby boomers are not a well-kept secret. They did not creep up on us like thieves in the night. The bulge in that generation has been working its way through society ever since they were born. When they needed schools, this country built them. When they needed housing, this country helped finance them. Their work through the years helped build the economy that we see today.

Now, they are on the doorstep of retirement, and some economists would like us to think this is an unexpected surprise that will plunge us into economic chaos and leave Generation X and those following behind in poverty. This could not be further from the truth. As a result of the changes that were enacted in 1983, Social Security will remain solvent until the youngest of the boomers is nearly 80 years old. Even without any changes at all, Social Security will pay all but about 25% of benefits thereafter.

Still, conservative economists and their supporters use the myth of boomer-generated catastrophe to fuel their unrelenting assault on the two enduring icons of the New Deal. It is clear that those of us who believe in the value of social insurance cannot afford to become complacent about the future.

Although many believe the battle against privatization has already been won, we must remember that millions of dollars still flow into the think tanks and conservative policy offices that support Social Security private accounts. We also must remember that Medicare is already well on its way to privatization. The Medicare Modernization Act of 2003 created a prescription drug benefit that is only available through private insurance companies. The legislation also created massive subsidies for Medicare Advantage, private health care sold to seniors under the umbrella of the Medicare program, where insurance companies receive an average 13% more per beneficiary than it would cost the federal government to cover those same seniors in traditional Medicare. And 2008 Republican Presidential nominee Senator John McCain, a strong supporter of private accounts, called Social Security's fundamental structure "a disgrace" (Denver, July 7, 2008) and named a long-standing champion of privatization, Martin Feldstein, as his surrogate spokesperson on the issue.

Proponents of privatization have spent years quietly planting the seeds of their propaganda in the press and in the public. President Bush frequently used words that fed the scare tactics of the privatizers—claiming the program will be "bust" or "flat broke" soon. Arguments such as these simply feed young people's belief that Social Security will not be there for them when they retire. What they do not fully understand is that the financial world they face is much riskier than that of previous generations, and they will absolutely need a guaranteed Social Security benefit and a program to cover their medical expenses when they reach late life.

In this book, Carroll Estes and her associates have gathered some of our leading scholars on social insurance to tell the story of the role of these programs in our country. They tell us how Social Security and Medicare came into being in the United States, discuss the ways the programs support economic and health security for all Americans, and emphasize especially how socially marginalized populations are affected by current policy and proposed changes. They discuss the politics involved in the debates about social insurance reform and suggest a variety of strategies to make reasonable changes to ensure the future viability of social insurance programs.

As I write this foreword, it is the 73rd anniversary of President Franklin D. Roosevelt's signing of the Social Security Act, and the fundamental promises we made to one another are under concerted attack. Now, more than ever, we must tell the story of how social insurance programs have assured basic economic and health security for millions of

Americans and how we can continue to fulfill the vital commitments that have made us a strong and caring nation. This book is a must-read for anyone who cares about these goals.

> *—BARBARA B. KENNELLY is the president and executive director of the National Committee to Preserve Social Security and Medicare. She served for 17 years in the U.S. House of Representatives from the state of Connecticut.*

Acknowledgments

The editors of this book first want to thank the authors who contributed to this volume for their dedication to research and teaching on social insurance.

We are especially grateful to Marilyn Hennessy of the Retirement Research Foundation and Bill Novelli, Betsy Sprouse, and Harry Moody from AARP for the support they have given to our work on social insurance, and to Paul Vandeventor and Community Partners, who have provided us with a nonprofit administrative home for Concerned Scientists in Aging and Students for Social Security. Additionally, we would like to thank Pamela Larson from the National Academy of Social Insurance, and Barbara Kennelly, Maria Freese, and Sandy Wise of the National Committee to Preserve Social Security and Medicare, who provided support and technical assistance regarding multiple policy issues.

We are grateful for the assistance and guidance of fellow members of Students for Social Security and Concerned Scientists in Aging, especially Melissa Shoshone Bartley and Marilyn Oakes Greenspan for their preliminary research on teaching social insurance.

We would like to thank our colleagues at the Institute for Health & Aging and the Department of Social & Behavioral Sciences at the University of California, San Francisco for their support, guidance, and assistance. In particular, Patrick Fox, Wendy Max, and Regina Gudelunas, were instrumental in arranging access to office space, phone lines, and printing facilities for the UCSF editors.

We also thank Minnesota State University, Mankato's College of Social and Behavioral Sciences and Department of Sociology and Corrections for their assistance and especially Karen Purrington and Kelsey Kruse for their administrative support.

And special thanks to our editor, Jennifer Perillo, and all the staff at Springer who tirelessly pushed this volume along.

Leah Rogne wants to acknowledge the support and encouragement of her family: Fred, Janos, Leslie, Beth, Kaja, Amara, and Sonja. She would like to give special thanks to her parents, Leslie and Katherine Rogne, for their ongoing dedication to a world in which people care about one another.

Carroll Estes would like to express her dedication of this work to her daughter, Duskie Lynn Estes, and her granddaughters, Brydie and MacKenzie. She would also like to dedicate this work to all future generations who will benefit from the nation's rededication to its vital and vibrant social insurance programs.

Brian Grossman would like to express his deep gratitude to Malcolm Haar, the man with whom he shares his life, for his emotional support and his services as a late-night proofreader. Brian thanks his family for their willingness to talk about the importance of this work: Linda and Henry Grossman; Sharon, Jason, Jake, Max, and Char Moses; Gail, Bob, Matthew, Haley, Alex and Kaitlin Haar; and Bernice Rothschild. Brian is also thankful to those family members who are no longer living but whose lives have been an inspiration: Rosie Grossman, Gertrude Marks, and Margot and Eddie North.

Brooke Hollister would like to dedicate this book to members of Students for Social Security and Concerned Scientists in Aging, who, since 2004, have tirelessly contributed to intergenerational efforts to educate the public on and advocate for the preservation and expansion of social insurance programs.

Erica Solway would like to acknowledge her grandparents, Leatrice Brawer, Bernie Brawer, Joan Brawer, Etta Solway, and Paul Solway, for their enduring love, encouragement, and support.

We all express our gratitude for the pioneering efforts of two of our most significant mentors and visionaries, the late Maggie Kuhn, cofounder of the Gray Panthers, and the late Tish Sommers, cofounder of the Older Women's League (OWL). They transformed our understanding of the intergenerational, structural, and global interconnections upon which the foundations of social insurance and social justice must be built. Their courage and actions continue to inspire and guide us.

In Memoriam: Mr. Social Security: The Extraordinary Contributions of Robert M. Ball

NANCY J. ALTMAN

This book is dedicated to the memory of Robert M. Ball, who died on January 30, 2008, at the age of 93. Ball has been called the spiritual leader of Social Security (Bethell, 2005) and was a key architect of and champion for the development of the Medicare program. In this essay, Nancy Altman, author of The Battle for Social Security: From FDR's Vision to Bush's Gamble, *outlines the influence Ball had on Social Security and Medicare in the United States, both as a Commissioner of Social Security under Presidents Kennedy, Johnson, and Nixon and as a lifelong advocate for social insurance programs in the United States. (Eds.)*

On January 30, 2008, when Robert M. Ball died, every single American, young and old, rich and poor, from every walk of life, and from every ethnic background, lost a tireless advocate. From the age of 24 until nearly his last breath, just short of his 94th birthday, Ball spent most of his waking hours dedicated to the successful pursuit of safeguarding and improving Social Security.

As a result of his 7 decades of dedication to Social Security, he is more responsible than any other person, living or dead, for all the good that Social Security does. He is more responsible than any other civil servant or presidential appointee, than any chairman of a congressional committee, than any president—more than Lyndon B. Johnson, more even than Franklin D. Roosevelt himself. Ball, more than anyone else, is responsible for the:

- 13 million seniors and 1 million children that Social Security currently lifts out of poverty (Sherman & Shapiro, 2005);
- 34 million seniors who are able to live with dignity, as a result of a guaranteed income and the independence that accompanies that guarantee (Social Security Administration, 2008a);
- 4 million widows and widowers who are able to maintain financial independence after the loss of a spouse (Social Security Administration, 2008a);
- 7 million Americans who receive Social Security benefits because their paychecks have been lost as a result of a serious disability (Social Security Administration, 2008a);
- 3.1 million children of deceased, disabled, and retired workers who receive Social Security benefits each month and another 3.4 million children who, while not receiving benefits themselves, live in the homes of relatives who do (Lavery & Reno, 2008);
- 164 million workers and their families who are currently insured by Social Security against the risk that they and their families might one day lose the security of their paychecks as a result of disability, old age, or death (Social Security Administration, 2008b).

Ball possessed an extraordinary and unusual set of strengths that allowed him to make such remarkable and far-reaching contributions to his fellow Americans. Throughout his life, he was a man of strong principles. At the same time, he worked hard to understand the views of others. He possessed a gentle spirit and warmth, with a light-hearted sense of humor. He was even keeled, rarely succumbing to anger or frustration. And his mind was razor-sharp. These qualities made him a natural and gifted negotiator—indeed a born master of the art.

Ball was able to bring people around to his position in a way that made them believe that they were getting *their* way. As a young man of just 31, he saved Social Security—the first of many times, throughout his life. In the late 1940s, more than twice as many senior citizens received means-tested welfare as received Social Security, and the average welfare payment was substantially larger than the average Social Security benefit. When politicians wanted to help their constituents, Social Security was not on their radar screen; the program was largely ignored.

Consequently, its benefits were not keeping pace with either inflation or increasing standards of living. Social Security was in danger of withering away.

In 1947, President Harry S. Truman and the Republican-controlled Congress agreed to establish an advisory council to study and make recommendations about the program. Ball became the Council's executive director. Through his astute and careful stewardship, the Council, which consisted of 17 distinguished members, representing a wide range of views, issued a report calling for the immediate expansion of the program. In 1950, Congress, which had by then fallen into Democratic hands, enacted the recommendations—a piece of legislation labeled by historians as a "new start" for Social Security (Berkowitz, 1998; see, also, Senate Finance Committee Report No. 1669, to accompany Social Security Act Amendments of 1950, 81st Congress, 2d Session, at 7 ["In order to have such a "new start" average wage, the individual . . . ."])

I personally witnessed a more recent example of Ball's skills as a master negotiator. In 1982, Ball was appointed to serve on the bipartisan commission established to solve Social Security's then-projected deficit. He became the de facto leader of the Democratic members and the representative of then-Speaker of the House, Thomas "Tip" O'Neill. I was the assistant to the commission's chairman, Alan Greenspan. That very successful commission today is frequently mentioned by prominent political leaders as a model to cope with Social Security's current projected deficit. I can attest, as a first-hand observer, the commission only succeeded because of Bob Ball. It would not have succeeded without him.

In addition to being a master negotiator, Ball was a highly skilled and extremely pragmatic administrator. Perhaps the best testament to his extraordinary abilities and extensive contributions is this: Having first been appointed Commissioner of Social Security by President John F. Kennedy in 1962, and reappointed by President Lyndon B. Johnson, this unabashedly liberal Democrat was reappointed yet again, this time by President Richard M. Nixon. Though Ball never concealed his liberal political views, President Nixon wanted to make sure that this important program ran smoothly, which meant keeping it in the hands of the most capable administrator around.

Ball's biggest and most complex administrative responsibility may have been the implementation in 1965 and 1966 of the just-enacted Medicare program, legislation that he helped draft and shepherd through Congress. Ball had the task of ensuring that Americans aged 65 and over had insurance to cover costs for services delivered by 6,600 hospitals, 250,000 physicians, and 1,300 home health agencies.

Adding to the complexity was the enactment—just the year before—of the Civil Rights Act of 1964. Hospitals could participate in Medicare only if they complied with the Civil Rights Act. Most southern hospitals at that time were racially segregated. The interaction of these two revolutionary changes in national policy effectively forced racially segregated hospitals throughout the south to integrate their hospital beds and staffs immediately. In a setting that involves the bathing of patients and other intimate details of life, generations-old policies and practices, based on deep-rooted racial prejudice, had to be changed overnight—and Ball was responsible to ensure that it was done.

Under Ball's leadership, Medicare got off to an incredibly efficient and successful start. In 1966, *The New York Times* reported about Medicare's first day, "The Medicare program, affecting Americans over 65, got off to a smooth start today. Some 160,000 patients already in hospitals from Guam to the East Coast and Puerto Rico automatically became Medicare eligible . . . Others were admitted during the day" (Schweck, 1966).

It is instructive to compare Ball's monumental achievement to the administrative nightmare produced a few years ago, in the implementation of the relatively simple job of adding one new benefit for prescription drugs to Medicare, an already smoothly running program. Here is what *The New York Times* reported about the new drug benefit's inaugural day: "[P]harmacists say beneficiaries may initially experience delays and frustrations as the promise of the new program is translated into practice. Tens of thousands of people who signed up . . . have yet to receive the identification cards that will permit them to fill prescriptions promptly at retail drugstores" (Pear & Freudenheim, 2006).

Unlike the implementation of the entire Medicare program, which involved thousands of hospitals, hundreds of thousands of physicians, and thousands of home health agencies, the implementation of the prescription drug benefit involved around 250,000 pharmacists and around 55,000 pharmacies nationwide. Moreover, Congress gave the Bush Administration over 2 years to do the job (Medicare Prescription Drug, Improvement, and Modernization Act of 2003). In contrast, despite the difficulty of the task, Congress gave the Johnson Administration less than a year to have Medicare up and running (Social Security Amendments of 1965). Moreover, unlike Ball, his counterparts today had the benefit of the information age, with its widespread computer technology, e-mail, faxes, and cell phones.

Ball, always scrupulous to avoid undeserved credit, would have said that the drug benefit scheme was poorly drafted, making implementation very difficult. If pressed, he might acknowledge that he had been responsible for the drafting of Medicare, had helped shepherd it through Congress, and had made sure that it could be implemented. Even then, Ball would be demonstrating undue modesty. Those of us not so reticent about his accomplishments know that his enormous talent, meticulous attention to detail, prodigious hard work, and devotion to public service are the primary reasons for the difference in results.

Perhaps Ball's most important contributions came in the area of policy development. Although the common stereotype is that as people age they become rigid and inflexible, this was decidedly untrue of Ball. He remained, until his death, an extraordinarily forward looking and imaginative thinker. In addition to his skills as a master negotiator and administrator, his flexible, inventive mind, together with his deep understanding of Social Security's philosophical underpinnings, and his hands-on experience with the program's operational side made him a policy genius. The plan he developed to eliminate Social Security's current deficit is a perfect example (see Altman, 2005). As was true of all Ball's policy contributions, his proposal is exceptionally sound policy and brilliantly astute politics. If the president and Congress are smart, they will quickly enact the plan, and resolve Social Security's financing for the foreseeable future. That would be a fitting, posthumous capstone to Ball's illustrious career.

Ball did not think of himself as religious and he had little interest in organized religion. Nevertheless, this minister's son embodied the most important spiritual lessons that religion teaches. He was extremely compassionate, particularly for the plight of the poor. He was extraordinarily generous with his time and energy—life's most important and scarcest gifts. He would spend endless hours with anyone interested in Social Security. He willingly reviewed manuscripts of anyone writing in the field, and he always did so with meticulous care and insight. Even when he had read a draft of a long article three or four times, he would always find something more, a new suggestion or insight he could contribute, which always strengthened the piece.

He possessed a deep respect for all fellow humans. Although he was born 5 years before women were granted the right to vote, he was a feminist to his core. He was completely devoid of prejudice. Indeed, in the months leading up to his death, he was genuinely thrilled at the idea that there might be an African American or female president of the United States. Moreover, he treated children with the same respect he treated everyone else.

Like those called to a ministry, he was devoted to the betterment of others, in his case, through Social Security. From the moment he first received the call, at age 24, he remained faithful to that calling until he took his final breath just 2 months shy of his 94th birthday.

Ball truly left the world better than he found it. He was a giant who cannot be replaced. But he left a vital legacy in the form of an organized and trained professional cadre. Knowing that he would not live forever, he conceived, organized, and nurtured the National Academy of Social Insurance, established in 1986. Today, the organization boasts a membership of more than 800 of the nation's leading experts on Social Security. Moreover, Ball personally inspired and educated hundreds of followers, now experts in their own right, who together must try to do a fraction of the good that this one man did single-handedly in preserving, strengthening, and expanding Social Security.

REFERENCES

Altman, N. J. (2005). *The battle for Social Security: From FDR's vision to Bush's gamble*. Hoboken, NJ: John Wiley & Sons, pp. 297–309.

Berkowitz, E. (1998). The transformation of Social Security. In S. Sass & R. K. Trieste (Eds.), *Social Security reform* (p. 25). Boston: Federal Reserve Bank of Boston.

Bethell, T. N. (2005). Roosevelt redux: Robert M. Ball and the battle for Social Security. *The American Scholar, 74*(2), 18–31.

Lavery, J., & Reno, V. P. (2008). *Children's stake in Social Security* (Social Security Issue Brief No. 27). Washington, DC: National Academy of Social Insurance.

Medicare Prescription Drug, Improvement, and Modernization Act of 2003. (2003, December 8). Part D drug program. Pub.L. 108–173.

Pear, R., & Freudenheim, M. (2006, January 1). As new drug plan begins, stores expect bumps. *The New York Times*, p. Front page.

Schweck, H. M., Jr. (1966, July 2). Medicare is off to smooth start: No overcrowding reported. *The New York Times*, p. Front page.

Sherman, A. (2005). *Social Security lifts one million children above the poverty line*. Washington, DC: Center on Budget and Policy Priorities.

Sherman, A., & Shapiro, I. (2005). *Social Security lifts 13 million seniors above the poverty line: A state-by-state analysis*. Washington, DC: Center on Budget and Policy Priorities.

Social Security Administration. (2008a). Monthly statistical snapshot. Washington, DC: Author.

Social Security Administration. (2008b). Social Security basic facts (Press Office Fact Sheets). Washington, DC: Author.

Social Security Amendments of 1965. (1965, July 30). Pub.L. 89–97.

Introduction: We're All in This Together: Social Insurance, Social Justice, and Social Change

CARROLL L. ESTES, LEAH ROGNE, BRIAN R. GROSSMAN, ERICA SOLWAY, AND BROOKE A. HOLLISTER

> *President Roosevelt in his message of June 8, 1934, to the Congress placed "the security of the men, women and children of the Nation first." He went on to suggest the social insurances with which European countries have had a long and favorable experience as one means of providing safeguards against "misfortunes which cannot be wholly eliminated in this man-made world of ours."*
>
> —(Secretary of Labor Perkins, February 25, 1935)

> *The convergence and interaction of liberating forces at work in society against racism, sexism, ageism, and economic imperialism are all oppressive 'isms' and built-in responses of a society that considers certain groups inferior. All are rooted in the social-economic structures of society. . . . All have resulted in economic and social discrimination. All rob American society of the energies and involvement of creative persons who are needed to make our society just and humane.*
>
> —(Kuhn, 1984, pp. 7–8)

> *Social justice exists in inverse proportion to serious harm and suffering. When social change designed to minimize serious harm is accomplished in a sustained way then social* progress *can be said to have occurred.*
>
> —(Doyal and Gough, 1991, p. 2)

Although "social insurance" is hardly a common household term in the United States today, social insurance programs such as Social Security,

Medicare, and Workers' Compensation are the foundation of economic and health security in this country. These programs provide for elders, younger people with disabilities, survivors, children, women, minorities and, indeed, all persons in the United States. By spreading the risk over a large pool of people, social insurance offers protection against devastating health care costs and protection against loss of income from such events as the death of a parent or spouse, the acquisition of a disability, or retirement.

WHAT IS SOCIAL INSURANCE?

There are diverse programs around the world that can be described as social insurance, and they all share two important characteristics: (1) they are government-sponsored insurance programs that protect citizens from predetermined outcomes that negatively impact their ability to participate in society (e.g., loss of income or loss of health); and (2) they have a communal orientation that considers the entire population, rather than just the individual, when identifying and mitigating risk (DeWitt, 2003). Unlike other forms of social support, social insurance programs do not use means testing (maximum income limits) to determine eligibility. Ideally, social insurance programs are funded by everyone and offer benefits to everyone.

As a concept, social insurance originated in the late 19th century when, in response to the effects of the Industrial Revolution on the German people, German Chancellor Otto Von Bismarck introduced a number of policies, including health insurance (1883), workers' compensation (1884), and compulsory old-age insurance (1889) (DeWitt, 2003) to safeguard his people from financial ruin. From a global perspective, the United States is a relative newcomer to social insurance. In 1911, Wisconsin was the first state to enact workers' compensation legislation, and other states followed suit until all states had such programs by 1959 (U.S. Department of Labor [US DOL], n.d.). It was not until 1935 that old age insurance (in the form of Social Security) was enacted by the U.S. Congress. Nearly 20 years later, in 1956, disability insurance was added to the Social Security program (Social Security Administration [SSA], 2005). Despite the introduction of the Medicare social insurance program for the elderly and Medicaid (not a social insurance program because eligibility depends on a person's income) in 1965 (Center for Medicare and Medicaid Services [CMS], 2006), the United States remains the only industrialized nation without some form of guaranteed health care for the population as a whole.

Social Security is the best-known social insurance program in the United States. Although it is arguably the most successful social program in American history, business and neoliberal interests in the United States have engaged in a concerted, decades-long campaign to undermine confidence in Social Security, especially among young people. Those favoring fundamental restructuring of the Social Security system have been largely successful in convincing many of the country's young people that Social Security will not be there for them when they retire. As a result, younger Americans are more likely to believe that "radical changes" are necessary, if not the only type of reform that will work (Cruikshank, 2003). Likewise, Medicare has come under attack, and claims about its economic instability have fueled efforts in Congress to restrict payments to beneficiaries and providers and to dismantle its fundamental social insurance principles.

Intergenerational Solidarity Under Siege

Clearly, threats to the programs that provide economic and health security affect Americans of all ages and generations. Retirement security and a solution to the potentially devastating costs of health care in later life are family and societal concerns, not just the concerns of old people. However, older persons are more directly dependent upon the substance of and changes in state policy emanating at the federal level than are most other age groups. This is because the economic and health security of elders is built upon retirement arrangements and the provision of medical and other old-age benefits that are guaranteed and secured through the nation state. Each of these systems is influenced by the strength and dominance of vested political, economic, and sociocultural interests in the U.S. nation state and in countries around the globe.

Separate from and in addition to the particular groups of individuals who are placed at greater risk, attempts to privatize and demolish state programs that guarantee health and income security threaten the larger ideal of social solidarity in the United States. Steeped in the neoliberal ideology of the "individual ascendant," these encroachments on social insurance programs ignore, downplay, and invalidate the interdependence of self and society (Twine, 1994) and recast multigenerational cooperative efforts to work together toward common social goals as unfair, antagonistic arrangements of exploitation. The result of this framing, of course, is the production of a constrained set of opportunities for action to address these injustices. Additionally, the consequences ripple further, providing both a political distraction from the truly exploitative nature of late/modern/global capitalism and an illusory cultural reflection of the United States as a nation of individuals rather than a nation of people working together collectively for the common good.

Increasingly, since the presidency of Ronald Reagan, the role and responsibility of the state has become contested as pressures have mounted on the state to roll back the social insurance gains of Roosevelt's New Deal and subsequent decades. Debates about the sustainability of entitlements and the responsibility of the state for upholding the historic social contract of Social Security and Medicare reflect the growing tension between the rising demands and increased power of market forces *versus* the diminished strength of those acting in the public interest in seeking to preserve and enhance the safety and security of all persons in the United States.

Ageism and the Attack on Social Security and Medicare

Ageism is a significant force that is manifested both structurally and ideologically. Structurally, ageism influences the agenda setting, formation, and implementation processes surrounding public policy. Ideologically, ageism bolsters the imagery of elders as undeserving persons who do not deserve the benefits that they have earned and paid for over many generations. Ageism is pernicious in its social and individual consequences (Butler, 2006; International Longevity Center-USA [ILC-USA], 2006; Estes & Portacolone, 2008). On the individual level, ageism extracts a high cost in terms of damaged self-esteem and diminished sense of personal control. In its contemporary form and at the collective structural level, ageism may be defined as the denial of basic and civil rights of elders (ILC-USA, 2006).

Familiar signs of ageism in policy debates are found in the crisis rhetoric that plays off the name-calling epithets of elders as Greedy Geezers, a "demographic tsunami" that the nation cannot afford, and as an undeserving lot who drain U.S. resources needed for capitalist development and productivity (ergo, profit) in the global economy. The name-callers have captured center stage, successfully employing the conservative think tanks and the media in framing its messages of the inevitability of "demography as destiny" and the construction of "apocalyptic demography" (Robertson, 1999). This portrayal runs directly counter to Friedland and Summer's (1999; 2005) evidence that "demography is not destiny."

This new ageism becomes a powerful tool of the New Right in its fight against social insurance and the U.S. welfare state. Blatant and subtle ageism and scare tactics around it are vehicles employed by finance capital and the U.S. state under multiple guises to privatize welfare states around the globe (Estes & Phillipson, 2002). If elders are conceived of as "the other," then threats to elders' well-being are not seen as current or potential threats to oneself, and programs benefiting elders are seen as fundamentally unfair to other generations. The demographic politics of ageism serves as an instrument of the interests of global financial capitalism and the global interests of a powerful medical industrial complex, obscuring the real forces driving the privatization debate.

The Interdependence of Social Insurance Versus the Independence of the "Free Market"

According to Estes, Biggs, and Phillipson (2003), older people in both the United Kingdom and in the United States have benefited from a commitment to interdependence as opposed to individualism, and a state policy that values "shared (as opposed to individual problem solving and responsibility)" and "pooling risks through social insurance (as opposed to individual risks)" (p. 141). In recent decades, however, the public discourse about the welfare state in general and about social insurance in particular has become increasingly negative, portraying successful and long-popular programs like Social Security and Medicare as failures (Marmor, Mashaw, & Harvey, 1990). An ideology of individualism that extols both the economic and moral superiority of the "free market" has come to dominate the policy debates. Alternative visions for programs based on interdependence and collective responsibility are devalued and ridiculed as outmoded and unsustainable.

The result is a move from a long-standing public commitment to intergenerational solidarity to an effort to "*responsibilize* a new senior citizenry to care for itself" (Katz, 2003, p. 26). Such efforts may be understood as part of the larger challenge to social justice and human rights for all citizens of the world. The major beneficiaries of this new climate of individualism (or what has been called the "ownership society") are the corporate members of the capitalist system. The interests that stand to gain most from privatization of social insurance programs are the private insurance industry, banking and investment interests, and the highly profitable medical industrial complex (see Estes, Biggs, & Phillipson, 2003; and Cruikshank, 2003).

Critical Gerontology and Public Social Science

This book is an outgrowth of efforts by an intergenerational group of gerontology scholars and students who came together in 2004 to develop and promote an alternative to neoliberal voices on the privatization debate. These scholars founded two groups, Concerned Scientists in Aging and Students for Social Security, with goals to (1) advance evidence-based knowledge concerning the role of social insurance (including Social Security and Medicare) as the foundation of economic and health security for all Americans and (2) provide public information and education with the aim of increasing the number of college and university conversations about social insurance as a universal human right.

Our objective is to expand the debate, which until now has been largely dominated by economists, to include a variety of disciplinary perspectives. The approach taken by participants in this initiative has invoked the frameworks of critical gerontology and public social science. Critical gerontology combines political economy, feminist theory, and a humanistic approach with a particular emphasis on empowerment (Estes & Phillipson, 2007; Estes & Grossman, 2007). From a critical perspective, scholars seek to "criticize and subvert domination in all its forms" (Bottomore, 1983, p. 183) and to examine and unmask the economic and political forces that shape and sustain the prevailing power arrangements and systems of inequality.

Public social science is a professional practice that calls on scholars and students to take their learning beyond the classroom and the scholarly journals to a wider public through critical conversations, civic engagement, and social movements. Expanding on his pivotal presidential address on public sociology at the 2002 American Sociological Association, sociologist Michael Buroway describes three goals of a public social science:

> The first is to empower subjugated communities in their relations to the structures of domination through collaborative relations between professionals and communities. The second goal is to transform common sense, turning private troubles into public issues. The third is to strengthen the legitimacy and power of the activist-professional and the public social scientists within the professional structures they inhabit (Burawoy, 2007, p. 132).

It is with that spirit that this collection of essays on social insurance is offered—to stimulate understanding as well as individual and collective action to support the goal of social solidarity as it is expressed in the fundamental principles of social insurance.

ORGANIZATION OF THIS BOOK

Featuring the voices of some of the most esteemed scholars in the field, this volume reviews the history of social insurance and provides a framework for understanding current policy debates and the moral and economic consequences of potential reform proposals. As attacks on social programs have increased over the last 2 decades, images of intergenerational division have dominated the public discourse. In contrast, the essays in this volume are oriented toward perspectives of intergenerational cooperation, interdependence, and collective responsibility. It is unlikely that people can make informed choices about the future when they are disconnected from the institutional history of the social and political contexts that energized the will of the people to establish social insurance programs in this country.

By filling a gap in our collective memory about the development and evolution of social insurance programs, the chapters may reconnect our consciousness and re-energize our commitments in the United States and in other nations to a larger and inclusive "commons" in which we embrace one another and the members of future generations. Further, an understanding of the basic principles through which national health care is provided for all members of a society, as it is in all other industrialized countries, is intended to advance discussions about the future of social insurance for universal health care for all persons in the United States.

The essays in this volume are organized into five parts. Part I provides an historical perspective on social insurance in the United States and in Europe and reviews the fundamental principles, values, and interests represented in the development of social insurance programs in the United States and abroad. The chapters in Part II are clustured around a discussion of what is at stake for various groups including women, people of color, and the working and nonworking poor. Part III focuses on the current debates about the future of social insurance and examines important aspects of the public discourses around its future. The chapters in Part IV provide critical perspectives on social insurance reform in the United States and Europe and explore economic dimensions of social insurance programs in the United States that have been largely left out of current debates. In Part V, scholars offer strategies to employ critical pedagogy as a means to empower students and the broader public to become active in society and aware of and informed about the importance of social insurance.

In significant ways, this volume builds on the insights and wisdom of Maggie Kuhn regarding the linkages between and the threats created by the social forces of ageism, sexism, racism, economic imperialism, war, and globalization. Maggie called for the convergence of liberating forces to address "the need for sweeping economic and social change in society" (Kuhn, 1984, p. 6). In the current sociohistorical moment, with a cascading meltdown of financial capital markets, a home mortgage crisis, a spiraling increase in unemployment, we are at a crossroads for social insurance in both developing and developed nations. In the wake of the current crisis, the highly interconnected nature of the global economy underscores the fact that we are indeed all in this together. In putting together this volume, we as editors seek to advance public understanding of social insurance within a framework that promotes a moral commitment to social justice and the awareness of the necessity for collective action and social change to provide for the common good.

REFERENCES

Bottomore, T. B. (1983). *A dictionary of Marxist thought*. Cambridge, MA: Harvard University Press.

Burawoy, M. (2007). Private troubles and public issues. In A. Barlow (Ed.), *Collaborations for social justice: Professionals, publics, and policy change* (pp. 125–133). Lanham, MD: Rowman and Littlefield Publishers, Inc.

Butler, R. N. (2006). Combating ageism: A matter of human and civil rights. In International Longevity Center-USA (Ed.), *Ageism in America* (pp. 1–5). New York: International Longevity Center-USA.

Center for Medicare and Medicaid Services (CMS). (2006). History. Retrieved October 29, 2008, from http://www.cms.hhs.gov/History/

Cruikshank, M. (2002). *Learning to be old*. Oxford, UK: Rowman and Littlefield.

DeWitt, L. (2003). Historical background and development of Social Security. Retrieved October 29, 2008, from http://www.socialsecurity.gov/history/briefhistory3.html

Doyal, L., & Gough, I. (1991). *A theory of human need*. New York: The Guilford Press.

Estes, C. L., & Grossman, B. R. (2007). Critical gerontology, aging, & health. In K. Markides (Ed.), *Encyclopedia of health and aging* (pp. 129–133). Thousand Oaks, CA: Sage Publications.

Estes, C. L., & Portacolone, E. (2009). Maggie Kuhn: Social theorist of radical gerontology. *International Journal of Sociology and Social Policy, 29*(1/2).

Estes, C. L., & Phillipson, C. (2002). The globalization of capital, the welfare state, and old age policy. *International Journal of Health Services, 32*(2), 279–297.

Estes, C. L., & Phillipson, C. (2007). Critical gerontology. In J. Birren. (Ed.). *Encyclopedia of gerontology* (pp. 330–336). New York: Elsevier.

Friedland, R. B., & Summer, L. (1999). *Demography is not destiny*. Washington DC: National Academy on an Aging Society.

Friedland, R. B., & Summer, L. (2005). *Demography is not destiny, Revisited*. Washington DC: Center on an Aging Society, Georgetown University.

International Longevity Center-USA (ILC-USA). (2006). *Ageism in America*. New York: International Longevity Center-USA.

Katz, S. (2003). Critical gerontological theory: Intellectual fieldwork and the nomadic life of ideas. In S. Biggs, A. Lowenstein, & J. Hendricks (Eds.), *The need for theory: Social gerontology for the 21st century* (pp. 219–243). Amityville, NY: Baywood Publishing Company.

Kuhn, M. (1984). Challenge to a new age. In M. Minkler & C. L. Estes (Eds.), *Reading in the political economy of aging* (pp. 7–9). Amityville, NY: Baywood Publishing Company.

Marmor, T. R., Mashow, J. L., & Harvey, P. L. (1990). *American's misunderstood welfare state*. New York: Basic Books.

Perkins, F. (1935). Social insurance for U.S. Social Security Administration (SSA). Retrieved October 29, 2008, from, http://www.ssa.gov/history/perkinsradio.html

Robertson, A. (1999). Beyond apocalyptic demography: Toward a moral economy of interdependence. In M. Minkler & C. L. Estes (Eds.), *Critical gerontology: Perspectives from political and moral economy* (pp. 75–90). Amityville, NY: Baywood Publishing Company.

Social Security Administration (SSA). (2005). Social Security: A brief history. Retrieved October 29, 2008, from http://www.ssa.gov/history/pdf/2005pamphlet.pdf

U.S. Department of Labor (US DOL). (n.d.). History, 6. Progressive ideas. Retrieved December 12, 2007, from http://www.dol.gov/oasam/programs/history/monoregsafepart06.htm

PART I

Social Insurance: History, Politics, and Prospects

Part I: Social Insurance: History, Politics, and Prospects

Introduction

BRIAN R. GROSSMAN

> *The basic purpose of all forms of social insurance is to replace a sufficient part of that wage income when it is lost as a result of any of these hazards—unemployment, accident, old age, or death of the wage earner—to insure not only that the individual may look forward to protection, but* that society as well may be protected against the hazards which it faces. [Italics added for emphasis]
>
> —Corson (1940)

Spanning over 7 decades, the history of social insurance in the United States begins with the approval of the Social Security program in 1935. However, just 4 years later, amendments were introduced that shifted the scope and structure of the program, moving Social Security from a program in which workers were only eligible to "take out" roughly as much as they had "put in" to one in which workers and their families were viewed as people who had earned the right to access benefits in the face of many of life's "hazards," to use Corson's word. Just 4 years after the program began, Social Security had been transformed into a symbol of interdependence and intergenerational cooperation.

Social Security began as a program based on a "contributory-contractual principle" (Berkowitz & McQuaid, 1988, p. 126). In such a system, laborers would contribute money to the program and upon retirement, could access money equal to the amount they had contributed. Berkowitz and McQuaid (1988) describe this initial structure of Social Security as a public sector program modeled on private sector concerns. The relatively restricted scope of the U.S. Social Security program at its inception is clear (see chapter 7). However, widespread fears about what the government could do with the large surplus that would accrue under this model of social insurance facilitated the introduction of the 1939 Social Security amendments and an expansion of both services offered and beneficiaries who could claim them (Berkowitz & McQuaid, 1988).

In particular, these amendments expanded benefits to the surviving children of deceased laborers and changed the benefit calculation formula so that older workers could more easily qualify for benefits and that workers who died young would pass on greater benefits to their survivors (Corson, 1940). Under this new model, Social Security contributions became a key way in which then current laborers were connected to people who were retired, the surviving spouses of laborers who had died, or workers with a permanent disability. By drawing the connection between the plight of the individual and the struggles faced by society in the quote above, Corson acknowledged the interdependence of human existence.

As a concept, interdependence recognizes that people, so frequently and misleadingly referred to as "individuals," are always enmeshed in dense sets of social relationships that implicate others in the course and content of the action of their lives. As Johnson (see chapter 3) illustrates, interdependence and intergenerational cooperation simultaneously operate at a number of social levels including within the family; between the family and the state; and across the generations of current laborers and those no longer, or unable to continue, laboring. Although the term *benefits* is used to describe the services provided through social insurance programs, the concept of interdependence allows for social insurance to be revisioned as providing benefits to society through multiple interconnected channels of self(ves), family(ies), and community(ies). Benefits can then be understood as the aggregate social goods that accrue from the financial contributions of current laborers; the continued financial[1] and social contributions of current beneficiaries; and the enduring

---

[1] One of the other points Corson (1940) makes is that social insurance helps retired workers (and other beneficiaries) retain their "purchasing power."

structures, social practices, and ideas with which these groups have interacted and to which they have contributed.

By virtue of being part of society, social insurance makes us all beneficiaries. In this way, social insurance in both its historical and contemporary forms represents an active step toward social justice. To the contrary, privatization efforts, even unsuccessful ones, represent a threat to social justice, replacing current levels of security with unknown quantities of risk in the guise of "saving" social insurance programs (Hacker, 2006). Privatization attempts recast the social boundaries of being human, reimagining people as decontextualized, autonomous individuals who need not be encumbered by the yoke of the state or the plight of others in society. Amidst these acrid politics, it can be difficult to discern the historical significance of social insurance programs and the legacy they represent to this generation and to those of the future.

In this first section, the authors revisit the history of social insurance and situate both the present moment for, and the future of, these programs in the wake of actions taken by generations past. In chapter 1, Robert Ball, former Commissioner of Social Security under Presidents Kennedy, Nixon, and Johnson, details the nine principles of social insurance that have helped Social Security to sustain its position as the most popular program in the United States. While reading this chapter, it is worthwhile to consider how these principles differ from those that structure other forms of social protection (see chapter 16).

In chapter 2, Ball provides his own analysis of these differences, comparing the principles that govern social insurance programs and those that operate in social assistance programs. Originally written in 1947, this chapter highlights the symbolic importance and material effects of continuing the social insurance component of Social Security. Ball explains the importance of social assistance programs, but identifies three key distinctions between these two types of programs. Consequently, he concludes that the effectiveness of Social Security as an income security mechanism would be greatly stymied if the program shifted from one that was part social insurance, part social assistance to one that was completely organized as a social assistance program.

In chapter 3, Malcolm Johnson responds to those who are questioning *if*, in fact, we are all still in this together. He addresses literature from around the world to document that, despite recent attempts to frame social policy discussions around intergenerational exploitation and greed, intergenerational equity is intact. Both across the life course and throughout the passage from one birth cohort to the next, the boundaries of the contract between the generations are continually shifting. Johnson argues that intergenerational cooperation must remain "open to renegotiation" as social, cultural, and economic practices change but that income and health security in old age must continue to be a guarantee.

Chapters 4 and 5 return the focus to the American experience with social insurance, focusing on Social Security and Medicare, respectively. In chapter 4, Domhoff suggests that the role of "corporate moderates," those business leaders of the 1920s and 1930s who supported Social Security, has been overlooked in the retelling of the history of Social Security. He contends that this lacuna is particularly detrimental as Social Security is currently being characterized as antithetical to business interests. Furthermore, Domhoff points to the potential utility of reclaiming the role of business leaders in the development of Social Security to provide space for a conservative political viewpoint that values this and other social insurance programs.

In chapter 5, Oliver and Lee provide a history of the development of the Medicare program, the "jewel in the crown" of President Lyndon Baines Johnson's Great Society programs introduced in 1965. The authors detail the changes in Medicare since its introduction, paying particular attention to those arising from the Medicare Modernization Act of 2003. Oliver and Lee are critical of these most recent changes as they signify an abandonment of the basic principles of social insurance. Moreover, the authors conclude that it was only due to a unique confluence of circumstances that these changes were allowed to occur in the first place. Indeed, they remind us it could have been otherwise.

In chapter 6, Kingson, Cornman, and Torre-Norton consider the future of social insurance in the United States by redirecting attention to the values that were reflected in the history of these programs. Although discussions about social insurance are cloaked in technical details and questions of economic efficiency, the authors encourage us to clarify, as a society, which values we wish to see endure. In particular, Kingson and his colleagues identify interdependence (and in particular intergenerational cooperation) as a value that has historically undergirded social insurance programs, is currently under attack in a climate that promotes hyperindividualism, and has the potential to be reestablished as central to the social insurance policy making of tomorrow.

REFERENCES

Berkowitz, E., & McQuaid, K. (1988). *Creating the welfare state: The political economy of twentieth-century reform*. New York: Preager.

Corson, J. J. (1940). Director's Bulletin No. 35, Reasons for the 1939 Amendments to the Social Security Act. Retrieved September 8, 2008, from http://www.ssa.gov/history/reports/1939no3.html

Hacker, J. (2006). *The great risk shift: The assault on American jobs, families, health care, and retirement and how you can fight back*. New York: Oxford University Press.

1

The Nine Guiding Principles of Social Security

ROBERT M. BALL

The following is an article written in 1998 by Robert M. Ball, Commissioner of Social Security under Presidents Kennedy, Johnson, and Nixon (see the dedication in this volume). We had hoped that Mr. Ball, whose service to and advocacy for social insurance spanned 70 years until his death on January 30, 2008, at the age of nearly 94, would contribute an original chapter to this volume. Instead, we share here his classic piece outlining the fundamental guiding principles of Social Security. (Eds.)

In the midst of the Great Depression, the founders of today's Social Security system took the bold step of establishing a new institution which they expected to be slow-growing but permanent. They wanted to make a decent retirement attainable for millions of Americans who would otherwise become dependent on their families or on public assistance when they grew too old to work or could no longer find employment. They wanted to protect workers' dependents by providing insurance to make the death of a breadwinner more financially manageable. They wanted to put an end to the poorhouse by distributing program income so as to provide at least a minimally adequate benefit for everyone regularly

From: Bethell, T. N. (Ed.). (2000). *Insuring the essentials: Bob Ball on Social Security* (pp. 5–10). New York: The Century Foundation Press, reprinted with permission.

contributing. And, foreseeing the inevitability of change—including the eventual need to insure against other major risks such as disability and illness—they sought to design an institution based on sustainable principles.

Accordingly, they took the long view. They gave major emphasis to estimating program income and expenses over a much longer period than was customarily done in other countries, and this is still true today. The time frame of 75 years that is now used for Social Security estimates is much longer than that used in almost all other contexts, from foreign social insurance programs to federal budgeting. The point, then and now, was not to try to pretend that anyone could really know precisely what would be happening in 75 or even 25 years; the point was that the planners of Social Security, in making exceptionally long-term commitments, wanted always to be looking far enough ahead to anticipate necessary improvements and make needed changes in ample time to preserve the integrity of the program.

That approach has served well. The legislation of 1935 and 1939 created the basic design of Social Security, and all major legislation since then can be seen as building on that design: extending coverage to more and more workers, improving the level of protection, adding protection against loss of income from long-term and total disability, providing protection for the elderly and disabled against the increasingly unmanageable cost of medical care, protecting against the erosion of income by inflation, and abolishing all statutory differences in the treatment of men and women.

These and many other accomplishments and adjustments have taken place within a framework consisting of nine major principles. Social Security is universal; an earned right; wage related; contributory and self-financed; redistributive; not means tested; wage indexed; inflation protected; and compulsory.

As with any framework, the stability of the entire structure depends on the contribution made by each part, so it is useful to review these principles and see how they work together.

1 *Universal*: Social Security coverage has been gradually extended over the years to the point where 96 out of 100 jobs in paid employment are now covered, with more than 142 million working Americans making contributions in 1997 [153 million in 2000]. And the goal of complete universality can be reached by gradually covering those remaining state and local government positions that are not now covered.

2 *Earned right*: Social Security is more than a statutory right; it is an earned right, with eligibility for benefits and the benefit rate based on an individual's past earnings. This principle sharply distinguishes Social Security from welfare and links the program, appropriately, to other earned rights such as wages, fringe benefits, and private pensions.

3 *Wage related*: Social Security benefits are related to earnings, thus reinforcing the concept of benefits as an earned right and recognizing that there is a relationship between one's standard of living while working and the benefit level needed to achieve income security in retirement. Under Social Security, higher-paid earners get higher benefits, but the lower-paid get more for what they pay in.

4 *Contributory and self-financed*: The fact that workers pay earmarked contributions from their wages into the system also reinforces the concept of an earned right and gives contributors a moral claim on future benefits above and beyond statutory obligations. And, unlike many foreign plans, Social Security is entirely financed by dedicated taxes, principally those deducted from workers' earnings matched by employers, with the self-employed paying comparable amounts. The entire cost of benefits plus administrative expenses (which amount to less than 1 percent of income) is met without support from general government revenues. [*Author's note:* This was true from 1935 until 2000, and the principle of funding Social Security largely from the earmarked contributions of workers and their employers remains desirable for the reasons stated. As of August 2000, however, it appears that in the future Social Security may be financed partially from general revenues, as are many foreign social insurance systems. The Clinton-Gore administration has made such a recommendation, as have several Republicans, including Sen. Phil Gramm (Texas) and Reps. Bill Archer (Texas) and Clay Shaw (Florida). The rationale for this approach, which was proposed in Social Security's early days, is discussed in chapters 17 and 18.][1]

---

[1] This is the author's note from the original publication. Contrary to what the author suggested might occur, no decision was made to finance Social Security from general revenues and Social Security continues to be funded from payroll taxes, not general revenues. The chapters cited in the author's note refer to chapters in Bethell, Thomas N. (Ed.). (2000.) *Insuring the essentials: Bob Ball on Social Security.* New York: The Century Foundation Press, in which Mr. Ball's article was republished. (Eds.)

The self-financing approach has several advantages. It helps protect the program against having to compete against other programs in the annual general federal budget—which is appropriate, because this is a uniquely long-term program. It imposes fiscal discipline, because the total earmarked income for Social Security must be sufficient to cover the entire cost of the program. And it guards against excessive liberalization: contributors oppose major benefit cuts because they have a right to benefits and are paying for them, but they also oppose excessive increases in benefits because they understand that every increase must be paid for by increased contributions. Thus a semi-automatic balance is achieved between wanting more protection versus not wanting to pay more for it.

5 *Redistributive*: One of Social Security's most important goals is to pay at least a minimally adequate benefit to workers who are regularly covered and contributing, regardless of how low-paid they may be. This is accomplished through a redistributional formula that pays comparatively higher benefits to lower-paid earners. The formula makes good sense. If the system paid back to low-wage workers only the benefit that they could be expected to pay for from their own wages, millions of retirees would end up impoverished and on welfare even though they had been paying into Social Security throughout their working lives. This would make the years of contributing to Social Security worse than pointless, since the earnings paid into Social Security would have reduced the income available for other needs throughout their working years without providing in retirement any income greater than what would be available from welfare. The redistributional formula solves this dilemma.

6 *Not means tested*: In contrast to welfare, eligibility for Social Security is not determined by the beneficiary's current income and assets, nor is the amount of the benefit. This is a key principle. It is the absence of a means test that makes it possible for people to add to their savings and to establish private pension plans, secure in the knowledge that they will not then be penalized by having their Social Security benefits cut back as a result of having arranged for additional retirement income. The absence of a means test makes it possible for Social Security to provide a stable role in anchoring a multi-tier retirement system in which private pensions and personal savings can be built on top of Social Security's basic, defined protection.

7 *Wage indexed*: Social Security is portable, following the worker from job to job, and the protection provided before retirement increases as wages rise in general. Benefits at the time of initial receipt are brought up to date with current wage levels, reflecting improvements in productivity and thus in the general standard of living. Without this principle, Social Security would soon provide benefits that did not reflect previously attained living standards.

8 *Inflation protected*: Once they begin, Social Security benefits are protected against inflation by periodic cost-of-living adjustments (COLAs) linked to the Consumer Price Index. Inflation protection is one of Social Security's greatest strengths, and one that distinguishes it from other (except federal) retirement plans. No private pension plan provides guaranteed protection against inflation, and inflation protection under state and local plans, where it exists at all, is capped. Without COLAs, the real value of Social Security benefits would steadily erode, over time, as is the case with unadjusted private pension benefits. Although a provision for automatic adjustment was not part of the original legislation, the importance of protecting benefits against inflation was recognized, and over the years the system was financed to allow for periodic adjustments to bring benefits up to date. But this updating was done only after a lag. Provision for automatic adjustment was added in 1972.

9 *Compulsory*: Social Security compels all of us to contribute to our own future security. A voluntary system simply wouldn't work. Some of us would save scrupulously, some would save sporadically, and some would postpone the day of reckoning forever, leaving the community as a whole to pay through a much less desirable safety-net system. With a compulsory program, the problem of adverse selection—individuals deciding when and to what extent they want to participate, depending on whether their individual circumstances seem favorable—is avoided (as is the problem of obtaining adequate funding for a large safety-net program serving a constituency with limited political influence).

In the middle of the Depression, it took courage to enact a system based on these principles. The Depression was a time of enormous and immediate needs, but Social Security was designed to be a slow-growing tree, one that could not provide much shelter in the near term. The point, however, was that, once grown, it would be strong enough to weather bad times as well as good.

A contributory retirement system takes a long time to develop since by definition, those who are already retired are not eligible for benefits. Fifteen years after the program was set up, only 16 percent of the elderly were receiving benefits, and it was not until the 1950s that politicians began to see much advantage in championing Social Security improvements. And it was only in the 1960s, three decades after enactment, that Social Security began having a major impact, paying benefits that were high enough and universal enough to significantly reduce poverty among the elderly, the disabled, and the survivors of beneficiaries. After the amendments of 1972 further increased benefits substantially and provided for automatic inflation protection, Social Security fully assumed the role planned for it, as the all-important base of a multi-tier retirement system in which private pensions and individual savings are added to Social Security defined protection.

The importance of that role would be difficult to exaggerate. Today Social Security is the only organized retirement plan—the *only* assured source of retirement income—for fully half of the total workforce. And it is the base upon which all who are able to do so can build the supplementary protection of pensions and individual savings.

Social Security continues to be the most popular and successful social program in America's history because its guiding principles enable it to work exactly as intended: as America's family protection plan.

DISCUSSION QUESTIONS

1. What are the three tiers of the U.S. retirement system? According to Ball, what role does Social Security play in this system?
2. Approximately what are the administrative costs of the Social Security program, according to Ball?
3. Ball says that Social Security is not "means tested." yet the program is "redistributive." Discuss the reasoning for and significance of these two guiding principles of Social Security.
4. How and why, according to Ball, did founders take the "long view" to the development of the Social Security system? How have the guiding principles Ball presents contributed to the longevity and success of the program?

2 Social Insurance and the Right to Assistance

ROBERT M. BALL

The following is an excerpt from a chapter written by Robert Ball (see the dedication) and was originally published in 1947. Ball outlines the differences between social insurance and social assistance as methods of income maintenance. His purpose was to highlight the inappropriateness of shifting the United States Social Security program from a joint social assistance/social insurance model to one that was structured solely on social assistance. Ball argues that such a move would be problematic for three reasons. In contrast to social insurance programs, social assistance programs (1) provide income maintenance on the basis of need rather than work performed, (2) rely on a means test to determine eligibility that results in a divisive split between those with more and those with less, and (3) offer benefits that raise people to at most, a minimum standard of living. (Eds.)

SOCIAL INSURANCE AS AN EARNED RIGHT

Each one of these points is in direct contrast to the social insurance approach. Social insurance payments are made to individuals on the basis of

---

From: Bethell, T. N. (Ed.). (2000). *Insuring the essentials: Bob Ball on Social Security* (pp. 5–10). New York: The Century Foundation Press, reprinted with permission.

a work record and are part of the reward for services rendered. Typically, the worker makes a direct contribution to the fund, but even if he does not "pay for his insurance" through an earmarked contribution which covers the cost of the risk, he earns the right to it through work. The insurance is part of the perquisites of the job. As in a private pension plan or group insurance, the question of who pays the cost is of the highest importance, but it is not the crucial one in determining whether there is an earned right to the payment. There is little hesitation in transferring to a payment for which one has worked all the feelings surrounding an earned right regardless of whether there has been a deduction from wages. Such a payment is a reward—something to be proud of—just as savings or high wages are. Private pensions, group insurance, and social insurance all belong, along with wages and salaries, to the group of work-connected payments, and it is this work connection, the fact that it is earned, which gives social insurance its basic character.

Public assistance in selecting people for payment because they are in need rests on an entirely different kind of right—the right to a minimum standard of living based on membership in a civilized community. As stated by Karl de Schweinitz (as of 1947) in *People and Process in Social Security*:

> The principle of self-help [in social insurance], however, is dominant. The individual is entitled to insurance by virtue of what he has done. Insurance is a positive experience. It is a measure of a person's success in the labor market. This is much more evident in old age insurance than in unemployment compensation, but the contrast in this respect between all forms of insurance and public assistance is marked.
>
> In public assistance the inherent factors are negative rather than positive. Entitlement is based not upon what the individual has done in payment or in work but upon his lack of any such resource. It is founded upon his need, upon what he has not. The individual applying for insurance points to the record of his wages. The applicant for assistance states that he is unable to maintain himself. The right to insurance is based on contributions which the prospective beneficiary has made in money or in work. The right to assistance is founded on the individual's kinship in a common humanity recognized by a community which has undertaken to see to it—and registered the fact in statute—that none of its members shall suffer if they are in need.

Although the fact that social insurance is an earned benefit does not depend on the employee contribution, this contribution does have great value in social insurance, private pension schemes, group insurance, and the like because it dramatizes the worker's direct interest in the fund. It makes it clearer to him and other people, as well, that he should have a real say in the planning and protection of the system from either undue liberalization or restriction. The contribution gives stability to the system by emphasizing both the earned right to the insurance and the proprietary interest of the worker in his benefit. To accomplish this it is of course not necessary that the entire cost of the benefit be paid for by earmarked contributions or that the benefit amounts be in direct proportion to the worker's own contribution. The basic character of the insurance as a work-connected payment remains, regardless of whether some groups are given a greater return for their money than others. In this respect, social insurance is similar to minimum-wage laws, which intervene in the "free play of economic forces" and insist that some people be paid higher wages than they would otherwise be able to get. The minimum wage and the "weighted" insurance benefit are earned payments, even though the amount is not what would have resulted from "free competition."

As an earned right, social insurance, unlike public assistance, is an integral part of the economic incentive system. Under social insurance, security is earned through work and is additional remuneration for working, while public assistance provides benefits without reference to work. Equally important, in social insurance the incentive to earn and save throughout one's working life is protected because any additional income, large or small, may be used to provide a higher standard of living. On the other hand, a private income from savings, since it must be deducted from the benefit, makes no difference in the total income of the public assistance recipient. In practice, it is true, even an income which has to be supplemented by public assistance may have real value in making the recipient feel less dependent, but it is the failure of public assistance to give the same satisfaction per dollar as an earned payment which makes this so. In strictly economic terms, a person who has little hope of accumulating enough to make him entirely ineligible for assistance has no reason to strive for a private income.

Even in New Zealand, which allows fairly substantial exempt amounts before reducing benefits, there is concern about the effect of the income test on incentives. It is recognized that the system works counter to general economic incentives for those who have any possibility of securing incomes above the exemption, for above this amount the benefits are larger the less one has been able to earn and save. The very liberalizations which make the receipt of a "means test" benefit in New Zealand less subject to stigma than anywhere else in the world intensify the danger that such benefits may weaken the desire to secure a private income above the amount which allows one to get a full benefit.

Partly because of the stigma attached to the receipt of public assistance in the United States, it is to be doubted that very many people deliberately avoid efforts at earning and saving in order to be eligible for a benefit or in order to get a higher benefit. However, the fear that a generous program administered in the spirit of right might be an inducement to some to work and save less is one of the reasons the community is reluctant to accept the full implications of a right to assistance and a standard of health and decency for assistance payments. Although incentives are a complex of many powerful motives in addition to the economic, no system of production can afford to ignore the relation of money payments to economic contribution. There are many faults in our present system of monetary incentives, and behavior contrary to the best interests of the community is frequently induced, but this fact argues for a closer connection between contribution and award, not for ignoring incentives in the provision of security. Some benefits must be paid on a "means test" basis, but it is important from the standpoint of economic incentives that primary reliance be placed on earned payments made without regard to need.

SOCIAL INSURANCE IS FOR ALL WHO WORK

Second, social insurance does not divide the community into two groups, putting those with enough money to support themselves in one group and those without enough money in another. It is true that certain foreign systems still have something similar to this in that they cover only lower-paid workers so that a certain class distinction does exist, but this is on the way out, and it never carried with it the same feelings as did a distinction based on a direct means test. In this country, of course, no coverage limitations based on income have ever existed. Thus, as in the case of a private pension plan, individuals of varying wage levels and varying standards of living receive payments from the same program. The low-paid wage-earner, the poor man without possessions, receives payments through the same mechanism as the highly paid salary worker or executive. There is none of the feeling in such a social insurance program, as there tends to be in assistance, that this program is for the "poor" or the "unfortunate," with all that such an attitude implies. It is not one part of the community caring for another, but the community meeting a universal need. Everyone has a stake in his earned pension and insurance benefits.

SOCIAL INSURANCE SUPPORTS A VARIABLE STANDARD OF LIVING

Finally, social insurance has as its purpose not only the maintenance of a minimum standard of living as set by the community but the underpinning of a higher-than-minimum standard of living for a large proportion of the workers under the program. This is inherent in the fact that it pays without regard to other resources, whether or not the benefits alone would allow a higher-than-minimum standard.

There is no question, for example, but that even the very low benefits of the present old-age and survivors insurance program enable many people to live at a standard considerably above what the community would consider a reasonable minimum for a "means test" program and that others who receive the payment would be able to live above such a minimum even without the benefit. This is not an accident of clumsy design but a major purpose of social insurance. As in the case of a private pension, one objective is to help people to have enough income not merely to be free from want, or to bring them up to a community minimum, but to help them to secure the economic bases for happiness and contentment. It is a program not only for the poor but for whoever is in danger of suffering a major reduction in living standards. It is a program of preventing destitution, as well as curing it.

Actually, there is nothing about social insurance to prevent payments which in themselves are more than enough to maintain minimum standards. Social insurance could never pay as much as the more liberal private pension systems, but it is by no means bound to pay only an amount will give the content of a community approved minimum applicable to all. The question is one of what the nation can afford and of how much of the national income we want to put into such benefits—not one of principle. When many current proposals would provide family benefits under old-age and survivors insurance as high as $120 a month and when some state unemployment insurance systems already pay over $100 a month to single persons, we are no longer dealing in community-determined minimums; many people in the community will have lower incomes than these and yet not be entitled to benefits under any program. When we combine this fact with the rough generalization that those who are entitled to the highest benefits are those who may be assumed to have the most income from other sources, since they had more to save from, it is clear that social insurance is not just another way of doing the same job that public assistance sets out to do.

A major purpose of social insurance is to keep people from having to apply for assistance, but it also performs for others who would not have been eligible for assistance under any circumstances the very valuable service of helping them to live above the community minimum. This objective would be unfair, discriminatory, and completely inappropriate in a program based upon need, but it is both right and proper in a program based upon work and earnings. Under a system of relating benefits to past wages, high benefits may be paid to highly paid wage-earners and the incentive system actually strengthened thereby, just as it is strengthened by differential payments in wages or in a private pension or disability system. There is little danger that the wage-earner will prefer the benefits to work, in those parts of the program where this is a factor, as long as his benefits are considerably below what he can earn while working. It is necessary to limit benefits for all to an amount below what the least skilled can earn only in a flat-benefit program.

DIFFERENCES IN TRADITION

These three important differences between social assistance and social insurance are inherent in the very nature of the two programs. They derive from the right to one being based on need, and the right to the other being based on work. Equally important at the present time and for a long time to come are differences in the two programs which are not inherent but which result from differences in origin and traditional attitudes toward the two programs. It is with respect to these differences that the concept of a right to assistance is making revolutionary changes.

One of the most striking contrasts between assistance and insurance in the United States at the present time is that what is freely conceded in the case of insurance requires a bitter, never completely won struggle in public assistance. For example, the right of the recipient to spend his benefit without restriction has seldom been questioned in the case of insurance but is a continual struggle in public assistance. In the same way, discretionary payments designed to enforce a code of conduct on the recipient different from that required of the rest of the community are not a problem in insurance. Yet, public assistance is carrying on a constant struggle against a tradition which used the payment as an excuse to reform or control the individual. There are probably many people who would still agree with Lewis Meriam (1946) when, speaking of those public assistance recipients whom he considers unable to manage their own affairs, he says:

> In such cases, the recipients of the benefits should be subject to the supervision of competent, professionally trained, public employees, and payments should be contingent upon suitable use and application of the public funds provided. . . . It seems reasonable to conclude that payment of public funds for persons whose need results from their personal limitations should be sufficiently contingent to make it necessary for the recipients to comply with minimum standards (Meriam, 1946, p. 867).

He is not speaking here, of course, of those who have been judged mentally incompetent under legal procedure but of people who have a way of ordering their lives which he considers undesirable and whose behavior he considers evidence of "personal limitation." This doctrine means, in effect, that to obtain minimum security an individual would have to give up freedom of action and submit to the dictates of others on how he should conduct his life in those essentials where other citizens are allowed to make their own decisions.

Leaving aside the question of whether such supervision is practical, whether in this way you can really get people to act the way you want, an equally important point is that making security contingent on the surrender of personal integrity and freedom of action is exactly what we want to avoid in a democracy. This issue goes to the heart of the central political problem of our time—how can people obtain economic security in a way which preserves individual freedom and human dignity? How can we avoid the false dilemma, beloved of totalitarians, of having to choose between a means of livelihood, on the one hand, and freedom on the other? There is little danger of the control of one person by another if the right to security is an earned right. It continues to be a danger in assistance as long as any important section of public opinion holds the traditional attitude, championed by Mr. Meriam, that a public assistance payment is not the recipient's own but a contingent gift from public funds.

Another important difference between the two programs, at present, is that the community frequently limits the amount of funds available for public assistance in such a way as to make a mockery of the concept of a right to a minimum standard of living. No feeling of contractual obligation to supply that minimum exists in fact, whereas a feeling of obligation to supply the amount written in the law does exist in social insurance. This is irrespective of whether the legal right to the two types of payments is equally strong.

Public assistance has arrived at the concept of right by way of a long, hard road. Its history is a combination of repression and punishment, on the one hand, and of humanitarian paternalism, on the other. While its worst features have been based on the idea that the individual was at fault and needed chastisement to make him better or that relief had to be made as unpleasant as possible or people would all refuse to work, equally destructive of the concept of right has been the paternalism which held that what the individual needed was reformation and help. Punitive or humanitarian, public assistance suffers from a history and tradition in which one group or class does something either to or for another.

Social insurance bypassed this tradition both of punishment and paternalism. Its origins are not in the poor law or in the voluntary activities of the wealthy and educated to improve the lot of the poor.

Its origins are in the sturdy efforts of self-reliant workmen to do things for themselves—in the sickness and death funds of the medieval guilds, the friendly societies, the fraternal orders, and the trade-unions. It borrows much from private pension plans and from private insurance and from a tradition of protective labor laws, frequently forced on an unwilling state by the power of workers' organizations. Here is no giving of one class to another but the development of institutions by those who are to benefit from them. Social insurance is firmly fixed in a tradition of self-help and earned right. Therefore, while assistance, in implementing the idea of right, must struggle to establish new attitudes, social insurance finds these attitudes ready-made.

To make use of these ready-made attitudes and to avoid the struggle which attends the reformation of an old tradition is highly important in social planning, now at least as important as preserving what is inherently different about the insurance approach. Part of the value of the contribution by the worker in social insurance and part of the value of connecting the benefits closely with the wage record lie in using the techniques which are readily identified with the tradition of self-help, with its accompanying freedom of action and freedom from the necessity of feeling grateful. They make doubly clear to all that this program has no connection with the tradition of the poor law.

CONCLUSION

There are, then, in spite of important similarities, very significant and real differences between public assistance and social insurance. From the standpoint of freedom, democratic values, and economic incentives, social insurance is greatly to be preferred wherever there is a choice. It is important that, through an extension of coverage and an increase in social insurance benefits, it be made clear that public assistance is not a rival to the insurance method but a supplement to it, performing the residual task that will always exist for a last-resort program that takes responsibility for meeting total need. The goal of a progressive Social Security program should be to reduce the need for assistance to the smallest possible extent and at the same time to enforce it as a legal and moral right, with an administration free from the controls and the humiliations and irritations of "poor law" procedures.

In attaining this goal, there is much to gain from the association of social insurance with assistance in the Social Security system. The fact that both devices are necessary, although different parts of a common program, reinforces the concept of assistance as a right. Insurance tends to be administered in the spirit of right, naturally and without question, and, through association, public assistance moves closer to an administration which is as firmly based in law and regulation and is as devoted to equity and definiteness as is insurance. The concept of public assistance as part of a broader Social Security program addressed to the total problem of income maintenance is important in the struggle to eliminate those undesirable features of assistance which are the result of tradition. There is no danger of assistance becoming too attractive and taking the place of social insurance, providing social insurance is made to fill its proper role. Quite the contrary, there is a long fight ahead to make assistance merely endurable in a democratic state. Assistance is never something to look forward to, since like a life-raft it performs the function of rescue and is the accompaniment of disaster—at its best, it is a necessary evil. Social insurance, on the other hand, can be a positive good, and in the preventing of disaster and in helping a family to maintain an accustomed standard of living is to be likened more to the devices and regulations which protect the safety and comfort of passengers and reduce the need for life rafts. As long as men value self-reliance, the alternative of earning one's security through work will be preferred to payments made because of need.

DISCUSSION QUESTIONS

1. What are the fundamental differences between social insurance and social assistance, according to Ball?
2. What are the reasons Ball gives that both systems of income maintenance—social insurance and social assistance—are necessary?
3. Select an example of a social insurance program and an example of a social assistance program. Create a poster with four sections: (1) Explain the social insurance program you selected and use Ball's article to justify why it is a good example of a social insurance program; (2) Explain the social assistance program you selected and use Ball's article to justify why it is a good example of a social assistance program; (3) Explain how your social insurance program would look different if it were a social assistance program; and (4) Explain how your social assistance program would look different if it were a social insurance program.

REFERENCES

Ball, R. M. (1947, September). *The Social Service Review, 21*(3), 331–344.

De Schweinitz, K. (1948). *People and process in Social Security.* Washington, DC: American Council on Education.

Meriam, Lewis. (1946). *Relief and Social Security*. Washington, DC: Brookings Institution.

3 Procession of the Generations: Are We Still Traveling Together?[1]

MALCOLM L. JOHNSON

INTRODUCTION

As the global implications of societal demographic aging gain heightened significance, with the emergence of large and previously poor nations on the world stage, issues of generational equity are close below the surface of new discourses. Nation states openly struggle to deal with a combination of economic downturn due to banking mismanagement and increased competition for petrochemicals and basic minerals. They blame the banks; the hedge funds; and the economic tigers of China, India, Brazil, and the resurgent countries of Eastern Europe. Rapidly, the domestic economic reappraisals turn to the unmanageable rising costs of pensions, Social Security, and health care for their retired populations. Not for the first time, justice between the generations and the commitment to social insurance is at risk.

Even a passing review of gerontological literature, however, reveals a larger body of generational relations studies that indicate shortfalls in family support for older people. Many social commentators have been

[1] This chapter is an edited, revised, and updated version of 'Interdependency and the Generational Compact' in Meredith Minkler and Carroll Estes (Eds.) (1999). *Critical gerontology: Perspectives from political and moral economy*. New York: Baywood.

and are ready to see the changed patterns as evidence of family failure and the abandonment of traditional obligations. They claim that modern societies will not be able to manage the costs of old age (Kotlikoff & Burns, 2004; Longman, 1987; Myles, 2002, 2003; Peterson, 2002).

In this chapter, we will reconsider the underlying principles of intergenerational equity within the context of a developing and growing body of evidence about how the younger generations relate to their parents as they enter later life. Part of the exploration will be to historically map and analyze the changing socioeconomic circumstances, patterns of living, and the impact of demographic change, as it affects the numerical and the economic balance between contiguous generations.

It is simply not acceptable to observe shifts in the way relationships unfold between adults and their parents and to characterize them as in decline. Too much irresponsible commentary has already placed into the political discourse the view that the growth in the numbers and proportion of older people is unsustainable. Immediately following this observation comes the cry from ideologues of the right and politicians of a timid and populist nature that the state must step back from its commitments to the old and poor, leaving them to the primary responsibility of their own resources and those of their families. In turn, families are chastised for failing in their responsibilities.

This narrative, neatly compressed into a few sentences, represents a bleak prospect for those who may have been given more life to live but not the resources to live it well. These debates take place alongside, rather than in intimate association with, others that deal with the supposed disintegration of social order. In particular, the ultimate theory of dissolution embodied in notions of postmodernism and the subset of them, post-Fordism,[2] has served to create a climate of despair about the continued willingness and capability of future generations to sustain the old and the infirm (Taylor, 1914).

The story line of this progression (or is it regression?) is that since the secularization of human values, individual rights have been through a series of reformulations which have been shaped by the modern state in league with organized religion. Industrial capitalism gives way to

[2] Post-Fordism is a term used to describe systems of economic production and consumption that are to be found in advanced economies in the late 20th century and beyond. It is distinguished from Fordism (the production line system of mass production introduced in automotive factories, by Henry Ford). It is characterized by a move away from standardized products, to flexible specialization which delivers diverse versions of products to suit the needs and tastes of different markets. In so doing it serves societies which are more individualistic and choice driven.

postcapitalism and to forms of economic and social disorder. Baudrillard (1983) extends the argument by claiming that the end of modernity is simultaneously the end of the social and the termination of bourgeois democracy, including the institutions of free speech and human rights (Turner, 1990). Zygmunt Bauman (2006), a respected interpreter of postmodernist theory, has recently addressed the endemic sources of uncertainty, which shape our lives, arising from the confusion of escalating social and economic change. He uses the term *liquid times* to characterize the shifting sands of morality and civil society.

Translating these interpretations of social fragmentation into the social welfare of older citizens requires a willingness to accept them as explanatory framework. It is abundantly clear, however, that Fordist influences created a post-World War II welfare state, which was essentially male, white, and geared to mass employment (Dora, 1988; Williams, 1994). It is also clear that major changes in employment patterns by gender, class, age, and race will have a marked and fairly rapid impact on health and social care provision and pensions. Williams concludes—and I concur—"that these issues and debates need to take account not only of the changing conditions of work but the changing conditions of the family, culture and nationhood" (p. 72). It is against the backdrop of this complex of dynamic social structures, ideas which undermine modernity and moralities that are equally fluid, that the procession of the generations takes place.

FAMILIES IN TRANSITION

The persistence of nuclear-family forms is indisputable, but mutations and new family forms in the past 3 decades have caused serious doubts about the capacity and commitment of domestic units to support all their members. So, inevitably, much of what follows will focus on the changing family. There is, however, another level of social obligation beyond that of kinship, which is also in flux. It exists at the societal level and is embedded in economic structures. On the one hand, there are reasons for some analysts to fear that the costs of the current arrangements for old and other dependent people are too great for governments to meet. On the other had, there is a progressive individualism in the political atmosphere which manifests itself in the work setting. Together, these perceived shifts away from formerly agreed obligations have stimulated a set of agitated responses.

Our task is to assess the veracity of the argument that changing social structures, demographic patterns, and ideologies of personal conduct have undermined the solidarity between people of different ages both at any point in time and across time. No assessment of the positive or negative consequences of change can be made without a point of reference.

So, we may start as Daniels (1988), Walker (1990), and Johnson and Falkingham (1988) did, among many, from the belief that there has operated in the past a generalized obligation on those who were young and fit enough to be economically active to make provision for those too young or too old to engage in the creation of income and wealth. In turn, these workers could expect that future cohorts of producers would sustain them in their need for income and services, to ensure their physical and social well-being. Such a statement would readily embrace the essence of the contemporary debate in North America, western Europe, and Japan. This debate focuses on the threatening inability of producers to go on delivering sufficient resources to maintain the level of economic transfer necessary to meet the rising claims of health, Social Security, and pension budgets for the retired population.

But despite its resonances of history and political economy, there are important missing dimensions. It makes too many assumptions about the sociology of the family and of the philosophical foundations of a contract between the generations, nor is there any hint of the seminal influence of the changing perceptions and roles of women as the principal caregivers. Even further away are the most recent environmentalist arguments, the prognostications of political economists, and the emergence of a subgroup of the young unemployed, who are captured in a new dependency.

GENERATIONS IN CONFLICT?

Propositions of universal family forms in the 1950s quickly led to a large body of empirical work (Bell & Vogel, 1968), which demonstrated a wide variety of patterns. These challenges to the universality thesis included Bettetheim's (1969) and Spiro's (1968) studies of kibbutzim, which presented both the strengths and the shortcomings of defamilied communal living. A range of anthropological research highlighted functioning matrifocal lone-parent families in the West Indies and Central America (Hannerz, 1969).

The debate then moved, first to a series of powerful assaults on nuclear-family living (Laing & Esterson, 1968; Leach, 1968; Toffler,

1971), which depicted it as pathological and harmful. Leach (1968) said, "Far from being the basis for a good society, the family with its tawdry secrets, is the source of all discontents." Then came a sustained focus on the role of women (Greer, 1970; Oakley, 1974), which gave rise to a new canon of feminist literature and gender studies that have both recorded and materially changed social perceptions of women. Running concurrently with the mass extension of paid employment among women, the two processes have affected the quantity, availability, and style of their contribution to household and caring activities (Finch, 1989). Such gender issues have become an important part of the generational debate because of the greater part played by women in the care of old and disabled people.

Specifically, gerontological interest in generational relations began to take form in the United States during the 1960s. It was prompted by the student uprisings based on protest movements concerning civil rights, student rights, anti-Vietnam War, rights for women, and the (hippie) counter culture. As Bengtson and Mangen (1988) put it, "These movements seemed to pit the young against the old. 'Don't trust anyone over 30' because a rallying cry that directly emphasized the counter culture's mistrust of the older generation." Leonard Cain (1967) had registered an early interest in the equity of a common retirement age for people of manifestly different life expectations, which led him to a broader examination of the new cohorts of older people in America. By the time Bengtson and Cutler (1976) came to review the literature for the first *Handbook of Aging and the Social Sciences,* the current shape of the dialogue had largely formed. Tracing ideas from Mannheim (1928), whose focus was on the understanding of what he called "generation units" as components of social change, they started with questions of definition and moved on to issues related to age–group differentiation, family and socialization, cohorts, political alienation of the young, age-connected patterns of Medicare usage, lineage and helping relationships, solidarity, and dependency ratios.

Solidarity of Care

The list of topics also formed the framework for the seminal studies conducted by Bengtson and Mangen, which began in 1970 and have continued up to the present day. They rely on two clear premises (1) that solidarity in intergenerational relations is complex and multidimensional rather than a unitary construct and (2) that the measurement tools for observing these phenomena required further elaboration. The emphasis on methodological refinement, using the LISREL statistical modeling technique,[3] has characterized the research. Such responses can be seen as both a natural progression in the sophistication of empirical research methods and as a reaction against the tide of opinion that had formed in that time as a result of the work of Townsend (1957) in the United Kingdom, Shanas (1962) in the United States, and their associates in Denmark (Shanas et al., 1968). These studies highlighted the high degree of family support to elderly people. Townsend (1957) goes as far as to say that "family obligations are taken more seriously than before" (p. 229). Yet, the indications of increasing loneliness and the uneven patterns of family support fueled an anxiety that these traditional caring arrangements were beginning to break down.

Bengtson and colleagues (1988) saw the need for a more clinically precise assessment that would enable a clearer differentiation of family and relationship types to emerge—and be studied over time, rather than at a fixed point in time. By 1988, he and his team had identified 13 family types which emerged from cluster analysis of their data. They fell into four main groups: (1) The "moderates," 50.1% of the sample; (2) the "exchangers," 12.6%; (3) the "geographically distant," 15.7%; and (4) the "socially distant," 18.5%. Falling into a kind of league table for helpfulness to the older generation, these groupings also represent clearly different formations. Families may be cohesive on one dimension but fragmented on others. The researchers conclude that, by their definitions of solidarity, only about half would exhibit solidarity.

While acknowledging that family solidarity is a multidimensional concept, of particular significance in this review is the extent of functional social exchange—the transfer of labor and helping skills—between the generations and within generations. On this dimension, the latest studies continue to confirm very high levels of commitment, even when the family has fractured in some way. Money flows largely from the old to the young, but care and support is given across the generations in all directions, with women in late-middle age being the major givers. Chatters and Taylor (1993), in their report of levels of assistance to elderly parents amongst American blacks conclude, "These findings are consistent

[3] LISREL is a sophisticated, specialist, high-level statistical software package that estimates structural equation models for manifest and latent variables. Bengtson and his colleagues began to use it to create models of generational relations soon after it came out in the mid-1970s—and ever since.

with previous work that indicates that intergenerational support is characteristic of black families."

In making this statement, they, too, found diverse patterns, based on region, physical proximity, marital status, and the degree of affectual closeness. Moreover, they highlight the emergence of widowed daughters as major caregivers to parents. Wellman's (Wellman & Wortley, 1989; Wellman, 1990, 1992) sequence of studies on Canadian samples extending over 2 decades provides further understanding of what kinds of help are provided by what kinds of kin. His main contribution is twofold: The identification of density and clustering in kinship networks, and the delineation of five basic "dimensions" of support (Wellman, 1992). The latter consist of Emotional Aid, Services, Companionship, Financial Aid, and Information supplied by close kin in that sequence of intensity. His longitudinal studies reveal extensive networks of kin and friends who supply high levels of aid. Sixty-one percent of network members provided emotional support and services, with the most immediate relations being primary providers. The cumulative impact of this data enabled Wellman (1990) to conclude, "While noting the strains in parent/adult child ties, my interest is in the high level of supportive resources they convey' who talked to us" (p. 211).

Recent studies indicate higher contributions than were previously reported and marked shifts as domestic roles modify in response to female employment and the regendering of work. From their own extensive research in Canada and international reviews of the literature, Chappell and Penning (2005) identified serious structural inequalities of gender, ethnicity, race, and class in the delivery of family care. They argue that the commodification of care around the world, in response to higher levels of female workforce participation, bear down most heavily on the poorest and most disabled. These findings confirm the results of other studies, such as Dilworth Anderson (2002) and complement the conclusions of Harper (2006), that worldwide care will increasingly come from spouses rather than children as more is demanded of women across the life course.

In a similarly wide-ranging distillation of family and generational research, Bengtson, Biblarz, and Roberts (2002) were able to report unexpected new strengths in the care equation. Generation Xers were significantly more positive than those of comparable parent families in the preceding baby boomer age group. Their data also shows that in the disintegration following divorce, not only do grandparents make a more significant contribution, but "families adapt by extending kin" (p. 161).

The long-term trend of the whole body of data indicates the remarkable persistence of family support and the very high level of personal responsibility accepted by family members. What we need to be aware of is the likely influence of secular changes in the population that could undermine these patterns, but which sometimes, paradoxically, provide solutions.

THE PROCESSION OF THE GENERATIONS

The nature of the solidarity between individuals and within the fabric of organized society has been the subject of philosophical examination throughout recorded history. In modem times, we look to the formative work of Locke and Rousseau. When Locke wrote of the social contract (Laslett, 1960) in the late 17th century, he drew on existing concepts of popular consent (Plamenatz, 1963). He refined them to provide an explanation of the legitimacy of government and the proper relationship between governments and their subjects in terms of the latter's obedience. Believing that government could only exist on the basis of consent, Locke declared that rulers were entitled to obedience but only if their subjects had actually consented to obey and so were committed to showing that they had consented and voluntarily agreed, even when it looked as if they had not. By linking consent with obligation as integral features of civil society, his writings served to fashion contemporary liberal political philosophy. In the context of the subject of this chapter, his contribution was to give greater credence to contractarian thinking, which Bentham and the utilitarians reinforced in the 19th century and John Rawls (1971) used as the point for departure of his *A Theory of Justice*.

As Laslett (1992) points out in his book with James Fishkin, *Justice Between Age Groups and Generations,* there are profound difficulties in articulating the contractual nature of intergenerational exchange, which in turn are magnified by attempts to consider the processional nature of justice over time. This is the essential conceptual element in the discourse about an intergenerational compact and the consequent issues of equity, which lie at the heart of this chapter. There are, of course, practical concerns about the willingness and capacity of governments and economic systems to deliver the resources to support elderly populations (see later discussion). In advanced societies, these are questions more of political conviction than of economic possibility. What will unlock the political uncertainty, based as it is on short-term strategies and misconceptions about the "burdens" of an aging population, is a newly refurbished notion of generational solidarity.

Moody (1992) goes on to argue that the character of generational giving and receiving is transitive, "We 'repay' the generosity of the preceding generation by giving in turn to our successors" (p. 229). Indeed, this apparent paradox is virtually universal. It is to repeat Laslett's term *processional*. But even if life can be metaphorically depicted as a procession, it is also one which stops at points in the life path to engage in a series of ritual exchanges.

Following nurture to adulthood, there may be a period of dependent "apprenticeship"—college or low earnings early in a career—and a parental transfer to enable the establishment of an independent household, perhaps through marriage. The appearance of grandchildren may prompt further gifts, as might financial misfortune or ill-health (Daniels, 1988). But as the journey leads the older generation to their last years, the often unspoken dialogue of emotional support and services in kind in the unspecified expectation of inheritance is acted out. Empirical evidence of this is to be found in long-term care where relatives seek to restrict expenditure to minimize diminution of their inheritance (Crystal, 1982).

Callahan (1987) has addressed these issues at the macro-level by proposing a set of criteria for delimiting the resources older people might claim from the health care system. For him, the bond between generations must respect limits that are at once humanistic, normative, and economically feasible. Although the fear he exposes is the unnecessary and undesirable use of scarce resources needlessly to extend life, it, too, is a metaphor for the boundaries that now exist in the gift relationship between generations.

Callahan's book provoked widespread criticism and hostility. Binstock and Post (1991) called it scapegoating. Moody (1991) called it a blunder. Many others were indignant. The American media were righteously angry. Yet, on maturer reflection, many of the critics have mediated their reactions and recognize, as I do, that Callahan has served us well by breaching the death taboo (Aries, 1977). *Setting Limits* is not only a compassionate book, it is intellectually courageous, for it gives systematic attention to the issue that could divide the young and the old, were it not honestly addressed. In his digest and response, Callahan makes few concessions to his critics, noting that the most vociferous of them (Jecker & Pearlman, 1989; Winslow & Walters, 1993) review the alternatives "and find them full of problems too" (p. 398).

Where I take issue with Callahan is with the prudentialism he shares with Rawls. It may "make good sense for the custodians of society" not to put its future well-being at risk by adopting rash policies which might undermine its cultural and financial wealth. But prudence should not extend to despair that the currently unfathomable problem is an unsolvable problem. However, I, too, am simply expressing a value-based judgment and revealing myself as more of an optimist than he. Indeed, the essence of the whole debate has not been about the quality of analysis but about the *politics* of generational equity—an issue taken up in the next section.

By contrast, the image of a procession is progressive, optimistic, and modern. Also at risk in the intergenerational debate is another metaphor—that of the contract. Human societies that are not subject to totalitarian regimes are founded on contracts, written (in law) and unwritten. The principal ingredients are consent and trust. There is an inescapable recognition of social exchange and reciprocity in those wider contracts between strangers. The compact between the generations is not only between unknown parties but also between the dead, the living, and the unborn. It is a moral responsibility to maintain the core of trust, even when the details of the agreement are under review—as they must be in the world of rapid and global change. So, if we are to join Laslett's procession, its value base needs to be reaffirmed.

So, the main issues are: If there is a contract between people and generations at large, is it a strong version (one where the conditions, duties, and reciprocal benefits are clearly known to all panics), or is it a weak version in which there is a broadly defined commitment for each generation to reward the preceding cohort for their lifetime contribution to the social good? If it is of this weaker sort, what latitude is there for redefinition in the light of current economic circumstances and prevailing ideas of solidarity? In short, is it acceptable for the quantity and quality of intergenerational transfers to be modified (reduced) in the light of new variables like the demographic revolution or the arrival of large-scale unemployment necessitating many people who are not old and not disabled to draw on the communal resource?

Laslett argues that it is the weaker form of contract that prevails in the modern world and that it is inevitably subject to renegotiation as cohort succeeds cohort and as social, economic, and political circumstances change. Some, like Epstein (1992), would argue that the only tenable response is to allow the market mechanism to determine what the generational contract can deliver. Although others would share Baybrooke's (1992) criticism that such an abandonment to market forces risks consigning some of our successors to effective slavery. In consequence, those who hold the authority of government are beholden to sustain the essence of the obligation to provide an adequate level of social and economic well-being for their older citizens. It is this very challenge to the social insurance principle that preoccupies governments across the world—not as a philosophical notion, but as an operational reality.

Gerontologists have largely selected their agendas—quite reasonably—from the empirical world around them in which old age and aging are still misunderstood. So, the emergence of a political economy of aging brought a new fusion of theoretical and policy issues which linked with but, until Callahan, did not fully embrace the issues raised in this section.

THE POLITICAL ECONOMY OF GENERATIONAL RELATIONS

The political economy of aging made its first significant mark in 1981 when Townsend (1981) published his seminal paper "The Structured Dependency of the Elderly: A Creation of Social Policy in the Twentieth Century.". In it, he drew attention, not simply to the socially and economically submerged position of elderly people as a group, but to the way society contrived to make and keep it so. In his own words, "I wish to put forward the thesis that the dependency of the elderly in the twentieth century is being manufactured socially and that its severity is unnecessary." Almost a decade later, the vigorous debate that Townsend provoked took another decisive turn, one which asserted that the old are taking too large a part of the national incomes of developed societies.

Led initially by Walker (1980) (who had foreshadowed these ideas), gerontologists welcomed the political statement Townsend had made and went on to offer their own elaborations of it. In Britain, Phillipson's (1982) research on U.K. pension policies over the past 100 years led to the publication of his influential book *Capitalism and the Construction of Old Age*. In the United States, Estes, Gerard, Zones, & Swan (1984) wrote convincingly and trenchantly about the oppression of older people in America and their labeling as a social problem in a way which purported to provide compassionately for its workers. Inevitably, others joined in, both from the United States (Myles, 1981) and Europe (Gaullier, 1982; Kohli, Rosenow, & Wolf, 1983).

Early critics of Townsend's thesis were hardly visible. The new orthodoxy gained a self-evident status. It took another new perspective on aging, which emerged fully in the mid-1980s—the history of aging and old age—to supply evidence that weakened some of the empirical support for "structured dependency." From France, there already existed the influential, if flawed, earlier work of Stearns (1977), which by showing the great variety of experience of older people in France, both supported and challenged the Townsend view. In North America, Achenbaum's (1986) concern with historical analysis of what constituted a "young" society cast further doubts on claims that the retired population in the past was ill-treated and deprived.

Other important historical contributions came from Laslett. His work on historical demography has made its own global impact. But it was probably the work of his colleague, Thomson (1984), that created the greatest controversy. In a paper on the decline of the welfare state, he both undermined the myth of the Victorian golden age in Britain and raised serious questions about the comparative economic treatment given to different generations and age groups.

Questions about the relative share of the national economic cake given to the old and the young started to come to the fore in the United States during Ronald Reagan's presidency. They arose from the reaction of commentators on the political right to the growing "burden" of health and Social Security payments to the expanding retired population. They saw the public cost of maintaining elderly people escalating at the same time as an observed growth in the discretionary income of people over the age of 55 amounting to one third of the national total. A view emerged in what Meredith Minkler (1987) called "corporate America" that the old constituted a group of developing wealth, whereas children and young people were suffering as a consequence of social programs for their elders.

In 1985, a new organization formed in America under the leadership of Senator David Durenberger and Representative James Jones. They called it Americans for Generational Equity (AGE). It defined itself as a nonpartisan coalition whose mission was to build an intellectual and mass-membership movement to promote the interests of the younger and future generations in the national political process. Its main targets were to increase the political power of young people and to reduce government expenditure on Social Security and Medicare. AGE claimed that as the elderly population grows bigger it becomes richer, demanding more costly public services and taking "more than its fair share." Children and young people were losing out. AGE claimed that although constituting only 11.5% of the U.S. population, those over the age of 65 consume 28% of the national budget and 51% of all government expenditure on social services. However, the objectives were not simply fiscal. Senator Durenberger is reported as saying, "The assumption that each working generation will take care of the one that preceded it is finished" (Minkler, 1972).

For a time, AGE sought to undermine social support for the old to relieve the young. Moreover, it challenged the social contract between the generations that a life of hard labor, which includes supporting the young, is repaid with income and care in retirement. Instead, it is everyone for themselves, from birth to death.

Contributors to the literature on aging are well aware that across Europe, one in three of the retired population are officially below the poverty line. On the other hand, we recognize that there is a growing subgroup of retired people who continue to be prosperous into old age (Victor, 1987). This latter group includes not only those with accumulated wealth but also those with inflation-proof pensions and lump-sum retirement bonuses. The elderly population is far from homogeneous. So, however distasteful its motives and publicity seeking its pronouncements, it is not possible to dismiss AGE (now defunct as an organization) and its imitators as having no case.

As Thomson's (1988) research on historical patterns of welfare spending in New Zealand pointed out, there are accumulated benefits to the elderly that leave young age groups gravely disadvantaged. The most obvious examples are the relative difficulty for younger people to enter the housing market as expenditure on public housing has been withdrawn. Similarly, the greatest burden of unemployment falls on those under the age of 25, while health care costs for the old have escalated. State pension levels have, in real terms, fallen in recent years, but the total cost continues to rise steeply.

Johnson and Falkingham (1988), observing the measurable disparities in generational shares in the United States, conducted an analysis of public expenditure in the United Kingdom. Their conclusions were that the British welfare state had been remarkably neutral in its allocation of resources between the generations, claiming that any discussion of intergenerational conflict for welfare resources in the United Kingdom would establish a false division. In their view, the inequalities lie along class lines in all age groups. Many other writers would see gender, at all ages, as a major variable, which, combined with class and ethnic origin, overshadows generation and cohort as the defining division (Arber & Ginn, 1991; Falkingham & Victor, 1991; Miller & Glendinning, 1989; Parker, 1993).

The publication of *Workers v. Pensioners: Intergenerational Justice in an Aging World* (Johnson, Conrad, & Thompson, 1989) attracted attention well beyond academic gerontology. The overt espousal of an intergenerational struggle for primacy and resources attracted widespread attention. But in the intervening years, the developed world has not experienced a contest between the generations. Indeed, nation states across the world have introduced antiage discrimination legislation and incorporated new dimensions into human rights legislation, which have set down parameters of social justice in old age.

The political economy discourse now continued at two levels: One concerned with distributive justice and the other with mechanisms politics. The economist Yung-Ping Chen (1993) addressed the long-term care component of the aging population "problem" by proposing that a "three-legged stool" of social insurance, private insurance, and Social Security should meet the costs, which were, at the time, estimated to total $108 billion a year (Vladeck, Miller, & Clauser, 1993). This approach focused on changing concepts of welfare (Hills, 1993) and the impact of the mixed economy of welfare, which has now invaded all the post–World War II welfare states. But even where pluralistic systems were long established, as in North America, the energy thrust and policymaking attention is with the economists concerned with pensions and Social Security. In the United Kingdom, Dilnot and colleagues' (1994) detailed economic projections and models of age-related income patterns over time, alongside alternative pension policies, represent the center ground. Their work and that of others in the field were heavily drawn on by the Social Justice Commission (1994) initiated by the Labor Party.

Parallel activity in the United States is exemplified by the work of Williamson and Pampel (1993), whose concerns mirror Dilnot's (1994). From their review of the policy alternatives studied in the United States, the United Kingdom, Germany, and Sweden, they recommend the new German and Swedish indexing formulas, both of which, they claimed, emphasized generational burden sharing. But their consideration of burden sharing made no reference to the ethical debate, only to that of contemporary criteria that will ensure a spread of responsibility for paying. It adds the novelty of proposing "tradable benefits" to allow holdings in one benefit (e.g., pension) to be transferred to another (e.g., long-term care).

During the last decade of the 20th century, it became evident that one of the key pathways forward for pension systems was for a reformulation of retirement. Johnson (1997) proposed—as had others—that flexible retirement should be made both possible and desirable, providing both a later pivotal retirement age and the opportunity to continue working without barrier. Such a reformulation of retirement would allow for what he called "third age portfolios." Of course, such arrangements have been in place in the United States for 2 decades. Not only does later and more flexible retirement allow for choice, but it also recognizes the necessity that continuing in employment is essential for many older people.

More recently, government-sponsored investigations have engaged in serious reviews of the evidence to establish the sustainability, Social Security, and pension systems. In the United States, an important study by the National Bureau of Economic Research (2004), and in the United Kingdom, the Pensions Commission delivered a substantial report (Pensions Commission, 2004). Both of these enquiries review the trends internationally deserving that longer lives and lower fertility rates are dramatically increasing the proportion of the population above current retirement ages. They proposed new partnerships between public and private pension systems, later retirement (in the United Kingdom, 68 years instead of 65), and the creation of new financial instruments, some of which would be obligatory forms of pension saving.

The focus of this analysis has been predominantly on North America, Europe, and the richer nations, but an expanding range of studies examining the impact of modernization (Burgess, 1969; Cowgill & Holmes, 1972, 1974) on erstwhile third world countries has explored shifting demography and solidarity between generations. It reveals that the "abandonment," sometimes attributed to African nations, is not empirically verified, but shortfalls in elder care are more a result of poverty and falling living standards (Aboderin, 2006; Apt, 1987, 1993). Similarly, in the Confucian world of East Asia, there are reports of a continuing commitment to the principles of filial piety. Research on Japanese, both at home and in America (Hashimoto, 1996; Hashimoto & Ikels, 2005), shows enduring determination to support the old, though new patterns are emerging. In China, where the single child policy introduced in the early 1970s has produced a dramatic imbalance between the generations known as the 4-2-1 family, there is both continuity and change. Young Chinese still accept their traditional responsibilities but cannot meet all the needs, so older spouses will have to take more of the weight in the future (Cai, 2007).

CONCLUSIONS

In reviewing each body of literature and ideas, my concern has been to draw out the main themes, evidence, and opinion rather than to make a comprehensive interdisciplinary assessment. In doing so, I am conscious of leaving many important associated themes unattended to. There is no assessment here of the disputes about what constitutes a cohort or a generation, communitarianism is given no more than a passing reference, and there is no detailed scrutiny of the economics of Social Security. Feminist critiques of social welfare and pension systems are underrepresented.

With David Selbourne (1994), I see the need for a renewal of citizenship, moral considerations, and a new disposition of freedom and duty. His anxiety about civic order is not one I can share in its entirety, but any involvement with justice between generations must pay regard to the robustness of the society which promises to provide for those who follow. This means that I also join in Laslett's procession, recognizing that the generational contract cannot be fixed for all time, but must be open to renegotiation.

Yet, the parameters of that new deal need to be set within a framework of secure knowledge that the central promise of the contract—adequate income and care of the old—is an enduring right. A greater recognition of finitude in old age and the need to talk about and plan for the dependency the fourth age might bring is one prerequisite for the new contract, but it will also serve as a necessary prologue to the continuing but largely silent dialogue between generations—at the personal and the societal levels. It is about the giving and receiving of nurture and dignity in old age and the ways in which these processes are transformed into a right through reciprocal giving in life and after its end. In this way, the necessary renegotiation of the details can proceed without crises and major generational conflicts.

The large literature on family formations and family caring leads me to believe that this most central agency in human society is not in terminal decline. On the contrary, its modification and diversification provide more options and more strengths. Intergenerational helping transfers are still empirically well-evidenced but different in kind, regularity, and format. Recent and more-sophisticated studies make it plain that a modern family, wherever it is in the world, is smaller and inevitably less resourced in direct person power to deliver intensive personal care to older persons. As Silverstein (2006) rightly summarizes, "If public provision to dependent populations has reached or surpassed its upper limit. At least for the time being, and before the baby boomers again change the world, there is good reason to believe that the generations still travel, if more uneasily, down the life path together."

DISCUSSION QUESTIONS

1. Summarize the empirical research Johnson shares about changing interfamily relations. Have the younger generations abandoned their elders?
2. Discuss what Johnson says about the concepts of family solidarity, social exchange, and the contract between generations.
3. What is a political economy perspective on generational relations?
4. What are a few changes occurring in interfamilial relations in the developing world?
5. In the title of this chapter, Johnson raises the question, "Are the generations still traveling together?" Using both empirical research cited by Johnson and the principles he says should guide intergenerational relations, prepare a short talk about the subject to a group of college students who are convinced that families no longer take care of one another.

REFERENCES

Aboderin, I. (2006). *Intergenerational support and old age in Africa.* New Brunswick, New York: Transaction Publishers.

Achenbaum, A. (1986). Aging of the first new nation. In A. Pifer & L. Bronte (Eds.), *Our aging society* (pp. 15–32). New York: W. W. Norton.

Apt, N. A. (1987). *Aging and, health, and family relations: A study of aging in the central region of Ghana.* Legon: University of Ghana.

Apt, A. (1993). The storm clouds are a grey. In K. Tout (Ed.), *Elderly care: A world perspective* (pp. 10–12). London: Chapman and Hall.

Arber, S., & Ginn, J. (1991). *Gender and later life: A sociological analysis of resources and constraints.* London: Sage.

Aries, P. (1977). *The hour of our death.* Paris: Editions du Seuil.

Baudrillard, J. (1983). *Simulations.* New York: Semiotext.

Bell, N. W., & Vogel, F. F. (Eds.). (1968). *A modern introduction to the family.* London: Collier Macmillan.

Bengtson, V., & Cutler, N. (1976). New generations and intergenerational relations. In E. H. Binstock & E. Shanas (Eds.), *Handbook of aging and the social sciences* (pp. 130–159). New York: Van Nostrand Reinhold.

Bengtson, V., & Mangen, D. (1988). Generations, families and interactions. In D. Mangen, V. Bengtson, & P. Landry (Eds.), *Measurement of intergenerational relations* (pp. 10–14). Newbury Park: Sage.

Bengtson, V., & Landry, P. (Eds.). *Measurement of intergenerational relations.* Newbury Park: Sage.

Bengtson, V. L., Biblarz, T. J., & Roberts, R. E. (2002). *How families still matter.* Cambridge: Cambridge University Press.

Bettellheim, B. (1969). *Children of the dream.* London: Thames and Hudson.

Binstock, R. H., & Post, S. G. (Eds.). (1991). *Too old for health care: Controversies in medicine, law, economics and ethics.* Baltimore: Johns Hopkins University Press.

Cai, R. Q. (2007). *Investigation of the consequences for public health and public health services of the demographic revolution in China and the single child family policy.* Unpublished doctoral thesis, University of Bristol, UK.

Cain, L. D. (1967). Age, status and generational phenomena: The new old people in contemporary America. *Gerontologist*, 7, 83–92.

Callahan, D. (1994) Setting limits: A response. *Gerontologist, 34*(3), 393–398.

Callahan, D. (1987). *Setting limits: Medical goals in an aging society*. New York: Simon and Schuster.

Chappell, N. L., & Penning, M. J. (2005). Family caregivers: Increasing demands in the context of the 21st century globalization. In M. L. Johnson, V. L. Bengtson, P. Coleman, & B. L. Kirkwood (Eds.), *The Cambridge handbook of age and ageing* (pp. 455–462). Cambridge: Cambridge University Press.

Chatters, L., & Taylor, R. (1993). Intergenerational support: The provision of assistance to parents by adult children. In J. S. Jackson, L. M. Chatters, & R. J. Taylor (Eds.), *Aging in black America*. Newbury Park, CA: Sage.

Chen, Y. P. (1993). A three legged stool: A new way to fund long term care. In Institute of Medicine (Ed.), *Care in the long term: In search of community security*. Washington, DC: National Academy Press.

Crystal, S. (1982). *America's old age crisis*. New York: Basic Books.

Daniels, N. (1988). *Am I my parents' keeper?: An essay on justice between the young and the old.* New York: Oxford University Press.

Dilnot, A., Disney, R., Johnson, P., & Whitehouse, E. (1994). *Pensions policy in the UK: An economic analysis.* London: Institute for Fiscal Studies.

Dilworth Anderson, P., Williams, I., & Gibson, B. E. (2002). Issues of race, ethnicity, and culture in caregiving research: A 20 year review (1980–2000). *Gerontologist, 42*(2), 237–272.

Dora, B. (1988). *From Taylorism to Fordism: A rational madness*. London: Association Books.

Epstein, R. (1992). Justice across generations. In P. Laslett & J. Fishkin (Eds.), *Justice between age groups and generations*. New Haven, CT: Yale University Press.

Estes, C. L., Gerard, L., Zones, J. S., & Swan, J. (1984). *Political economy, health and aging*. New York: Little, Brown.

Falkingham, J., & Victor, C. (1991). *The myth of the woopie?: Incomes, the elderly and targeting welfare*. London: London School of Economics.

Finch, J. (1990). *Family obligations and social change.* London: Polity.

Gaullier, X. (1982). Economic crisis and old age: Old policies in France. *Ageing and society*, 2, 165–182.

Greer, G. (1970). *The female eunuch.* London: Paladin.

Hannerz, U. (1969). *Soulside: Inquiries into ghetto culture and community*. New York: Columbia University Press.

Harper, S. (2006). *Ageing societies*. London: Hodder Arnold.

Hashimoto, A. (1996). *The gift of generations: Japanese and American perspectives on ageing and the social contract*. Cambridge: Cambridge University Press.
Hashimoto, A., & Ikels, C. (2005). Filial piety in changing Asian societies. In M. L. Johnson, V. L. Bengtson, P. Coleman, & B. L. Kirkwood (Eds.), *The Cambridge handbook of age and ageing* (pp. 437–442). Cambridge: Cambridge University Press.
Hills, J. (1993). *The future of welfare*. York: Joseph Rowntree Foundation.
Jecker, N., & Pearlman, R. A. (1989). Ethical constraints on rationing medical care by age. *Journal of American Geriatrics Society, 37*, 1067–1075.
Johnson, M. L. (1997). Generational equity and the reformulation of retirement. *Scandinavian Journal of Social Welfare, 6*(3), 162–167.
Johnson, P., & Falkingham, J. (1988). Intergenerational transfers and public expenditure on the elderly. *Ageing and Society, 8*(2), 129–146.
Johnson, P., Conrad, C., & Thomson, D. (Eds.). (1989). *Workers v. Pensioners: Intergenerational justice in an aging world*. Manchester: Manchester University Press.
Kohli, M., Rosenow, J., & Wolf, J. (1983). The social construction of aging through work: Economic structure and life world. *Ageing and Society, 3*, 23–42.
Kotlickoff, L., & Burns, S. (2004). *The coming generational storm: What you need to know about America's economic future.* Cambridge: MIT Press.
Laing, R. D., & Esterson, A. (1979). *Sanity, madness and the family*. Harmondsworth, England: Penguin.
Laslett, P. (1960). *Locke's two treatises of government*. Cambridge: Cambridge University Press.
Laslett, P., & Fishkin, J. (Eds.). (1992). *Justice between age groups and generations*. New Haven, CT: Yale University Press.
Leach, E. (1968). *A runaway world*. London: BBC Publications.
Longman, P. (1987). *Born to pay: The new politics of aging in America.* Boston: Houghton Mifflin.
Mannheim, K. (1928). The problem of generations. In P. Kecskemeti (Ed.), *Essays on the sociology of knowledge*. London: Routledge and Kegan Paul.
Miller, J., & Glendinning, C. (1989). Gender and poverty. *Journal of Social Policy, 18*(3), 363–381.
Minkler, M. (1987). The politics of generational equity. *Social Policy*, Winter.
Moody, H. R. (1991). Allocation, yes; age-based rationing, no. In R. H. Binstock and S. G. Post (Eds.), *Too old for health care. Controversies in medicine, law, economics and ethics.* Baltimore: Johns Hopkins University Press.
Moody, H. R. (1992). *Ethics in an aging society*. Baltimore: Johns Hopkins University Press.
Myles, J. F. (1981). Income inequality and status maintenance. *Research into Aging, 2*, 123–141.
Myles, J. F. (2002). A new contract for the elderly. In G. Esping-Anderson, D. Gallie, A. Hemerijk, & J. Myers (Eds.), *Why we need a new welfare state* (pp. 130–174). Oxford: Oxford University Press.
Myles, J. F. (2003). What justice requires: pension reform in ageing societies. *Journal of European Social Policy, 13*, 264–270.
National Bureau of Economic Research. (2004). *Who wins and who loses? Public transfer accounts for US generations born 1850 to 2090*. Cambridge, MA: National Bureau of Economic Research.

Parker, H. (1993). *Citizen income and women*. London: Basic Income Research Group.
Pensions commission. (2004). *Pensions: challenges and choices*. London: Stationery Office.
Peterson, P. (2002). The shape of things to come: Global ageing in the 21st century. *Journal of International Affairs*, *56*, 198–210.
Phillipson, C. (1982). *Capitalism and the construction of old age*. London: Macmillan.
Plamenatz, J. (1963). *Man and society*. London: Longman.
Rawls, V. A. (1971). *A theory of justice*. Cambridge: Harvard University Press.
Selbourne, D. (1994). *The principle of duty: An essay on the foundation* of *civic order*. London: Sinclair Stevenson.
Shanas, E. (1962). *The health of older people*. Cambridge: Harvard University Press.
Shanas, E., Townsend, P., Wedderburn, D., & Friis, H. (1968). *Old people in three industrial societies*. London: Routledge and Kegan Paul.
Silverstein, M. (2006). Intergenerational family transfers in social context. In R. L. Binstock, & L. K. George (Eds.), *The handbook of aging and the social sciences* (pp. 165–180). Amsterdam/Boston: Elsevier.
Social Justice Commission. (1994). *Strategies for national renewal.* London: Vintage.
Spiro, M. E. (1968). Is the family universal? In N. W. Bell, & E. F. Vogel (Eds.), *A modern introduction to the family*. London: Collier, Macmillan.
Stearns, P. (1977). *Old age in European society*. London: Croom Helm.
Taylor, F. W. (1914). *Principles of scientific management*. New York: Harper.
Thomson, D. (1988). *The welfare state and generational conflict: winners and losers*. Paper presented at the Conference on Work, Retirement and Intergenerational Equity, St. John's College, Cambridge, England.
Thomson, D. (1984). The decline of social welfare: Failing support for the elderly since early Victorian times. *Ageing and Society*, *4*, 451–482.
Toffler, A. (1971). *Future shock*. London: Pan.
Townsend, P. (1957). *The family life of old people*. London: Routledge and Kegan Paul.
Townsend, P. (1981). The structured dependency of the elderly: A creation of social policy in the twentieth century. *Ageing and Society*, *1*(I), 5–28.
Turner, B. S. (Ed.). (1990). *Theories of modernity and postmodernity*. London: Sage.
Victor. C. (1987). Income inequality in later life. In M. Jefferys (Ed.), *Growing old in the twentieth century* (pp. 115–127). London: Routledge.
Vladeck, B. C., Miller, N. A., & Clauser, S. B. (1993). The changing face of long term care. *Health Care Finance Review*, *14*(4), 5–23.
Walker, A. (1990). The economic burden of ageing and the prospect of intergenerational conflict. *Ageing and Society*, *10*(4), 377–396.
Walker, A. (1980). The social creation of poverty and dependency in old age. *Journal of Social Policy*, *9*(5), 45–75.
Wellman, B. (1990). The place of kinfolk in personal community networks. *Marriage and Family Review*, *15*(1/2), 195–228.
Wellman, B. (1992). Which types of ties and networks provide what kinds of social support? *Advanced Group Processes*, *9*, 207–235.
Wellman, B., & Wortley, S. (1989). Brothers' keepers: Situating kinship relations in broader networks of social support. *Sociological Perspectives*, *32*(3), 273–306.

Williams, F. (1994). Social relations, welfare and the post-Fordism debate. In R. Burrows, & B. Louder. *Towards a post-Fordist welfare state* (p. 72). London: Routledge.

Williamson, J. B., & Pampel, F. C. (1993). Paying for the baby boom generation's social security pensions: United States, United Kingdom, Germany and Sweden. *Journal of Aging Studies*, 7(1), 41–54.

Winslow, G. R., & Walters, J. W. (Eds.). (1993). *Facing limits: Ethics and health care for the elderly*. Boulder, CO: Westview Press.

4

The Little-Known Origins of the Social Security Act: How and Why Corporate Moderates Created Old-Age Insurance

G. WILLIAM DOMHOFF

INTRODUCTION

In an era when the governmental old-age social insurance program created by the Social Security Act of 1935 is under constant attack by big-business organizations and business-financed think tanks, it may come as a surprise when I claim that the basic principles behind old-age insurance were created and actively supported by the corporate moderates who owned and controlled the biggest and most powerful corporations of the 1920s and 1930s, companies such as Standard Oil of New Jersey, General Electric, International Harvester, and Metropolitan Life Insurance. This suggests that the corporate establishment's current negative stance toward old-age pensions may not be inevitable. In fact, old-age social insurance made enormous business and political sense to corporate moderates from the 1930s to the early 1970s. They only turned against it as part of a more general ideological and political attack on "big government" that began in the mid-1970s in the face of a new set of economic and political problems caused by skyrocketing oil prices, stagflation, and the pressures put on government budgets by the social movements that arose in the 1960s (Piven & Cloward, 1982).

The corporate moderates of the 1920s and 1930s did not act without the advice and help of the experts on social insurance they financed and directed in the fledgling think tanks of that day, especially the first human resource counseling firm in American history, Industrial Relations Counselors, Inc. (Kaufman, 2003). They also worked with experts who were brought together by the Social Science Research Council, founded in 1923 by the Laura Spelman Rockefeller Memorial Fund to generate new policies on a wide range of issues (Bulmer & Bulmer, 1981; Karl, 1974). These efforts were financed over the next decade and longer by the handful of new charitable foundations that corporate moderates created to shape policy proposals in the era before World War I, led by the Rockefeller Foundation and the Carnegie Corporation.

The corporate moderates and their allies insisted that government old-age insurance had to be based on three principles they developed during several years of experience with private pension plans, especially in conjunction with the major life insurance companies of the time (Klein, 2003). First, the level of benefits must be tied to salary level, thus preserving and reinforcing the values established in the labor market. Second, unlike the case in many countries, there could be no government contributions from general tax revenues. Instead, there had to be a separate tax for old-age pensions, which would help to limit the size of benefits. Third, there had to be both employer and employee contributions to the system, which would limit the tax payments by the corporations.

One of the experts who worked with the corporate moderates in designing old-age social insurance, J. Douglas Brown, a professor of economics at Princeton who specialized in industrial relations within a special program created by John D. Rockefeller, Jr., summarized what he called the "American philosophy of social insurance" in a retrospective book. His emphasis was on "the need for a perpetual corporation to assure a flow of effective and well—motivated personnel for the year-by-year operation of the company" (Brown, 1972, pp. 90–91). More specifically, "retirement programs with adequate pensions became necessary to prevent an excessive aging of staff or the loss of morale that the discard of the old without compensation would involve;" thus, old-age insurance was simply "a charge on current production to be passed on to the consumer" (Brown, 1972, p. 90).

In formulating their social insurance plans, the corporate moderates even enjoyed the tentative support of some ultraconservative business leaders, as demonstrated by a somewhat favorable report by a committee of the National Association of Manufacturers in December 1934. However, they lost that support in the spring of 1935 when the ultraconservatives went into all-out opposition against the New Deal due to issues related to support for union organizing and higher taxes on the wealthy (Brents, 1984; Jenkins & Brents, 1989). Furthermore, these ultraconservatives had little or no impact on the old-age provisions of the Social Security Act because their main political allies, the conservative Republicans, had no power in Congress due to the overwhelming Democratic electoral victories of 1930, 1932, and 1934. Nonetheless, the plans of the corporate moderates were modified in a conservative direction through the elimination of agricultural workers from the social insurance plan. This elimination was a result of the great power of Southern plantation capitalists due to the seniority system in Congress and the close ties that Southern Democrats enjoyed with President Roosevelt (Alston & Ferrie, 1999; Quadagno, 1988).

In placing so much emphasis on rival segments of the ownership class in explaining the origins and shaping of old-age insurance, I am indeed saying there was little direct impact from organized labor, liberals, or leftists. By the late 1920s, organized labor was small in numbers and weak in organization, with the important exception of several railroad unions, whose insistence on government pensions for retired railroad workers in 1933 and 1934 helped set the stage for the Social Security Act. Other than that, organized labor's most important contribution to old-age insurance was its decision to drop its long-held opposition to government pension programs in the face of the failure of their own meager and actuarially unsound pension plans and growing concern about corporate-controlled pensions. This cleared the way for organized labor activists to back the plan that finally emerged.

As for the liberals and social workers of that era, they found themselves playing second fiddle to what they called the "insurance crowd," even though they had access to the New Deal through Eleanor Roosevelt and the Department of Labor, where Frances Perkins was the secretary of labor. They were fully represented by their most prominent spokespersons in discussions of what became the old-age social insurance plan at the Social Science Research Council (SSRC), but their desire for a pension for everyone older than age 65 funded by general tax revenues and without demeaning qualifications did not prevail. Nonetheless, they worked very hard for the passage of the Social Security Act once the New Deal put its stamp of approval on the corporate moderates' formulations (Gordon, 1994, pp. 261–263).

As for the activists who were to the left of the New Deal liberals, their agitation, writing, and lobbying helped to create a more favorable climate for "doing something" about old-age pensions, and it was their phrase—"social security"—that came to designate what had been called "economic security," "social insurance," or "industrial pensions" (Klein, 2003, pp. 78–80). Like liberal New Dealers, they advocated protection for everyone without qualification and wanted to finance social security out of general tax revenues. However, none of these leftist advocates was hired by the government or put on an advisory committee despite their visibility and prominence, to the great annoyance of their admirers. At a later stage in the legislative process, when the bill was already formulated, a highly visible social movement called the Townsend Plan generated pressure for an extremely generous pension for everyone older than age 60, which was used by liberals and moderates as a bogey man in an attempt to neutralize the scare tactics generated by ultraconservative opponents of the corporate moderate program (Amenta, 2006).

THE ROAD TO GOVERNMENT OLD-AGE PENSIONS

The program that became old-age social insurance in 1935 had its origins in private pension plans developed in the second half of the 19th century by a handful of corporations, especially railroads (Graebner, 1980; Sass, 1997). Private pensions then received an indirect boost in the first 15 years of the 20th century, when corporate leaders asked life insurance companies to create a plan to insure against industrial accidents as a way to avoid both government insurance and continuing liability suits (Fishback & Kantor, 2000; Klein, 2003). Led by Equitable Life and Metropolitan Life, the insurance companies gradually came to see that they also could develop group life insurance plans that paid small pensions to an employee's survivors for a few years. This in turn reinforced the idea that these companies could do a better job with private pensions than the corporations themselves if contributions were made by both the companies and their employees (Klein, 2003; Sass, 1997). But the biggest corporations of the era were not prepared to abandon their own plans, which they believed to be helpful in controlling their workforces and limiting strikes.

However, private corporate pension plans, paid for entirely by the company, which was not legally bound to pay the pension in any case, did not have the effects corporations hoped they would and were actuarially unsound. These shortcomings became especially clear to those who worked on social benefit issues for Industrial Relations Counselors, Inc. (IRC), which had been created and funded out of his own pocket by

John D. Rockefeller, Jr., in 1921 as a subgroup within the law firm that provided him with advice on labor relations. This consulting firm was formally incorporated in 1926 to make careful studies of labor relations at specific companies and provide advice to management (Gitelman, 1988; Kaufman, 2003).

The IRC and Early Social Insurance Research

The work by IRC was carried out for the most part by Murray Latimer and Bryce Stewart, who later joined with the aforementioned J. Douglas Brown of Princeton as major figures in the drafting of the old-age insurance provisions of the Social Security Act. At the time he was hired in 1926, Latimer was a 25-year-old instructor in finance at the Harvard Business School after receiving his master's in business administration from there in 1923. During his years at IRC, he helped to establish pension plans at Standard Oil of New Jersey as well as three other Rockefeller oil companies and an independent steel company, American Rolling Mill. His 1932 book for IRC, *Industrial Pension Systems in the United States and Canada*, which explained the inadequacies of most private pension plans, especially in the face of the financial problems created for many companies by the Great Depression, was well-known and respected at the time. It is still frequently cited in historical accounts.

Stewart, a Canadian with vast experience in employment and labor issues, worked as director of the National Employment Service of Canada from 1914 to 1922 after his large role in its establishment. He came to the United States in 1922 to develop and administer the Amalgamated Clothing Workers' unemployment insurance fund, jointly financed by labor and management, but controlled by the union. He joined the staff of IRC in 1927 at the age of 44 and served as the director of research from 1930 until his retirement in 1952, except for a return to Canada as deputy minister of labor during World War II. Like Latimer, he was widely known in the early 1930s for his work on social insurance. He also did important work for the SSRC and state agencies in Minnesota, Wisconsin, and New York before serving the New Deal in various capacities (Domhoff, 1996, pp. 133–141).

In late 1933, Stewart, Latimer, and Brown were asked by the federal coordinator of transportation to create a sound social insurance system for the growing number of aging and retired railroad workers, whose well-organized agitation and lobbying had led to a proposed railroad retirement act written in good part by the leadership of the railroad labor unions (Brown, 1965; Graebner, 1980). It was this experience, in the context of the growing problems with company-funded private pension plans, that gradually led them to understand the possibilities for using the group pension policies developed by the insurance companies as a model for government old-age pensions that would be compatible with the major concerns of corporate leaders. Lacking the information needed for the actuarial studies necessary for a sound system, they used a $300,000 grant from the recently established Civilian Works Administration to put 1,500 people to work collecting records on 400,000 railroad employees and 110,000 pensioners; they then hired a staff of 500 in New York, many who were unemployed railroad clerks, to analyze the data (Brown, 1965; Latimer & Hawkins, 1938). Because of this work, Latimer was appointed chairman of the three-person Railroad Retirement Board in the summer of 1934 upon passage of the railroad retirement bill and remained in that position until 1946.

The Creation of the Social Security Act

By November 1933, the experts at IRC who had been working on issues related to social insurance for nearly 4 years felt confident enough about their ideas for transitioning from private to public social insurance, including old-age pensions, to bring them to the formal attention of experts just outside their circles. Using a grant from the Rockefeller Foundation and working under the auspices of the SSRC, which by then had its own committee on unemployment and social insurance issues, they invited 18 people representing a wide range of social service organizations to attend a conference on social insurance. Five were social workers, including Edith Abbott, one of the most famous women reformers of the Progressive Era and dean of the School of Social Service Administration at the University of Chicago since 1921. Notably, the most important government official was Harry Hopkins, a former social worker who headed the Federal Emergency Relief Administration.

The starting point for the discussions at the SSRC conference was a document prepared by Stewart listing the kinds of studies needed to decide some of the issues that had to be resolved in designing a social insurance program. Although the attendees were unanimous in encouraging the SSRC to move forward in refining Stewart's proposal, Abbott did express disagreements based on her preference for "one welfare statute," paid for out of general tax revenues and "available to all without stigmatizing qualifications" (Gordon, 1994, p. 261; Witte, 1963). The same group met for a second SSRC conference in early April 1934 to consider a second version of Stewart's proposal. Once again, there was general approval, so Stewart and a coauthor, an economist from the SSRC who was working temporarily in the Department of Labor, revised the report to emphasize the need for a unified plan based on careful studies by the federal government. That is, they wanted unemployment insurance and old-age pensions to be the two main provisions in a larger package that became the Social Security Act. As they explained in a report to the SSRC in relation to their original grant:

> In a draft report, revised following the April conference, the unified character of the task of planned protection was developed, and the several phases of relief and social insurance were considered in terms of (a) the problems of planning, administration, and coordination, (b) the present state of knowledge in each field, and (c) further work specifically required for the proper integration of each major segment into a unified program (Stewart & Givens, 1934b p. 1).

Stewart and other experts then sent Perkins and Hopkins copies of their report in an effort to convince them that general, not piecemeal, legislation was necessary to deal with issues of social insurance. From their point of view, their efforts were successful in influencing the creation of the Cabinet-level Committee on Economic Security (Stewart & Givens, 1934b, p. 1). There is evidence for this belief in that the planners had many personal interactions with Perkins and Hopkins in relation to this program, but it also should be noted that one of the most prominent corporate moderates of the era, Gerard Swope, the president of General Electric, directly discussed the program with Roosevelt in the spring of 1934 (Loth, 1958). I think the following quotation is strong evidence that the corporate-supported planners from the IRC and SSRC had a major impact on the direction taken by the Roosevelt Administration:

> At the request of officials of the Department of Labor and the Federal Emergency Relief Administration, these materials were made informally available in the formulation of plans for a government inquiry. A draft plan for such an inquiry, developed upon the basis of the exploratory study, was placed in the hands of a Cabinet committee, and these plans have eventuated in the establishment by Executive Order, June 29, 1934, of the Committee on Economic Security. Thus the original project became merged in a major planning venture at the Administration (Stewart & Givens, 1934b, p. 1).

The cabinet-level Committee on Economic Security was chaired by Perkins and included Hopkins, as well as the attorney general, the secretary of treasury, and the secretary of agriculture. The committee was assisted by a large staff of experts drawn from the IRC, the SSRC, and a number of government agencies (several of the "government" experts had until recently been employees of foundations, think tanks, and universities). It also had input from an Advisory Council made up of 23 private citizens, including all of the prominent corporate moderates, labor leaders, and social welfare advocates. The structure and process for the committee's work, and much of the research agenda, came from the report that was written after the second SSCR conference (Schlabach, 1969, p. 99; Witte, 1963, pp. 15–16). Stewart was asked to lead the entire research staff, but he turned the job down; instead, he accepted the position as head of unemployment studies (Quadagno, 1988, p. 111; Witte, 1963, pp. 13–14, 31).

The importance of the corporate moderates' ideas to the development of old-age pensions is seen in the fact that Latimer and Brown were the first two people asked to head the research staff on this issue. As the executive director of the staff explained in a work diary that he gave to the SSRC Committee on Social Security in late 1935 to aid its efforts to improve the act, "It was agreed by everyone consulted that the best person in the field was Murray Latimer, who was unavailable because he was chairman of the Railroad Retirement Board" (Witte, 1963, p. 29). However, Latimer was able to serve as chair of an oversight Committee on Old Age Pensions, an important policy role in itself, and worked closely with the research staff in drafting the proposal. Latimer was also given the opportunity to recommend a leader for the staff; his suggestion was one of his collaborators on the railroad retirement study, Brown, whom he also knew through Brown's work for IRC and annual conferences at Princeton on social insurance (Witte, 1963, p. 30). When Brown decided that he could only give part of each week to the work at hand, Professor Barbara Nachtrieb Armstrong of the School of Law at the University of California, Berkeley, was placed in charge of the old-age study (Armstrong, 1965, p. 36). She was a strong admirer of Latimer and Brown, who worked very closely with her, along with Otto Richter, an actuary on loan from AT&T. (The impressive details of Armstrong's career and advocacy for old-age pensions can be found in Domhoff (1996, pp. 151–153).)

The plan prepared by Armstrong and her colleagues sailed through the Committee on Old Age Pensions, but two features of the plan made

Perkins and the other members of the CES a little nervous, its national scope and the insistence on employee contributions. However, the original plan prevailed on both issues. Thus, the process produced a clear victory for the corporate moderates in terms of policy preferences. However, the plan next faced a different kind of challenge. There may have been some inclination on the part of Witte, Perkins, and Roosevelt to wait for a year to send it to Congress because unemployment insurance was considered more important and less controversial. Perkins and staff director Edwin Witte later denied there was any such move afoot, but Armstrong, Latimer, and Brown, were convinced there was and spoke off the record to reporters to that effect after an ambiguous line in a speech to a national conference by Roosevelt. The uproar in the newspapers, along with an outcry from grassroots movements for old-age pensions, led to the assurance by all concerned that old-age pensions would be included in the legislative proposal (Armstrong, 1965, pp. 88–89; Brown, 1965, p. 13; Schlabach, 1969, p. iii).

Shortly after this dust-up, the moderate corporate leaders came into the picture in a supporting role through their membership on the Advisory Council. According to Armstrong (1965, pp. 82–83) and Brown (1972, p. 21), these businessmen were critical in convincing Roosevelt and Perkins to retain the old-age provisions in the legislation. As Brown (1972, p. 21) put it:

> The likelihood of gaining the support of the Cabinet Committee for our proposals was still in doubt. At this critical time, December, 1934, help came from an unexpected source, the industrial executives on the committee's Advisory Council. Fortunately included in the Council were Walter C. Teagle of the Standard Oil Company of New Jersey, Gerard Swope of General Electric, and Marion Folsom of Eastman Kodak, and others well acquainted with industrial pension plans. Their practical understanding of the need for contributory old-age annuities on a broad, national basis carried great weight with those in authority. They enthusiastically approved our program. Just as the newspaper writers had carried us through the November crisis, the support of progressive industrial executives in December ensured that a national system of contributory old-age insurance would be recommended to the President and Congress.

There were many twists, turns, and amendments once the Social Security Act reached Congress, which are too detailed and convoluted to deal with here (Quadagno, 1988; Witte, 1963). The important point in terms of this chapter is that the IRC and SSRC experts expected the act to be imperfect and had already written a proposal calling for a large SSRC study paralleling the government effort (Stewart & Givens, 1934a, p. 1). This proposal became the basis for another SSRC conference, this time directly under the auspices of the Rockefeller Foundation, on March 22–23, 1935, in Atlantic City, New Jersey, while Congress was considering the report from the Committee for Economic Security. This conference unanimously recommended funding for two committees of the SSRC that would work with the Social Security Administration in developing its staffing and procedures. The committees would also discuss ways to improve on the legislation. The Rockefeller Foundation then gave the SSRC's Advisory Committee on Public Administration $386,000 between 1935 and 1940, with most of the money going for studies of the new Social Security Board during the first 2 years (Fisher, 1993, p. 139). These studies were done in conjunction with a new Committee on Social Security, which received its own 3-year grant for $225,000 from the Rockefeller Foundation.

The Clark Amendment

Then, just when it seemed that there was general agreement on the main outlines of the old-age provisions of the Social Security Act, a proposal was made by a Philadelphia insurance man, who did a brisk business installing retirement programs for corporations, to allow corporations with their own stable pension plans to opt out of the system if they so desired ("contracting out"). He convinced Bennett Champ Clark, a conservative Democratic Senator from Missouri, to introduce this amendment, and it became known as the Clark Amendment. The Senate passed it, but Roosevelt sent word that it was unacceptable because it would make it impossible to determine how much the government would have to collect from employers and employees in the government program, among many actuarial and administrative problems. The Clark Amendment caused a 2-month delay in the signing of the bill. The deadlock was broken in August when it was agreed that the amendment would be reconsidered the following year after experts had a chance to see if contracting out could be made compatible with the overall system.

However, it turned out that few corporate moderates, even those from large insurance companies who had been somewhat hesitant about the IRC planning (even though they had involvement in it through their actuaries), had any interest in this amendment. This fact becomes clear through Brown's letters to Latimer and other IRC experts concerning his discussions with executives across the country and at the annual meetings of the American Management Association (Domhoff, 1996, pp. 168–169).

Even more authoritatively, the SSRC's Committee on Social Security commissioned a study to determine the extent of corporate interest in the Clark Amendment. The author, who had first worked on old-age pensions for the Carnegie Corporation 20 years earlier, reported that he could find only a few corporate executives who supported the Clark Amendment once they understood it. Building on this report, Latimer wrote a report for the Social Security Board on March 23, 1936, in which he said, "With the possible exception of Standard Oil Company of New York, I know of no industrialists favoring the Clark Amendment, if such amendment has all or most of the following features" (Latimer, 1936, p. 1). The memo then lists several basic features, such as being at least as favorable as the Social Security Act.

The conclusion was obvious to Brown, Latimer, and other corporate-oriented planners: Companies should focus their old private programs on white-collar workers and executives to make employment at their companies all the more lucrative and attractive. Most corporate executives caught on fast, although a few ultraconservatives used the passage of the Social Security Act as an opportunity to shrink their plans (Quadagno, 1988, p. 118). As for most large insurance companies, they enthusiastically backed Latimer and Brown on this issue and spoke of the new act as a likely boost for the private pension plans they marketed (Klein, 2003, chap. 3).

Amendments to the Social Security Act

Once the Social Security Act had passed and the Clark Amendment was buried, corporate moderates, liberals, and advocates of the Townsend Plan began to argue about how to improve the act, with much of the discussion taking place within the SSRC committees. All parties agreed that the system should be financed on a pay-as-you-go ("paygo") basis rather than by building up a pension reserve, as the act had mandated at the insistence of the secretary of treasury. Furthermore, they could agree to a payment schedule that gave a slight boost to low-income retirees and restrained benefits at the top. These changes were favored by liberals, labor, and Townsendites because of their concern that low-income people have enough money to live on. They suited Keynesian economists because they put money into the hands of those most likely to spend it and avoided the drag on the economy that a government pension fund would create.

On the corporate side of the divide, insurance companies pushed for such a plan because it left plenty of room for their profitable private plans for those with higher incomes, especially for the corporate executive plans that were their biggest customer target. Indeed, this desire was so great that one insurance company even helped finance the liberal reformers who pushed for "adequacy" in old-age pensions (Sass, 1997, p. 282, ftn 17). As for the corporate moderates, they favored paygo in good part because they did not want the government to have any investment funds to manage, which they considered a dangerous precedent that might tempt the Social Security Administration to push for even better pensions.

Several other reforms to the 1935 act, which I do not have the space to discuss here, were carried out in 1939 based on recommendations by a Social Security Advisory Committee headed by Brown and including several members from the SSRC committees (Fisher, 1993; Manza 1995). With the passage of the 1939 amendments, Social Security had reached the form it would have for the next 40 years.

CONCLUSION

If my claims are as solidly grounded in archival research as I think they are, it is worth asking why this version of events is not better known. There are several reasons. First, policy formulation is one thing in the United States and the politics of enactment are another. The planners and experts recede into the background and the politicians take over. This point is all the more important in the case of the Social Security Act because it was formulated by moderate Republicans and embraced by the New Deal. As the years passed, the Republicans did not want to admit any role in it and liberals wanted to claim it as their own.

Second, just as the plan was being discussed in Congress, a Supreme Court ruling in May 1935 almost undermined the rationale for the new legislation and endangered its constitutionality. In a case concerning the new government retirement program for railroad employees, the court ruled that pensions and unemployment relief are not "proper objects" of legislation under the constitution. Nor are the alleged positive effects of pensions on the efficiency and morale of the workforce an acceptable reason. The preamble justifying the social security proposal therefore had to be rewritten. The new version emphasized that such legislation would contribute to the "general welfare" of the country, which is permissible under the constitution. In other words, an ideology based in social welfare had to be constructed that stressed "needs," not efficiency and control of labor markets. This change in justification caused the labor market and industrial relations bases of the plan to be lost from sight and contributed to the belief that social workers, liberals, and unions had created the Social Security Act (Graebner, 1980; Graebner, 1982).

Third, many prominent ultraconservative business leaders were highly visible in their opposition, including Congressional testimony against the bill. On the other hand, moderate business supporters were less outspoken, which left experts from Industrial Relations Counselors, Inc., the Social Science Research Council, and the government's Committee on Economic Security as its main defenders as the act moved through Congress. Fourth, some of the key archival records upon which my assertions are based only became available through the Rockefeller Archives in the 1990s, including the papers of the Social Science Research Council (Domhoff, 1996, chap. 5). Fifth, most of the standard histories of the New Deal are focused on Roosevelt, party politics, and the legislative process, with little or no concern for the possible role of business leaders and the foundations and think tanks they directed.

Explaining the role of the corporate moderates in the origins of government old-age pensions might be useful to those who want to preserve and enhance the current Social Security program. Perhaps supporters of Social Security could win over rank-and-file moderate Republicans if they could show them that business leaders did not always see governmental old-age pensions as a threat to freedom and liberty. An understanding of the role of moderate corporate leaders also might be of use to moderate Republicans in Congress in answering those ultraconservatives who say that the Social Security Act of 1935 is strictly a liberal-labor program.

DISCUSSION QUESTIONS

1 Why is Domhoff's argument important to the understanding of Social Insurance in the United States?
2 Why should corporate moderates today be in support of Social Security and social insurance programs?
3 According to Domhoff, why has the history of the enactment of Social Security been forgotten?

REFERENCES

Alston, L. J., & Ferrie, P. (1999). *Southern paternalism and the American welfare state*. New York: Cambridge University Press.

Amenta, E. (2006). *When movements matter: The Townsend Plan and the rise of social security*. Princeton: Princeton University Press.

Armstrong, B. N. (1965). Oral History. In *New Deal oral history project*. New York: Columbia University.

Brents, B. (1984). Capitalism, corporate liberalism and social policy: The origins of the social security act of 1935. *Mid-American Review of Sociology, 9*, 23–40.

Brown, J. D. (1965). Oral History. In *New Deal oral history project*. New York: Columbia University.

Brown, J. D. (1972). *An American philosophy of social security: Evolution and issues*. Princeton: Princeton University Press.

Bulmer, M. & Bulmer, J. (1981). Philanthropy and social science in the 1920s: Beardsley Ruml and the Laura Spelman Rockefeller Memorial, 1922–29. *Minerva, 19*, 347–407.

Domhoff, G. W. (1996). *State autonomy or class dominance? Case studies on policy making in America*. Hawthorne, NY: Aldine de Gruyter.

Fishback, P. V., & Kantor, S. E. (2000). *A prelude to the welfare state: The origins of workers' compensation*. Chicago: University of Chicago Press.

Fisher, D. (1993). *Fundamental development of the social sciences*. Ann Arbor: University of Michigan Press.

Gitelman, H. M. (1988). *Legacy of the Ludlow massacre*. Philadelphia: University of Pennsylvania Press.

Gordon, L. (1994). *Pitied but not entitled*. New York: Free Press.

Graebner, W. (1980). *A history of retirement*. New Haven: Yale University Press.

Graebner, W. (1982). From pensions to social security: Social insurance and the rise of dependency. In J. N. Schact (Ed.), *The quest for security*. Iowa City, IA: Center for the Study of the Recent History of the United States.

Jenkins, J., Brents, C., & Brents, B. (1989). Social protest, hegemonic competition, and social reform. *American Sociological Review, 54*, 891–909.

Karl, B. (1974). *Charles E. Merriam and the study of politics*. Chicago: University of Chicago Press.

Kaufman, B. (2003). Industrial Relations Counselors, Inc.: Its history and significance. In B. Kaufman, R. Beaumont, & R. Helfgott (Eds.), Industrial relations to human resources and beyond: The evolving process of employee relations management (pp. 31–112). Armonk, NY: M.E. Sharpe.

Klein, J. (2003). *For all these rights: Business, labor, and the shaping of America's public-private welfare state*. Princeton: Princeton University Press.

Latimer, M. (1936). Memorandum to members of the Social Security Board. In *Altmeyer Papers*, (Vol. Box 2), Folder on the Clark Amendment. Madison: Wisconsin State Historical Archives.

Latimer, M., & Hawkins, S. (1938). Railroad retirement system in the United States. In *Murray Latimer papers*. Washington George Washington University Library, Special Collections.

Loth, D. (1958). *Swope of GE*. New York: Simon and Schuster.

Manza, J. (1995). *Policy experts and political change during the New Deal.* Unpublished Doctoral dissertation, University of California, Berkeley.

Piven, F. F. & Cloward, R. A. (1982). *The new class war: Reagan's attack on the welfare state and its consequences*. New York: Pantheon Books.

Quadagno, J. S. (1988). *The transformation of old age security: Class and politics in the American welfare state*. Chicago: University of Chicago Press.

Sass, S. A. (1997). *The promise of private pensions: The first hundred years*. Cambridge: Harvard University Press.

Schlabach, T. F. (1969). *Edwin E. Witte: Cautious reformer*. Madison, WI: State Historical Society of Wisconsin.

Stewart, B., & Givens, M. (1934a). *Planned protection against unemployment and dependency: Report on a tentative plan for a proposed investigation.* New York: Social Science Research Council.

Stewart, B. & Givens, M. (1934b). Project report: Exploratory study of unemployment reserves and relief (economic security). New York: Social Science Research Council.

Witte, E. E. (1963). *The development of the social security act*. Madison: University of Wisconsin Press.

5 The Medicare Modernization Act: Evolution or Revolution in Social Insurance?

THOMAS R. OLIVER AND PHILIP R. LEE

HISTORICAL SHIFTS IN MEDICARE POLICY DEVELOPMENT

Medicare is one of the largest and most popular social programs administered by the U.S. federal government. It provides direct benefits to 44 million Americans. Medicare spending now exceeds $420 billion annually, accounting for 14% of the federal budget and over 17% of all national health spending (Kaiser Family Foundation, 2008; Keehan, Sisko, Truffer, Smith, Cowan, Poisal & Clemens, 2008).

The enactment of Medicare has been described as the "jewel in the crown" of Lyndon Johnson's Great Society (Bernstein, 1996). It was created in 1965 to reduce the economic burden of illness on the elderly and their families. President Johnson described its importance in a speech in June 1966, just before the program became operational. Medicare, he said, "Will free millions from their miseries. It will signal a deep and lasting change in the American way of life. It will take its place beside Social Security and together they will form the twin pillars of protection upon which all of our people can safely build their lives and their hopes" (Health Care Financing Administration, 1996, i).

Although Medicare aimed to alleviate the special situation of the elderly—they incurred higher medical expenses, earned less income than workers younger than 65 and thus were less likely to have health insurance—the economic protection of the program and its institutional design was also meant to appeal to younger people who would be contributing to the program during their working years. The intergenerational contract of social insurance was meant to run both ways. President Johnson framed its meaning at the signing ceremony in July 1965, "No longer will older Americans be denied the healing miracle of modern medicine. No longer will illness crush and destroy the savings they have so carefully put away over a lifetime so they might enjoy dignity in their later years. No longer will young families see their own incomes, and their own hopes, eaten away simply because they are carrying out their deep moral obligations" (Health Care Financing Administration, 1996, I).

The principal architects of the program were not merely focused on health care for the elderly; Medicare was the vessel on which to commence the passage toward universal health insurance for all Americans. Medicare's structure and benefits, indeed, were quite limited and not tailored to the chronic care needs of the elderly. This reflected the view of its founders that Medicare was to serve as the foundation for a more comprehensive system of public health insurance in this country (Ball, 1995; Marmor, 2000; Oberlander, 2003).

More than 4 decades later, Medicare is seen by many Americans and policy makers in a very different light. Beginning in the last half of the 1990s, the usual concerns about slowing program spending were joined with an unprecedented battle over the size and role of government, as well as maneuvering for a series of critical elections. Medicare, as the largest available source of budget "savings," became a main focus in a partisan showdown between President Clinton and the new Republican majorities in Congress.

But spending *per se* was not the only issue; the fundamental nature of the entitlement to senior citizens was being challenged, as was the division of responsibilities between the public and private sectors. "It was not consensus politics being practiced in Washington, or even conservative politics as previously defined. This was ideological warfare, a battle to destroy the remnants of the liberal, progressive brand of politics that had governed America throughout most of the twentieth century" (Johnson & Broder, 1996, p. 569). Medicare had entered into the realm of electoral and ideological politics for the first time since 1964, and the simplistic and polarizing policy debate and political deadlock that ensued was regarded as a symptom of a broader breakdown in American politics.

Proposals for Medicare reform since 1995 have generally reflected the bitter politics ignited by President Clinton's health care financing and reform proposal in 1993–1994. In the end, the debate over the Clinton plan became a polarized, partisan struggle that Republicans pursued for political gain, which contributed to their capturing majority control in the House of Representatives and Senate in the 1994 election. The stage was set in 1995 for a showdown on the budget, including proposals for substantial reductions—"savings" or "cuts," depending on one's perspective—in the future growth of Medicare spending. Congressional proposals were blocked by presidential vetoes, and the ensuing policy differences contributed to a temporary shutdown of the U.S. federal government in late 1995. The public reaction to the stalemate reflected doubts about some of the Republican initiatives and had the effect of slowing change in Medicare as well as other programs.

Despite marked differences in political philosophy and policy priorities, the Clinton administration and Republican congressional leaders cooperated to push through a set of reforms in Medicare financing and coverage as part of the Balanced Budget Act of 1997. This legislation introduced additional insurance options for Medicare beneficiaries, modified payments for health plans and providers, and created a separate State Children's Health Insurance Program. The individual policy changes were relatively modest, yet the combined package authorized a reduction of an estimated $115 billion in projected spending on Medicare and established the basis for further restructuring in later years (Etheredge, 1998).

The historical shifts are a reminder that the state of the Medicare program cannot be understood apart from developments in American politics. Hacker and Skocpol (1997) argue that the Republican surge represented a dramatic turn in American politics with its three-fold strategy: First, reduce spending in existing programs and lower taxes to prevent future spending; second, transfer authority for federal-state programs such as AFDC and Medicaid to the states while retaining sufficient federal control over eligibility and benefits; and third, replace publicly provided services with public purchasing of privately provided services. All three strategies were on display in the 1995 Republican proposals for Medicare reform. Hacker and Skocpol (1997, p. 315) observe:

> [D]espite the similarities between the Truman and Clinton health security efforts, overall contexts of government and politics are much less hospitable to governmentally funded reforms today than they were after Truman's defeat. Back then, market transformations and political dynamics were both pushing toward expanded access to health services and insurance coverage.

> Today, by contrast, both push in the opposite direction. The private insurance market is fragmenting, federal budgetary constraints stymie new programs, and the deficit dominates debate over existing programs. Equally important, a stable reform coalition like that of Truman's day has yet to emerge, while a new and fiercely conservative corps of Republicans is championing coherent programmatic alternatives based on antigovernment premises.

Thus, the politics of entitlements and privatization became the contemporary context for policy debates over the substantive design of the Medicare program. Nearly all participants in the health policy community asserted the need to "modernize" the Medicare program. Modernization meant different things to different participants, however:

- A more comprehensive package of benefits in line with the current technological capabilities of pharmaceuticals and medical care
- Program operations administered primarily by private companies rather than the federal government
- Renegotiating the social contract with the elderly in time to avoid intergenerational conflict and financial collapse of the entire social insurance system, and economic ruin from forcing workers to sustain the entitlements of an aging population.

These competing interpretations of modernization and the policy prescriptions that accompanied them, were a constant source of tension: The first definition implied the need for considerable expansion of the program, while the latter two definitions implied the need to rein in the broad regulatory and redistributive roles of this large public program.

By 2000, there were three major, unresolved issues within the policy debate: (1) the proposed addition of a Medicare benefit for outpatient prescription drugs; (2) the role of managed care and market competition in the future of Medicare; and (3) the proposed transition from the current guarantee of "defined benefits," under which the government covers all covered services for a Medicare beneficiary regardless of cost, to a "defined contribution," under which the government would pay a fixed amount for a beneficiary to enroll in private insurance coverage. Solutions to these issues did not appear to be mutually compatible, but by the fall of 2003, a confusing and controversial political process culminated in reforms to both expand the scope of the Medicare entitlement and expand the role of private companies in administration of the Medicare program (Oliver, Lee, & Lipton, 2004). This episode of "modernization," notably, did not rein in either the short- or long-term costs of the Medicare program; instead, the new reforms created a much costlier program.

In late 2003, both houses of Congress narrowly passed and President George W. Bush (R) signed the Medicare Prescription Drug, Improvement, and Modernization Act (P.L., 108-173), which authorized Medicare coverage of outpatient prescription drugs as well as a host of other changes to the program. The statute, commonly known as the Medicare Modernization Act (MMA), included the following major provisions (Health Policy Alternatives, 2003; Congressional Budget Office, 2004, 12–13; Kaiser Family Foundation, 2004):

- It offered Medicare beneficiaries temporary drug discount cards sponsored by private firms with federal approval, with modest subsidies for low-income beneficiaries.
- It required most beneficiaries to choose whether to maintain any existing prescription drug coverage or to join a new Medicare Part D program, beginning in January 2006. The Part D drug benefits would be offered through stand-alone drug plans or through comprehensive plans under Part C, renamed the Medicare Advantage program. The standard Part D benefits would have an estimated initial premium of $35 per month and a $250 annual deductible. Medicare would pay 75% of annual expenses between $250 and $2,250 for approved prescription drugs, nothing for expenses between $2,250 and $5,100 (the "donut hole") and 95% of expenses above $5,100. Private plans could alter the specific benefits as long as they remained actuarially equivalent to the standard benefits.
- It mandated that all individuals who are eligible for both Medicare and Medicaid would now receive their drug coverage through Medicare. The government would cover the premiums, deductibles, and coinsurance for beneficiaries who are eligible for Medicaid and provide substantial subsidies for other beneficiaries based on income and asset tests. States would be required to pass back to the federal government most of the funds they would save on Medicaid drug coverage.
- It prohibited beneficiaries who enroll in Part D from purchasing supplemental benefits to insure against prescription drug expenses not covered in the program.

- It provided over $86 billion in subsidies for employers and unions to encourage them to maintain their prescription drug coverage for retirees.
- It allowed new Part D prescription drug plans to use formularies approved by the government and to negotiate independently with drug manufacturers but it prohibited any direct governmental price negotiation.
- It maintained the current ban on reimportation of prescription drugs from other countries and authorized the Food and Drug Administration to study the potential effects of reimportation from Canada.
- It committed $14 billion to boost payments to managed care plans in the Medicare Advantage program. At least temporarily, managed care plans would for the first time be paid more per enrollee than the average cost per enrollee in the traditional fee-for-service program.
- It authorized new, tax-free health savings accounts for individuals younger than age 65 (not for Medicare beneficiaries).

The new drug coverage represented a major new federal entitlement for Medicare beneficiaries, who were spending an average of $2,864 per year on prescription drugs (Kaiser Family Foundation, 2005). The drug assistance and other provisions of the new law were projected to cost taxpayers as much as $724 billion from 2006 to 2015 (Kaiser Family Foundation, 2005). Senate Majority Leader Bill Frist (R-TN), one of the chief negotiators and political investors behind the initiative, hailed its passage: "Today is a historic day and a momentous day. Seniors have waited 38 years for this prescription drug benefit to be added to the Medicare program. Today they are just moments away from the drug coverage they desperately need and deserve" (Pear & Hulse, 2003).

Yet, in the wake of this political breakthrough, public opinion on the final product was surprisingly unsupportive:

> After years of fierce campaigning, lobbying, and legislating over the issue, a landmark agreement finally emerged in Congress this week to provide Medicare prescription drug benefits. Among the key stakeholders in the legislation, there were definite winners and losers. But the group that should have come out on top—America's seniors—was reeling and confused at the prospect of limited help, while watching industry groups count their booty. In fact, members of Congress from both parties contended that some seniors

> struggling to pay for prescription drugs may actually end up worse off than they are now (Serafini, 2003, p. 3590).

In a poll taken the week President Bush signed the new Medicare law, 47% of senior citizens opposed the changes and only 26% voiced their approval. Among individuals of all ages who said they were following the Medicare debate closely, 56% said they disapproved of the legislation, although 39% supported it (ABC News/Washington Post, 2003). Their disappointment reflected high expectations as well as the upside-down politics that produced the new reforms:

> Even before Bush's ink on the bill was dry, the two political parties prepared to make the issue a focus of the 2004 elections. Bush, who defied conservatives in the Republican Party by backing a massive increase in a federal program long championed by Democrats, heralded the act as a strengthening of "compassionate government." And Democrats, calling the legislation inadequate and harmful to many seniors, drafted substantially more generous prescription drug coverage and vowed to "take back our Medicare" (Milbank & Deane, 2003, p. A1).

IS THE MEDICARE MODERNIZATION ACT EVOLUTIONARY OR REVOLUTIONARY?

Does the turmoil surrounding the enactment and implementation of the MMA reflect only the political dynamics of that moment, or does it reflect more fundamental changes in the nature of the policy process and the substance of the policies themselves? Is this a revolutionary change in Medicare—at least potentially—or does the MMA follow the patterns established throughout the history of the program? The following sections examine how the MMA fits with the long-term evolution of Medicare as a health care program, a social insurance program, and as a source and reflection of broader political developments.

We will focus our attention on the following three main areas: (1) changes in the key actors in Medicare policy—institutions, officials, policy experts, interest groups, and beneficiaries—and their resources and understandings; (2) changes in the nature of the policy process from the early 1960s to the present; and (3) changes in the state of the health care system and the substantive issues and alternatives debated in the health policy community.

Key Actors in Medicare Policy

One means of assessing the historical significance of the MMA is to determine whether that episode represents a departure in terms of political mobilization and partisan maneuvering. Were the political actors and the resources they devoted to the issue similar to earlier episodes of Medicare reform?

Perhaps the most obvious anomaly regarding the MMA is that the greatest expansion of Medicare since its inception was pushed through political institutions controlled by Republicans. An unexpected window of opportunity opened when Republicans regained majority control of the Senate and maintained control of the House after the 2002 elections. At that point, President Bush made Medicare reform one of his administration's highest domestic priorities. Two of his party's most powerful legislators, Senate Majority Leader Frist and House Ways and Means chairman Bill Thomas, considered Medicare reform to be a high priority and were in a position to shepherd it through the Congress. Republican leaders concluded that they could claim credit for a prescription drug benefit or, because they controlled both the legislative and executive branches of government, they could face negative consequences at the polls in 2004 if they failed to deliver on President Bush's pledge to deliver drug benefits in the 2000 campaign. Medicare reform, in their view, could take a major issue away from the Democrats and help ensure President Bush's re-election and Republican domination of national politics (Oliver, Lee, & Lipton, 2004; Jaenicke & Waddan, 2006).

The MMA is also exceptional by other standards. President Bush's activities, from his agenda-setting proposals in March 2003 to his early-morning lobbying over the Thanksgiving holiday, represented the most extensive involvement by a president in Medicare policy since President Johnson's original battle with Republicans and the American Medical Association to establish the program in 1965. The involvement of party leaders in both houses of Congress was exceptional as well. Frist, Hastert, and the chairmen of the two principal committees—Bill Thomas of House Ways and Means and Charles Grassley of Senate Finance—were the chief framers and negotiators of the legislative package.

However narrow its final passage, the MMA was only possible due to historic shifts by two key interest groups. In contrast to past episodes, the Pharmaceutical Research and Manufacturers of America (PhRMA) was not unalterably opposed to prescription drug benefits under Medicare. Instead, the industry group publicly advocated a prescription drug benefit "as part of a Medicare program that is modernized to allow beneficiaries to choose among qualified private-sector health plans" (Holmer, 1999, p. 24). Industry leaders appeared to recognize that if some drug benefits were on the horizon, it would be better to help craft those benefits than to oppose them outright.

The prospects for reform increased dramatically when, very late in the process, AARP appeared to go against the tide of public opinion and announced its support for the conference committee report: "The endorsement provides a seal of approval from an organization with 35 million members. Republicans also hope it provides political cover against charges by some Democrats that the bill would undermine the federal insurance program for the elderly and disabled" (Pear & Toner, 2003b). AARP committed $7 million dollars to a weeklong newspaper and television advertising campaign aimed at Medicare beneficiaries and wavering members of Congress who were about to vote on the bill. It was a coup for Republicans, some of whom had previously referred to AARP as a "wholly owned subsidiary" of the Democratic Party. The AARP endorsement, in turn, infuriated its usual allies in the Democratic leadership, labor, and consumer groups (Broder, 2004; Broder & Goldstein, 2003; Carey, 2003a; Pear & Toner, 2003b; Stolberg, 2003; Vaida, 2004).

However, these historic shifts by key actors did not assure sufficient votes for the reform package. Liberal opponents such as the AFL-CIO; Association of Federal, State, County, and Municipal Employees; Consumers Union; Families USA; and the American Nurses' Association criticized the inadequacy of the drug benefits, the threat to retiree benefit programs, the boost it gave to private health plans, and the lack of any meaningful price controls (Pear & Toner, 2003a; Pear & Toner, 2003b; Dionne, 2003). At the same time, conservative groups such as the Heritage Foundation and the National Taxpayers Union attacked the new benefits as a burden to taxpayers and the economy. They criticized what they regarded as an inevitable replacement of employer-sponsored retiree coverage with a massive new public prescription drug program (notwithstanding its administration through private contractors). They also opposed any Medicare legislation that did not establish direct price competition between the managed care and fee-for-service programs (Agan, 2003; Butler, Moffit, & Riedl, 2003; Chen, 2003).

In the end, there was much anguish by supporters and opponents as legislative leaders repeatedly rescued the reforms from apparent defeat. Ultimately, it was the "sheer force" of Republican leadership—House Speaker Hastert and Senate Majority Leader Frist, in concert with

President Bush and DHHS Secretary Tommy Thompson—that maintained sufficient party discipline to nudge the reform package over the finish line in 2003 (Goldstein, 2003; Koszczuk & Allen, 2003; Schuler & Carey, 2004).

The Process of Medicare Policy Making

There are two major ways in which the process of Medicare policy development in 2003 differed significantly from earlier periods of reform. First, in the 2003 reform efforts, health policy was not subservient to fiscal policy, and President Bush and congressional leaders were not constrained by the commitment to budget containment that had dominated Medicare policy for over 2 decades. The nearly perennial federal budget deficit, which grew dramatically after the tax cuts proposed by President Ronald Reagan and adopted by Congress in the early 1980s, was a dominant influence until the short-lived budget surpluses of the late 1990s (Oberlander, 2003; Oliver, Lee, & Lipton, 2004; Marmor, 2000; Mayes & Berenson, 2006). The federal budget process had influenced Medicare policy in two ways. First, it provided a powerful context for framing health policy issues, forcing debates to focus on the problem of cost containment more than on access or quality of coverage, and to focus more on incremental regulatory solutions than more comprehensive reforms. Second, it established powerful procedures—in particular, budget reconciliation—to facilitate those solutions.

During the 1980s, Medicare policy became closely intertwined with federal budget policy. Authorization to develop the Prospective Payment System (PPS) for hospital services, for example, was included in a broad deficit-reduction measure, the Tax Equity and Fiscal Responsibility Act of 1982 (TEFRA, P.L. 97-248), in response to both general concerns about the federal budget deficit and more specific concerns about Medicare cost increases in the hospital sector (e.g., Moon, 1996, 53–55). As deficits continued to grow despite TEFRA and the Deficit Reduction Act of 1984 (DEFRA, P.L. 98-369), Congress adopted a series of changes in budget procedures, building on rules enacted in the post-Watergate era that were designed to reduce the deficit and control both entitlement and discretionary spending. The Gramm-Rudman-Hollings legislation (the Balanced Budget and Emergency Deficit Control Act of 1985, P.L. 99-177), established deficit targets for each year through Fiscal Year (FY) 1991 and a sequestration procedure under which budget resources would be canceled if the estimated deficits exceeded the targets (Schick, 1995,

p. 39). To avoid this consequence, under "reconciliation" procedures, the House and Senate Budget Committees issued instructions to designated committees to report legislation to reduce the projected deficit by the required amount.

Medicare became a frequent target for deficit reduction under these procedures and in the budgets submitted by the Executive Branch: Every budget submission by President Reagan and President George H.W. Bush contained proposals for substantial cuts in Medicare (Moon, 1996, p. 2). Frequent changes to PPS formulas intended to reduce hospital reimbursements and cuts in reimbursements for durable medical equipment are only two of many examples of legislative efforts to rein in Medicare costs in the general budget deficit reduction effort, and the process became one of congressional micromanagement of Medicare spending (Moon, 1996, p. 78). The new benefits enacted in the Medicare Catastrophic Coverage Act of 1988, including prescription drug coverage, were also in part the victim of these budget procedures, as they effectively required prefunding of the new program. This feature contributed to the hostility of the Medicare population to the legislation following its enactment, and the resulting political pressure ultimately led to its repeal in 1989 (Moon, 1996, pp. 115–144).

Legislation implementing the 1990 budget "summit" agreement (the Omnibus Budget Reconciliation Act [OBRA] of 1990, P.L. 101-508) changed the budget procedures in several ways. First, it abandoned fixed deficit reduction targets and substituted targets based on projected increases in program expenditures. Second, it introduced annual limits in federal spending for "defense and nondefense" spending, "discretionary" spending, and violent crime reduction. Finally, it instituted "paygo" rules for entitlement spending, which required that legislation increasing such spending be offset to avoid an increase in the deficit (Schick, 1995, p. 39). In addition to these procedural changes, the 1990 legislation provided for tax increases and spending cuts, once again targeting Medicare spending. Following the pattern established in previous budget bills, the Medicare changes largely involved freezes or reductions in updates to formulas for payments to hospitals, physicians, laboratory services, and other Medicare providers.

By the late 1990s, the fiscal context for Medicare policy had shifted considerably. The payment reforms made in the Balanced Budget Act of 1997 and an accompanying crackdown on fraud led to an unprecedented slowdown in the growth of Medicare spending; indeed, in 1999, Medicare spending actually declined for the first time in the program's history

(Congressional Budget Office, 2004, p. 137). Also, economic prosperity and a booming stock market erased annual federal budget deficits and produced sizable budget surpluses for the first time in decades. From FY 1998 through FY 2001, annual surpluses ranged from $69 to $236 billion (Congressional Budget Office, 2004, p. 129). These two developments extended the projected life of the Part A hospital trust fund from 2001 to 2029 and greatly reduced the pressure to seek further efficiencies in Medicare.

The projected budget surpluses, in fact, made it more necessary for political leaders to answer why the government could not help cover prescription drugs for all beneficiaries. Political support was also easier to muster now than in the past because the "paygo" requirements of OBRA 1990 expired in 2002. As a result, policy makers were not forced to create a costly prescription drug benefit within a zero-sum financial game, which would force them to pay for the new coverage by imposing higher costs on seniors themselves, increasing taxes, or making cuts in other parts of Medicare or other domestic programs. The willingness to spend new federal revenues made it far less likely that policy makers would see a repeat of the revolt that led to the repeal of the Medicare Catastrophic Coverage Act and its drug benefit.

The second major change was the transformation of Medicare policy making from a deliberative, pragmatic, and bipartisan process into a highly polarized, deadlocked debate. Paul Sabatier and Hank Jenkins-Smith (1993) argue that on many policy issues the competing coalitions are not temporary alliances—"strange bedfellows"—but rather individuals and organizations who share common values and beliefs about what constitutes appropriate and effective public policy. They hold "deep-core" normative beliefs and "near-core" policy beliefs that are highly resistant to change. In addition, they hold a variety of "secondary" beliefs that are more tactical than strategic and are more subject to change over time. Building on these beliefs, they develop long-standing relationships with other members of the advocacy coalition and exhibit a high degree of coordination on political strategy.

For most of the Medicare program's history, the principal advocacy coalitions were organized around the interests of providers, beneficiaries, and governmental officials (Oliver, 1993, pp. 128–130). The core values centered on professional autonomy (and economic interest) for providers, preservation of meaningful entitlements for beneficiaries, and protecting the public purse for governmental officials. Within the governmental coalition, especially in the congressional committees of jurisdiction, there was considerable bipartisanship, which was useful when countering beneficiaries' and providers' shared interests in expanding services and when instituting regulatory regimes for cost containment (Oberlander, 2003, p. 106, 133; Oberlander, 2007, p. 195; Oliver, 1993, pp. 132–141).

The politics of the Clinton health plan drastically changed the politics of Medicare. Although President Clinton had seized on "managed competition" as a synthesis of liberal goals and conservative methods (Starr, 1992; Hacker, 1997), the health insurance industry, small business groups, pharmaceutical companies, and other opponents successfully attacked the reforms on the grounds that they represented heavy-handed intrusion on individual choice and created sizable new bureaucracies to manage the system and constrain costs if competition failed to do so (Johnson & Broder, 1996; Skocpol, 1996). In the mid-1990s, the advocacy coalitions around Medicare policy fractured, dividing providers and governmental officials in particular; the new coalitions are much more aligned with the Democratic and Republican parties and, as a result, the debates over adding prescription drugs and other strategies to "modernize" Medicare became highly polarized.

In contemporary politics, conservative Republicans and liberal Democrats often hold fundamentally different deep-core beliefs about individual responsibility, the role of government, and the capacity of the private sector for meeting social needs. They also have very different near-core beliefs that shape their policy preferences. Democrats tend to favor a government-financed system of national health insurance. They consider Medicare, along with Social Security, as the central components of a social insurance system that provides universal protection to all of the nation's senior citizens. Where health care is purchased privately, Democrats still favor a strong hand for federal and state regulation of providers, health plans, and the rest of the health care industry.

In contrast, Republicans tend to advocate individual, not collective, responsibility for securing most goods and services. They accept a minimal governmental role in Medicaid, welfare, and other safety net programs for the poor, but generally oppose expansion of universal entitlements. Republicans have stressed the superiority of markets over government in the allocation of resources and thus want to preserve a major role for private business and health systems in the provision of health care services.

These distinct approaches are deeply entrenched. Robin Toner (2003) notes how intertwined politics has become with policy prescriptions:

> In fact, the divisions over health care—specifically, how much to trust private markets, how much to rely on government—are among the most profound in politics today. Republicans and their allies say turning Medicare into more of a private health care market place, in which numerous health plans compete for the elderly's business, will give the program's beneficiaries more choices and modernize its bureaucratic structure before the baby boom generation hits.... Democrats and their allies say Medicare was created because the private health insurance market failed to meet the needs of the elderly. They charge that what some Republicans are ultimately aiming for is replacing the guaranteed benefits of Medicare with a voucher.

The different approaches of Republicans and Democrats depend largely on whether one views medical care as a market good or as a medically determined need (Svihula, 2008; White, 2007, pp. 229–231). According to Sherry Glied (1997, p. 26), there are sharp contrasts between "marketist" and "medicalist" advocates of health care reform. "Marketists" see health care as just another good or service. They object to government financing of health care because it distorts the market (despite abundant evidence that the market does not function properly in health care). For "medicalists," allocation should depend on needs determined by expert providers, whose diagnosis and treatment should be guided entirely by medical science and not costs (despite abundant evidence that practice patterns of health care providers are often unscientific and excessively costly). She argues that the ideological differences contribute to political deadlock and undermine even incremental reform, because "every such change increases the likelihood that either the marketist or medicalist view of health care will ultimately prevail."

Between 1999 and 2003, initiatives to add prescription drug coverage to Medicare reached an impasse—even when it appeared the coverage could easily be funded by federal budget surpluses—because of divided government and ideological conflict between the dominant advocacy coalitions in Medicare policy. The impasse was due, more than anything else, to the seemingly irreconcilable core beliefs guiding public policy in general and Medicare in particular. Even when Republican leaders accepted the need for governmental subsidies of prescription drug costs, they almost exclusively favored the marketist approach in policy design, rejecting standard benefits and central administration. This was especially true for Rep. Thomas and his colleagues in the House of Representatives. Most Democratic leaders strongly favored the medicalist approach, albeit with a heavy dose of governmental oversight. Similarly, AARP focused on adequate benefits for all beneficiaries—ruling out a strictly marketist approach—although PhRMA vetoed any steps that could easily lead to price controls in what was by far the most lucrative segment of its market.

The MMA was enacted despite strong partisanship at a level not seen even in the original enactment of Medicare in 1965, nor at any other moment in the program's history. The process began with a degree of bipartisan cooperation in the Senate Finance Committee. The final package approved by the committee reflected the goals of improving the scope and quality of Medicare services and making them available to all Medicare beneficiaries (instead of using new benefits as a carrot only for beneficiaries who joined managed care plans). It authorized new preferred-provider organizations to offer both catastrophic coverage and preventive services in addition to standard Medicare benefits and new prescription drug coverage (Toner & Pear, 2003; kaisernetwork.org, 2003). In addition, it required the federal government to offer "fallback" drug coverage in the event that private plans were not available in some areas of the country. In June 2003, the full Senate passed S.1 by a margin of 76 to 21. It had substantial bipartisan support, as key Democrats such as Edward Kennedy and Minority Leader Tom Daschle felt it was best to accept the new $400 billion commitment as "money in the bank" toward a more comprehensive program (Toner & Pear, 2003).

The level of cooperation deteriorated from that point on, however. In the wake of Senate action, the full House narrowly passed H.R. 1 by a vote of 216 to 215 only after an abnormally long roll call. The bare winning margin came despite intense lobbying by the White House in support of the bill and a visit by Vice President Dick Cheney (R) to the House floor (Goldstein & Dewar, 2003; Angle, 2003). House leaders had to persuade several GOP representatives to switch their votes at the last moment to save the measure. Many conservatives were reluctant to commit such large sums to a new federal entitlement, and they also felt that the bill did not go far enough in creating incentives for beneficiaries to switch from the traditional fee-for-service program to private health plans. To hold some conservative votes, House leaders attached a provision not germane to Medicare, an expansion of tax-exempt health savings accounts for uninsured or self-insured individuals and families—a move that was projected to add $174 billion more to the federal deficit over 10 years (Toner & Pear, 2003; Congressional Budget Office, 2003, p. 5).

House and Senate leaders convened a conference committee in August 2003 and initially planned to complete their work by the end of the summer. The conference committee deviated from normal procedures and was heavily stacked in favor of Republican priorities. The chair, Thomas, allowed only two Democratic senators to participate in the day-to-day discussions—Max Baucus, who was working side-by-side with Finance Committee chair Grassley, and John Breaux, who had long supported market-oriented reforms with Frist and Thomas. Minority Leader Daschle, who voted for the original Senate bill, was excluded entirely from the discussions. The three Democratic conferees from the House were also excluded, which reduced their participation to signing or not signing the conference committee report (Carey, 2003b; Pear & Toner, 2003c).

At several points, participants close to the conference committee negotiations believed that another opportunity for reform would be missed. In November 2003, however, the conferees reached agreement on a new version of H.R. 1, the Medicare Prescription Drug, Improvement, and Modernization Act of 2003. The 678-page conference report included many of the features that had come to be widely accepted in earlier proposals, such as the discount card, additional assistance for low-income beneficiaries, a substantial gap in benefits for individuals with high drug costs ("doughnut hole"), and the use of private pharmacy benefit managers in lieu of direct governmental regulation. Yet, the bill reflected "concession" more than "compromise," with the final provisions on some of the most controversial issues watered down so as to become almost meaningless to their proponents. This deepened rather than resolved cleavages that pitted Democrats against Republicans and, at times, Republicans against Republicans (Goldstein, 2003; Rapp, 2003).

The House vote on the conference report came at 3:00 AM on November 22. The reforms appeared to be dead when, at the end of the normal 15 minutes allowed for voting, the bill was losing by 15 votes. At that point, Hastert and the rest of the Republican leadership went into action and eventually reduced it to a razor-edge margin of 216 to 218. It stuck there while DHHS Secretary Thompson, defying House custom, moved onto the floor and the leaders roused President Bush to make another half-dozen calls to convince a handful of their colleagues to change their votes. A Republican who was retiring in 2004 claimed he was offered $100,000 to help his son run for his seat, on the condition that he switch his vote (Schuler & Carey, 2004). After holding open the vote for nearly 3 hours—by far the longest known roll call vote in the history of the House—H.R. 1 passed by a margin of 220 to 215. The vote closely followed party lines: Only 16 Democrats supported the final package, whereas 25 Republicans opposed it (Broder, 2003; Carey, 2003a; Koszczuk & Allen, 2003).

On November 25, the Senate leadership brought up H.R. 1 for final action and again the outcome was far from certain for many hours. A vote to close off debate prevailed by a wide margin, but it appeared that opponents would succeed in blocking the legislation on a budgetary point of order. The Congressional Budget Office officially projected a net cost of $395 billion for the reform package. Democrats, however, contended that the budgetary impact of the tax-free health savings accounts was not fully counted and, if it was, the cost of the full package would exceed the $400 billion limit allowed by the Senate budget resolution several months earlier. After colleagues beseeched him to support the president and his party, former Republican majority leader Trent Lott gave in and cast the deciding vote to waive the budget rules and proceed to an up or down vote on the Medicare bill itself. He then voted against the bill along with eight other Republican senators, but 11 Democrats and one independent voted in favor of the reforms, and the final version of H.R. 1 was approved by a margin of 54 to 44 (Carey, 2003b; Koszczuk & Allen, 2003).

An editorial in the *Washington Post* summarized the chaotic conclusion to the debate on H.R. 1:

> For sheer political drama, it would be hard to beat the past few days on Capitol Hill. Between the normally apolitical hours of 3 and 6 on Saturday morning, the House voted, by the tiniest of margins, to pass a hugely controversial Medicare bill. During the vote, which was of unprecedented length, the House Republican leadership, cajoled, berated and twisted arms, barely controlling a conservative revolt, while President Bush, jet-lagged from his trip to Europe, called up recalcitrant members one by one. On Monday it was the Senate's turn. Opponents of the bill used a bag of parliamentary tricks in an attempt to defeat what Sen. Edward Kennedy (D-Mass.) has called an "attack on Medicare as we know it." Nevertheless, two attempts to waylay the bill were defeated by some of the bribes and threats that won the day in the House, along with the fears of some Democratic senators of blocking a big new entitlement bill so soon before an election (Washington Post, 2003).

What happened to overcome the ideological and political impasse in 2003? The critical changes were external to the ongoing legislative battles. First, the contextual conditions shifted with Republicans in control of both houses of Congress and the White House, and a decision by President Bush to invest heavily in reaching a prescription drug program in order to take that issue away from Democrats in his 2004 re-election campaign. The president and the Republican leadership in Congress intensely lobbied legislators and the pharmaceutical industry to concede some of their market-oriented agenda on Medicare in order to strengthen their broader political agenda.

Second, a broadly constructed set of evidence and arguments emerged to challenge the practices of the pharmaceutical industry. Drug manufacturers were accused of charging Medicare beneficiaries prices that were many times higher than prices for the identical drug in other countries, obtaining unwarranted extensions of patents to pad profits and delay the introduction of generic competitors, and making multimillion dollar investments in me-too drugs and direct-to-consumer advertising. Criticism of those practices, combined with the spectacular rise in drug spending per beneficiary and consequent erosion of supplemental coverage through employers and the existing Medicare + Choice managed care program, led Republicans to take responsibility for moving legislation that previously would never have been a high priority for them.

Third, the decision of AARP to endorse H.R. 1 broke up the long-standing alignment of the competing coalitions and gave lawmakers political cover to vote for the reform package and if necessary disregard their ideological convictions. The unprecedented momentum for action forced members of both advocacy coalitions into concessions in policy design that challenged their core values. Conservatives won a heavy role for the private sector in providing drug coverage. They were unable to dramatically strengthen the overall role of private health plans in Medicare, however, and agreed to provide beneficiaries who choose to remain in the fee-for-service program with comparable benefits to managed care enrollees. Many liberals supported the original Senate bill and a critical few ended up voting for the final version of H.R. 1, despite the fact that it introduced means-testing of benefits and income-related premiums for the first time in Medicare's history. They may have believed that helping the neediest beneficiaries—those with low incomes and those with extraordinary drug expenses—is their core priority. If so, it was preferable to waiting for a more favorable political climate in which to adopt a more universal and generous program. They may have also believed that once the government is providing some prescription drug assistance, if that assistance proves inadequate for large numbers of beneficiaries then policy makers will be forced to improve the program rather than neglect it.

A final departure from the conventional policy process was also instrumental in the narrow passage of MMA. In March 2004, the chief actuary of the Centers for Medicare and Medicaid Services revealed that, as early as the previous summer, his office had estimated higher costs for the proposed reforms than the congressional budget analysts. The actuary's superiors in the Bush administration, however, had ordered him to withhold the estimates from members of Congress and warned him that "the consequences for insubordination are extremely severe" (Goldstein, 2004; Stolberg, 2004). Members of both parties acknowledged that if the administration's estimates had been known to legislators and the public, significant changes would likely have been required in the final provisions of H.R. 1. Otherwise, it would have faced even stronger opposition from conservatives in the House, and opponents in the Senate may well have succeeded in blocking the bill on a budgetary point of order (Schuler & Carey, 2004; Stolberg & Pear, 2004; Washington Post, 2004).

The Goals and Instruments of Medicare Policy

The course of policy development leading up to passage of the MMA reveals significant discontinuities in the patterns of political mobilization and in the legislative process. A final area for inquiry concerns the nature of the MMA reform package itself: What does the MMA represent in terms of continuity and change over the 40-year history of Medicare? Are there also significant departures from past policies significant enough to produce revolutionary rather than evolutionary changes in the Medicare program and the American health care system as a whole?

One can begin by examining the scope and types of policy change envisioned by the statute. The MMA is most notable for offering, after 38 years, some coverage of outpatient prescription drugs for Medicare beneficiaries. The dominance of drug coverage in the public debate was a relatively new phenomenon. From the late 1960s to the late 1990s, prescription drug coverage for Medicare beneficiaries was always linked to the fate of other proposals for health care reform, and only at the end of the Clinton administration did the issue take on a life of its own. But the MMA includes many other provisions aimed at restructuring the basic health insurance program and even the nature of private health insurance.

A number of episodes in the evolution of Medicare are significant for one or more of the following reasons: (1) they have a material impact on resource allocation, (2) they establish a new role for government in policy and regulation; or (3) they shift the manifest purpose of the program. Although minor changes in the Medicare program are relatively routine, the following list focuses primarily on innovations establishing coverage for new populations, new areas of benefits, new methods of financing, or new methods of paying for services.[1] These policy shifts tend to fall somewhere in between the major change wrought by the creation of Medicare itself and the frequent fine-tuning of program benefits and financing.

1965–1966 Enactment of Medicare (along with Medicaid), program implementation.[2] Johnson administration officials require that hospitals must abide by the 1964 Civil Rights Act to receive Medicare payments, accelerating the end of racial segregation in hospital care.

1972 Amendments extending Medicare benefits to Social Security Disability Insurance beneficiaries, creating End Stage Renal Disease program, allowing research and demonstration projects, authorizing PSROs, and establishing the Medicare Economic Index (MEI implemented in 1975).

1982 Authorization of Medicare risk contracts with Health Maintenance Organizations (implemented in 1985).

1983 Adoption of the Prospective Payment System for Medicare hospital services, replacing cost-based reimbursement with new fixed payments for diagnosis-related episodes of care.

1984–1996 Series of changes in the Medicare physician payment system, especially provisions in the 1989 budget legislation to establish a Medicare Fee Schedule for physician services, limits on balance billing of

[1] Rowland (1991), for example, provides an extensive list of legislation between 1965 and 1989 affecting health benefits for senior citizens.

[2] The presence of Medicaid, especially its coverage for nursing home care, has been a critical complement to the Medicare program. The availability of nursing home care, prescription drugs, and other services for low-income Medicare beneficiaries ("dually-eligible") has served as a political safety valve, taking pressure off of policy makers to expand Medicare benefits. We do not delve further into Medicaid policy in this paper, nor the relationship between the Medicare and Medicaid programs.

beneficiaries, and volume performance standards (implemented from 1992–1996).

1988–1989 Enactment and subsequent repeal of Medicare catastrophic health insurance program and prescription drug benefits.

1990 Adoption of requirement that "Medigap" policies (private insurance for benefits not covered by Medicare) must conform to ten standardized benefit packages approved by the National Association of Insurance Commissioners (implemented in 1992).

1997 Enactment of the Medicare + Choice program (Part C) to expand options for enrollment in managed care, adoption of changes in the financing of home health services and graduate medical education, and authorize medical savings accounts for Medicare beneficiaries.[3]

2003 Enactment of a new Medicare Part D prescription drug assistance program through private drug plans or Medicare Advantage managed care plans, subsidies to employers to maintain retiree prescription drug benefits, subsidies to aid managed care plans, adoption of a "trigger" or cap on proportion of program financing from general revenues, and demonstration of price competition between traditional fee-for-service and managed care options.

Peter Hall (1993) distinguishes types of policy change according to whether policy makers have changed the basic *goals* of the policy, changed the basic *instruments* for achieving those goals, or changed the *setting* of those policy instruments. What Hall describes as "third order change"—altering goals, instruments, and settings all at once—is rare in the evolution of Medicare. Those episodes are limited to:

- The creation and implementation of Medicare in 1965–1966.
- The 1972 legislation, expanding the population and services covered by the program; establishing a variety of cost containment mechanisms such as Professional Standards Review Organizations

---

[3] Among its health initiatives, the Balanced Budget Act of 1997 also established the State Children's Health Insurance Program and increased state flexibility in restructuring Medicaid programs.

(to conduct peer review of the quality and cost of care), the Medicare Economic Index, and authority for research and demonstrations for alternative systems of delivery and payment.

- The 1988 legislation, setting boundaries on beneficiaries' financial liability, devising income-related premiums and drug utilization review, and increasing the scope of benefits with drug coverage (later repealed).
- The 2003 legislation, establishing new benefits for prescription drug coverage, creating novel risk-bearing private drug plans, increasing payments to managed care plans, and establishing new subsidies to employers for retiree benefits, a potential structure for direct competition between the fee-for-service and managed care programs, and vastly expanding the availability of health savings accounts for the population not eligible for Medicare.

From this perspective, the MMA is clearly third-order change and takes its place alongside only a handful of other major reforms in the history of Medicare. The addition of prescription drug coverage was not tinkering, but a fundamental commitment to a new role for the entire program on behalf of beneficiaries. New instruments in the form of private drug plans, a "soft" cap on program financing from general revenues, and competition between the fee-for-service and managed care program (Medicare Advantage) varied in their immediate impact, but laid the foundation for a potentially dramatic transformation of the program over time.

The most prominent initiative in the MMA depends on the emergence and sustainability of risk-bearing, drug-only insurance plans to serve the vast majority of beneficiaries in the traditional fee-for-service program. This was a significant departure from the logic of risk pooling and integrated benefits; from 1965–1994, all proposals to add prescription drug benefits contemplated a straightforward expansion of the Medicare Part B program (Oliver, Lee, & Lipton, 2004).

It was also a significant political turnabout because, in the past, the insurance industry opposed this approach. In 2000, the then-president of the Health Insurance Association of America, Charles Kahn III, had argued that no insurer would provide drug-only coverage because "it would be like providing insurance for haircuts": Only those seniors with high out-of-pocket costs would be motivated to join the new plans. If insurers were not free to set premiums, they could easily lose money on such plans (Morgan, 2000; Pear, 2000, 2003).

Since a Clinton administration proposal in 1999, a separate drug benefit administered by private organizations had been the dominant approach. Under the Clinton proposal, however, the federal government would have been the insurer under a new Medicare Part D, whereas the economic risk fell primarily on private plans under the legislative proposals in 2003 (Oliver, Lee, & Lipton, 2004). Perhaps the most important impact in the long term is the further fragmentation of Medicare financing and administration because beneficiaries choosing to stay in the fee-for-service program will be enrolled in up to three separate parts of Medicare (Parts A, B, and D). The types of oversight and regulation that the Centers for Medicare and Medicaid Services exercises over Part A and Part B are, at least for the time being, barred for Part D.

Even the modest re-setting of payment rates to Medicare Advantage plans was novel. It reversed the economic analysis underlying the Balanced Budget Act of 1997, when officials recognized that payments to managed care plans *unintentionally* exceeded the true costs of services for the plans. The MMA subsidies represented the first time that the federal government was *intentionally* paying health plans more than the projected costs for treating beneficiaries in the traditional fee-for-service program (Biles, Nicholas, & Cooper, 2004). The new policy was at odds with the basic argument in favor of market competition, namely, that it was more efficient and would help contain the Medicare budget over time. One critic commented on the ironic turn of events: "Here's another bit of insanity: The bill pays private insurance companies to take elderly patients. You know how one of the tenets of conservative philosophy is that private companies can always deliver a product better and cheaper? So why does the Medicare bill offer billions in subsidies to private insurers to induce them into the market? That's not competition; that's corporate welfare" (Tucker, 2003).

Another milestone in the MMA was the institution of means-testing of benefits and income-related premiums for the first time in Medicare's history. Income-related premiums were first enacted in the Medicare Catastrophic Coverage Act in 1988, but were detested by beneficiaries and became a focal point for the campaign that ultimately repealed the law the following year (Himelfarb, 1995). Means-testing of benefits is an even more profound change, as it threatens the universality of the entitlement and makes it easier for political leaders and the general public to equate Medicare with Medicaid and other "welfare" programs. These two elements threaten some of the most important founding principles of Medicare, as articulated by Robert Ball, former Commissioner of the Social Security Administration and one of the program's architects. In particular, they undermine the principles that:

- All participants should have a guaranteed set of benefits—a defined benefit package—not just a defined contribution plan or premium subsidy.
- All participants regardless of race and income should be treated the same.
- Although persons with higher wages pay more of the costs of the program through Part A contributions during their working lives, there is no means test for benefits once they sign up for Medicare.
- The use of general revenues in addition to premiums to finance Part B would heavily subsidize services not only for the poor but also for well-off Medicare beneficiaries.

The overriding policy objective since Medicare was created has been to maintain the original entitlement and benefits. Despite continual escalation in program costs and budgetary pressures from outside the program, policy makers have seldom even considered reducing benefits. Although the aggregate costs of health care coverage have increased for Medicare beneficiaries, policy makers have also kept increases in cost-sharing to a minimum. Part B premiums were indexed to inflation rather than program costs, until they slipped to the point that they were covering only 25% of program costs. A significant component of the physician payment reforms in the 1980s limited balance billing of beneficiaries or eliminated it altogether by increasing physician acceptance of Medicare assignment. An increase in beneficiary cost-sharing was considered and rejected in the 1990 budget agreement between the President Bush and congressional leaders.

When necessary, policy makers have reduced payments to health care providers rather than impose explicit burdens on beneficiaries (Janus & Brown, 2007; Oliver, 1993; Smith, 1992; White 2007). The basic social contract has always been with voters, not the health care industry. The MMA, through a variety of policy innovations, has the potential to severely undermine that social contract (Oberlander, 2007).

THE DURABILITY OF MEDICARE AND LIMITS TO THE MEDICARE REVOLUTION

In many respects, the most notable feature of Medicare is the persistence of its basic purposes and structure even in the face of dramatic changes in politics, public policy, and the health care system. Prior to 2003, many outside observers understood the political power of the elderly to be the chief obstacle to significant restructuring of Medicare. Pointing to Medicare beneficiaries as the "third rail" of American politics is insufficient, however, to explain the development of Medicare over time. We suggest that the Medicare program has been a "conservative" program for *many* reasons:

First, it is difficult to make significant changes due to a variety of population groups and organizations protecting their interests. Once a group or industry has gained material benefits through public policy, it is difficult to reduce those benefits (Stigler, 1971; Wilson, 1973). Medicare, like most other areas of American public policy, suffers from "organizational sclerosis" (Olson, 1989). This applies to senior citizens and the disabled, health care providers, private health insurers selling Medigap, and the pharmaceutical industry. Thus, even as policy makers adopted new means testing of both benefits and premiums, whether for pragmatic reasons (arbitrary spending limits) or ideological reasons (attacking social solidarity) those restraints were only possible because at the same time they were broadening the scope and value of benefits for nearly all participants in the Medicare program (Oberlander, 2007, p. 192). "Organizational sclerosis" in Medicare also plays out in the form of pressure for more equal access to benefits and services across all geographic regions of the country, usually driven by members of the Senate representing states with large rural populations. The most important manifestation of this is that, even though it subverted their ideological predispositions and policy preferences, Republican leaders elected not to force the overwhelming majority of Medicare beneficiaries out of the traditional fee-for-service program, and they made participation in the Part D drug benefits voluntary. The 2003 reforms cannot be said to strengthen the fee-for-service program, but they do not appear to greatly accelerate its demise, either.

Second, the history of Medicare provides ample evidence that even small changes to a big program have large, unpredictable consequences. Lindblom (1959; 1979) and Braybrooke and Lindblom (1963), among others, argue that disjointed incrementalism occurs because the "branch" method of decision making (Where do we go from here?) is typically *easier* than the "root" method of decision making (How do we get back to first principles?); it is difficult to gain sufficient agreement among interested parties, particularly when the knowledge base is weak as was the case in the MMA effort to establish private, stand-alone drug plans and other market-oriented policies. Incrementalism may also be *preferable* because the branch method avoids large-scale mistakes; yet Medicare provides many examples of how cautious, segmented problem solving creates new problems in other areas of the program and also sets a course of action that proves to be ineffective, yet hard to undo. Thus, although policy makers are properly cautious in formulating reforms, from a historical perspective they are often too ready to tinker with dysfunctional systems at the margin. If policy makers find in the near future that the reforms under MMA, particularly the separate drug plans and ban on government negotiation of prices, make it difficult to contain that part of the Medicare budget, they will be hard pressed to impose regulatory solutions without rebuilding the institutional infrastructure first.

Third, policy change is difficult because of transformations in American political institutions. Medicare came into being during a brief period of highly partisan, unified government; yet there was less hostility within Congress, little hostility between the branches of government, and little hostility between the private sector and governmental officials. Over time, however, Medicare policy has come to reflect an era of commonly divided government, increased hostility between political parties and branches of government, federal budget deficits and resistance to tax increases, and multiple committee jurisdiction over the program. All of these factors affect the capacity for policy change: Fiscal constraints actually facilitate small to midlevel policy change, but serve to deter major reforms, especially any that would, in the short term, increase program spending. Proponents of the MMA were fortunate to have a political window of opportunity for reform at the very moment that concerns over federal spending were at their lowest level in decades. But after tax cuts and a sluggish economy eliminated the surplus revenues that could have funded new Medicare benefits, the federal government faced record budget deficits of $375 billion for FY 2003 and $477 for FY 2004, exacerbated further by the invasion and occupation of Iraq and hundreds of billions of dollars in additional tax cuts (Congressional Budget Office, 2004; Weisman, 2003). Many conservative Republicans were growing anxious about further expanding commitments for mandatory federal spending

(Grier, 2003). So, although the MMA squeezed through because of raw political muscle, the emerging budgetary constraints suggested that easy fixes to new and ongoing problems in Medicare would face greater barriers. Indeed, after Democrats regained slim majorities in both houses of Congress after the 2006 elections, leaders re-instituted the "paygo" rules that require proposals with additional spending to be offset with budget cuts elsewhere. In addition, a new package of Medicare legislation (the Medicare Improvement for Patients and Providers Act of 2008), adopted when Congress overrode a veto by President Bush, scaled back payments to Medicare Advantage plans so they have a less obvious competitive position in relation to the traditional, fee-for-service side of the program.

Finally, the highly contingent and controversial adoption of the MMA makes clear that, although Medicare beneficiaries are well-positioned to preserve their basic benefits, that constituency alone does not have the capacity to gain *improvements* in the program. It took the rarest of alignments of political leadership, partisan control of political institutions, strategic positioning of several important interest groups, and a green light for new federal spending to set these new policies into place.

The price of "modernizing" Medicare by making it more comprehensive and appropriate for chronic health conditions was to abandon, at least in part, the framework of social insurance where new benefits for retirees and the disabled are financed by younger workers. Because the new benefits come with potentially thousands of dollars of out-of-pocket costs each year, instead of being secured through a basic entitlement "earned" during one's working years, the diverse economic and health conditions of beneficiaries make it difficult to maintain the equity and social solidarity long supplied by Social Security and Medicare. What that means for the future of the program and American politics is unclear at this moment, but it puts even greater pressure on those who defend Medicare as a relative island of security and fairness in a society rife with health and social inequalities.

DISCUSSION QUESTIONS

1 How did the original architects of the Medicare program see the implementation of health care coverage for older adults fitting into a plan for health care coverage for people of all ages? What happened to that dream?

2. Describe how the political climate has changed in relation to programs like Medicare and discuss the contours of the debate surrounding the enactment of the Medicare Modernization Act of 2003.
3. In what ways, according to Oliver and Lee, did the Medicare Modernization Act abandon fundamental principles of social insurance? What interests benefited from the passage of the Act and how?
4. How and in what ways did AARP influence the passage of the MMA? What other issues has AARP been involved in as of late? What are the implications of AARP's political sway for future reform efforts?

REFERENCES

ABC News/Washington Post Poll. (2003). Poll released on December 8. Retrieved October 3, 2008, from http://abcnews.go.com/images/pdf/883a37Medicare.pdf

Agan, T. (2003, August 26). Dangerous interaction: How mixing a drug benefit with Medicare could mean an overdose of federal spending. National Taxpayers Union Foundation Policy Paper 143. Retrieved October 3, 2008, from http://www.ntu.org/main/press_papers.php?PressID=164&org_name=NTUF

Angle, M. (2003). Difficult Medicare conference looms after narrow house passage. *Capitol Spotlight*, June 30.

Ball, R. (1995). What Medicare's architects had in mind. *Health Affairs, 14*(Winter) 62–72.

Bernstein, I. (1996). *Guns or butter: The presidency of Lyndon Johnson*. New York: Oxford University Press.

Biles, B., Nicholas, L. H., & Cooper, B. S. (2004). *The cost of privatization: Extra payments to Medicare advantage plans*. New York: Commonwealth Fund.

Braybrooke, D., & Lindblom, C. E. (1963). *A strategy of decision*. New York: The Free Press.

Broder, D. S. (2003, November 23). Time was GOP's ally on the vote. *Washington Post*, p. A1.

Broder, D. S. (2004, March 18). AARP's tough selling job. *Washington Post*, p. A31.

Broder, D. S., & Goldstein, A. (2003, November 20). AARP decision followed a long courtship. *Washington Post*, p. A1.

Butler, S. M., Moffit, R. E., & Riedl, B. M. (2003, November 10). Cost control in the Medicare drug bill needs premium support, not a trigger. *Backgrounder,* No. 1704. Washington DC: The Heritage Foundation.

Carey, M. A. (2003a, November 22). Medicare deal goes to wire in late-night house vote. *CQ Weekly*, p. 2879.

Carey, M. A. (2003b, November 29). GOP wins battle, not war. *CQ Weekly*, p. 2956.

Chen, L. J. (2003, August 26). What seniors will lose with a universal Medicare drug entitlement. *Backgrounder* No. 1680. Washington, DC: The Heritage Foundation.

Cohen, R. E., Victor, K., & Baumann, D. (2004, January 10). The state of congress. *National Journal*. Retrieved March 8, 2004, from http://nationaljournal.com

Congressional Budget Office (CBO). (2003). Cost Estimate for H.R. 1, Medicare Prescription Drug and Modernization Act of 2003, as passed by the House of Representatives on June 27, 2003 and S. 1, Prescription Drug and Medicare Improvement Act of 2003, as passed by the Senate on June 27, 2003 with a modification requested by Senate conferees. 22 July.

Congressional Budget Office (CBO). (2004). The *budget and economic outlook: Fiscal years 2005 to 2014*. Washington, DC: CBO, January.

Dionne, E. J., Jr. (2003, November 18). Medicare monstrosity. *Washington Post*, p. A25.

Etheredge, L. (1998). The Medicare reforms of 1997: Headlines you didn't read. *Journal of Health Politics, Policy, and Law, 23*(June), 573–579.

Glied, S. (1997). *Chronic condition: Why health reform fails*. Cambridge, MA: Harvard University Press.

Goldstein, A. (2003, November 30). For GOP leaders, battles and bruises produce Medicare bill. *Washington Post*, p. A8.

Goldstein, A. (2004, March 19). Foster: White House had role in withholding Medicare data. *Washington Post*, p. A2.

Goldstein, A., & Dewar, H. (2003, June 27). Medicare bills would add drug benefits. *Washington Post*, p. A1.

Grier, P. (2003, September 25). Shift against drug benefits in Medicare. *Christian Science Monitor*, p.1.

Hacker, J. S. (1997). *The road to nowhere: The genesis of President Clinton's plan for health security*. Princeton, NJ: Princeton University Press.

Hacker, J. S., & Skocpol, T. (1997). The new politics of U.S. health policy. *Journal of Health Politics, Policy, and Law, 22*(April), 315–338.

Hall, P. A. (1993). Policy paradigms, social learning, and the State: The case of economic policymaking in Britain. *Comparative Politics*, (April), 275–296. Health Care Financing Administration. (1996). *Profiles of Medicare*. Washington, DC: Author.

Health Policy Alternatives. (2003, December 10). *Prescription Drug coverage for Medicare beneficiaries: A summary of the Medicare prescription drug, improvement, and modernization act of 2003*. Prepared for the Henry J. Kaiser Family Foundation.

Himelfarb, R. (1995). Catastrophic *politics: The rise and fall of the Medicare catastrophic coverage act of 1988*. University Park, PA: Pennsylvania State University Press.

Holmer, A. F. (1999). Covering prescription drugs under Medicare: For the good of the patients. *Health Affairs, 18*(July–August), 23–24.

Jaenicke, D., & Waddan, A. (2006). President Bush and social policy: The strange case of the Medicare prescription drug benefit. *Political Science Quarterly, 121*(2), 217–240.

Janus, K., & Brown, L. D. (2007). Medicare as incubator for innovation in payment policy. *Journal of Health Politics, Policy and Law, 32*(2), 293–306.

Johnson, H., & Broder, D. S. (1996). *The system: The American way of politics at the breaking point*. Boston: Little, Brown.

Kaiser Family Foundation. (2004). *The Medicare prescription drug law*. Menlo Park, CA: Author.

Kaiser Family Foundation. (2005). *Medicare chartbook* (3rd ed.). Menlo Park, CA: Author.

Kaiser Family Foundation. (2008). *Medicare and the president's fiscal year 2009 budget proposal*. Menlo Park, CA: Author.

Kaisernetwork.org. (2003, June 27). Senate, House approve separate Medicare bills that call for new coverage option, drug benefit. *Daily Health Policy Report*.

Keehan, S., Sisko, A., Truffer, C., Smith, S., Cowan, C., Poisal, J., & Clemens, M. K. (2008, February 26). Health spending projections through 2017: The baby boom generation is coming to Medicare. *Health Affairs 27*(Web Exclusive), 145–155.

Koszczuk, J., & Allen, J. (2003, November 29). Late-night Medicare vote triggers some unexpected alliances. *CQ Weekly*, p. 2958.

Lindblom, C. E. (1959). The science of muddling through. *Public Administration Review 19*, 79–88.

Lindblom, C. E. (1979). Still muddling, not yet through. *Public Administration Review 39*, 517–526.

Marmor, T. R. (2000). *The politics of Medicare* (2nd ed.). New York: Aldine de Gruyter.

Mayes, R., & Berenson, R. (2006). *Medicare prospective payment and the shaping of U.S. health care*. Baltimore: Johns Hopkins University Press.

Milbank, D., & Deane, C. (2003, December 9). President signs Medicare drug bill. *Washington Post*, p. A1.

Moon, M. (1996). *Medicare now and in the future* (2nd ed.). Washington, DC: The Urban Institute Press.

Morgan, D. (2000, July 3). Bitter pill for health policy pro: Drug bill put head of insurer group at odds with old allies. *Washington Post*, p. A17.

Oberlander, J. (2003). *The political life of Medicare*. Chicago: University of Chicago Press.

Oberlander, J. (2007). Through the looking glass: The politics of the Medicare prescription drug, improvement, and modernization act. *Journal of Health Politics, Policy and Law, 32*(2), 187–220.

Oliver, T. R. (1993). Analysis, advice, and congressional leadership: The physician payment review commission and the politics of Medicare. *Journal of Health Politics, Policy and Law, 18*(Spring), 113–174.

Oliver, T. R., Lee, P. R., & Lipton, H. L. 2004. A political history of Medicare and prescription drug coverage. *Milbank Quarterly*, *82*(June), 283–354.

Olson, M. (1989). Is Britain the wave of the future? How ideas affect societies. *LSE Quarterly*, *3*(Winter), 279–304.

Pear, R. (2000, January 27). House Republicans to draft bill on Medicare prescription drugs. *New York Times*, p. A18.

Pear, R. (2003, July 1). Private health insurers begin lobbying for changes in Medicare drug legislation. *New York Times*, p. A20.

Pear, R., & Hulse, C. (2003, November 25). Senate removes two roadblocks to drug benefit. *New York Times*, p. A1.

Pear, R., & Toner, R. (2003a, November 17). G.O.P. begins push for Medicare bill. *New York Times*, p. A18.

Pear, R., & Toner, R. (2003b, November 18). Medicare plan covering drugs backed by AARP. *New York Times*, p. A1.

Pear, R., & Toner, R. (2003c, November 20). Counting votes and attacks in final push for Medicare bill. *New York Times*, p. A25.

Rapp, D. (2003, November 22). Editor's notebook: An imperfect art. *CQ Weekly*, p. 2870.

Sabatier, P, A., & Jenkins-Smith, H. C. (Eds.). (1993). *Policy change and learning: An advocacy coalition approach*. Boulder, CO: Westview Press.

Schick, A. (1995). *The federal budget: Politics, policy, process*. Washington, DC: Brookings Institution.

Schuler, K., & Carey, M. A. (2004, March 20). Estimates, ethics, and ads tarnish Medicare overhaul. *CQ Weekly*, p. 699.

Serafini, M. W. (2003, November 22). No cure-all: Key provisions of the Medicare bill. *National Journal*, p. 3590. Retrieved December 1, 2003, from http://nationaljournal.com

Skocpol, T. (1996). *Boomerang: Clinton's health security effort and the turn against government in U.S. politics*. New York: W.W. Norton.

Smith, D. G. (1992). *Paying for Medicare: The politics of reform*. New York: Aldine de Gruyter.

Starr, P. (1992). *The logic of health care reform*. Knoxville, TN: Whittle Books.

Stigler, G. (1971). A theory of economic regulation. *Bell Journal of Economics and Management, 3*(1), 3–21.

Stolberg, S. G. (2003, November 23). An 800-pound gorilla changes partners over Medicare. *New York Times*, Section 4, p. 5.

Stolberg, S. G. (2004, March 19). Senate Democrats claim Medicare chief broke law. *New York Times*, p. A14.

Stolberg, S. G., & Pear, R. (2004, March 19). Mysterious fax adds to intrigue over the Medicare bill's cost. *New York Times*, p. A1.

Svihula, J. (2008). Political economy, moral economy, and the Medicare modernization act of 2003. *Journal of Sociology and Social Welfare, 35*(1), 157–173.

Toner, R. (2003, January 11). Political memo: Weapon in health wars: Frist's role as a doctor. *New York Times*, p. A12.

Toner, R., & Pear, R. (2003, June 27). House and Senate pass measures for broad overhaul of Medicare. *New York Times*, p. A1.

Tucker, C. (2003, December 1). Prescription drug plan is expensive boondoggle. *Baltimore Sun*, p. 15A.

Vaida, B. (2004, March 13). Lobbying—AARP's big bet. *National Journal*. Retrieved March 17, 2004, from http://nationaljournal.com *Washington Post*. (2003, November 25). The grand finale. Editorial, p. A28. *Washington Post*. (2004, March 15). Dealing drugs. Editorial, p. A24.

Weisman, J. (2003, July 15). Budget deficit may surpass $450 billion: War costs, tax cut, slow economy are key factors. *Washington Post*, p. A1.

White, J. (2007). Protecting Medicare: The best defense is a good offense. *Journal of Health Politics, Policy and Law, 32*(2), 221–246.

Wilson, J. Q. (1973). *Political organizations*. New York: Basic Books.

6

The Future of Social Insurance: Values and Generational Interdependence[1]

ERIC R. KINGSON, JOHN M. CORNMAN, AND AMANDA L. TORRE-NORTON

The debate over the future of Social Security, usually presented as a financial issue or an issue of affordability, is really a debate about societal values and the balance between how much risk should be addressed through individuals and individual families and how much risk should be addressed through social mechanisms such as social insurance programs. Simply put, the debate is about how much added risk society, through public policies and private practices, wants to place on families now and into the future, and the place of our country's current social insurance programs like Social Security and Medicare in that balance.

Much like the dissonance between the competing values of majority rule and protection of minority rights, the debate over the balance between individualism and interdependence has been with the country for many generations. In the past decade, the pendulum has swung in the direction of placing greater risk on individuals and their families. This shift is evident in:

- The belief that a free market approach is the answer to restraining health care costs, an approach that has resulted in rising health

[1] This chapter draws upon work previously authored by Jack Cornman and Eric Kingson in Cornman, J. C., Kingson E. R., & Butts D. (May/June 2005). Should we be our neighbors' keeper? *Church and Society,* journal of the Presbyterian Church USA (Special Issue on the Social Compact), pp. 34–41.

insurance premiums, an erosion of insurance protections, a decline in corporate sponsorship of retiree health benefits, and an increase in the numbers of Americans without health insurance.

- The move from defined benefit to defined contribution occupational pension plans, making private pensions income more dependent on employee investment decisions, stock market fluctuations, and economic conditions than is the case with benefit-defined plans.
- The restructuring of the workforce from one in which employees could expect steady employment to one of job and economic uncertainty due to the outsourcing and job elimination and/or restructuring. Today's employees are more likely to hold many different jobs during their working lives and are likely to experience greater volatility of family income.
- The growing income gap, which finds the rich getting richer and the medium and lower income workers barely holding their own.
- Retrenchments and cuts in Medicare, Medicaid, Food Stamps, higher education and other federal and state social welfare programs that have come as the result of large and growing annual deficits, primarily driven by tax cuts benefiting well-off Americans and war expenditures.

Clearly, the debate is taking place at a time when stresses on many families have increased and will continue to increase into the foreseeable future.

The proposal to privatize Social Security—the Old-Age Survivors and Disability Insurance program (OASDI)—is an example of efforts to shift risks experienced over the course of life even more onto individuals and individual families. Advocates of privatizing Social Security are challenging the traditional *inter*dependent, social insurance approach to providing widespread protection against loss of income due to retirement, disability, or death of a working person. Consistent with the "Ownership Society" framework, where individualism prevails over collective responsibility, they advocate privatizing some, or all, of the program. This approach would undermine Social Security's traditional structure and underlying values (Cornman, Kingson & Butts, 2005).

Moreover, tilting the balance more toward individualization of risk also raises the prospect of unraveling the intergenerational cohesion—compact, if you will—inherent in social insurance programs and critical to societal well-being and progress in general.

Yes, a number of the country's social insurance programs are in need of fixes, starting with Social Security and Medicare. However, there is ample time, and there are viable options for making Social Security financially sound well into the next century (Altman, 2005; Ball, 1998; Ball, 2006; Diamond & Orszag, 2005; Herd & Kingson, 2005; Reno & Lavery, 2005; Schulz & Binstock, 2006; Steuerle & Bakija, 1994; White, 2001). Dealing with the finances of Medicare in the long run likely depends on reforming the entire approach to health care in the United States.

The debate on how to fix these critically important programs should begin with and focus on what values the American people want the programs to reflect. In our view, the debate should give great weight to the importance of collective responsibility and the interdependence of generations to the long-term well-being of society.

To make our case, we will define the "social insurance" approach to economic security and discuss the philosophy of social insurance, highlighting values driving social insurance policy and how those values are reflected in the structure, function, and benefits of social insurance. Using Social Security as an example, we then discuss how social insurance policy gives expression to and strengthens the reciprocity and interdependence of generations, and how proposals to privatize, in whole or part, are based on and advance the view that individualization of risk is more fundamental to social progress than shared risk and cohesion among generations. We conclude with a call to educate policy makers, analysts, and the general public about the values that will be at stake in future discussions about the future of social insurance. Indeed, the values the nation wishes to promote should have at least equal standing to analysis of the financial and benefit implications of various reform proposals.

But first, we offer a brief and, we trust, a compelling statement of why intergenerational cohesiveness is basic to the well-being and improvement of society.

THE INTERDEPENDENCE OF GENERATIONS

The notion of individual independence has broad acceptance in this country even though no individual or generation has ever succeeded entirely on his or its own. Most so-called self-made people have parents, teachers, coworkers, the benefits of knowledge passed on from previous generations, customers, and others, all of whom had a hand in their success. The current information economy, for example, that provides employment for many of today's workers and individual wealth for many investors is the product, in part, of government expenditures for research and development of computers and the Internet.

Ironically, one reason the country is debating the future of Social Security—the growth and longevity of the older population—is itself the product of intergenerational transfers current and previous generations have made in research, public health, economic development, education, and other areas of critical importance.

Public education and programs serving older people are the most talked about exchanges between generations, but intergenerational transfers occur in the private as well as public domain, at the family as well as the societal levels. Intergenerational public transfers include expenditures for education, health care, public roads and other infrastructure, research, environmental protection, and the common defense. Indeed, it is difficult to think of a public expenditure that does not involve the exchange of resources and benefits across more than one generation.

At the societal level, generations pass on the benefits of economic development; cultural norms; and great art, knowledge, and technology compiled over time. At the family level, generations within families raise children, care for grandchildren, provide care to older family members, and leave inheritance.

In short, the United States is a highly interdependent society in which individuals and families have needs throughout their lives that can only be met by other individuals or social institutions, and a society in which intergenerational transfers are crucial to the continuity and progress of individuals and the nation over time.

In summary, exchanges of resources, knowledge, and values across family and societal generations (intergenerational transfers) are required for individuals, families, and societies to advance and prosper. Robert Ball, the leading figure in the development of Social Security from the late 1940s until his death in 2008, makes this point most succinctly:

> We owe much of what we are to the past. We all stand on the shoulders of generations that came before. They built the schools and established the ideals of an educated society. They wrote the books, developed the scientific ways of thinking, passed on ethical and spiritual values, discovered country, developed it, won (and protected) its freedom, held it together, cleared its forests, built its railroads and factories and invented new technology ... Because we owe so much to the past, we all have the obligation to try to pass on a world to the next generation which is a little better than one we

inherited so that those who come after, standing on our shoulders, can see a little further and do a little better in their turn (Kingson, Hirshorn & Cornman, 1986, p. 24–25).

THE SOCIAL INSURANCE APPROACH AND PHILOSOPHY

All people face risks related to major life events—death of a parent or spouse, illness, unemployment, old age, workplace injury. All people and all societies address such risks through a variety of private and public mechanisms. At the most fundamental level, these risks are borne privately by individuals themselves or by the care and support families provide to members experiencing major difficulties.

In the private sector, individuals may purchase private insurance or be fortunate enough to receive protection through their employers. The public sector, in turn, utilizes a number of mechanisms to help protect against such risks, including, for example, mandates to individuals to purchase health insurance as in Massachusetts, mandates and/or incentives to employers (e.g., private pension tax expenditures) to provide protections to their employees, welfare programs such as Supplemental Security Income and Medicaid, and social insurance.

The social insurance approach to economic security provides protections against identifiable risks that could overwhelm the finances of individuals and their families. In contrast to welfare programs that give immediate relief to extreme financial problems, social insurance programs—Medicare, Social Security, Unemployment Insurance, and Worker's Compensation—seek to prevent financial distress over time. Built on the principle of universal coverage, social insurance provides a social means of pooling risks. Utilizing insurance principles, the costs and risks of coverage (e.g., for health, life insurance) are spread across a broad population (e.g., almost all working Americans). In exchange for making relatively modest work-related contributions over many years, social insurance provides individuals and their families with a floor of protection against predictable risk (Altman, 2005; Ball, 1998; Diamond & Orszag, 2005; Schulz & Binstock, 2006; Steuerle & Bakija, 1994; White, 2001).

Benefit receipt is usually tied to contributions made by an employee and/or employer. The right to a social insurance benefit is considered "earned." Unlike welfare programs (e.g., SSI, Medicaid), eligibility does not require a means test—that is either a test of income and/or assets. By preventing dependency and providing benefits as an "earned right" while simultaneously protecting individuals and their families against economic insecurity, Social Security enhances the dignity of beneficiaries (Ball, 2000; Kingson & Schulz, 1997; Schulz & Binstock, 2006).

Social insurance differs from private insurance in an important way—participation is compulsory. It must be this way to simultaneously provide both widespread adequate protection and to maintain the financial stability of a social insurance program. Of necessity—the need to make a profit—private insurance companies try to "cherry pick" the "best risks" (i.e., the potentially most profitable clients) and, to the extent possible, keep the potentially "worst risks" (i.e., expensive) out of their insurance pools. Unlike private insurance, social insurance programs do not turn away "bad risks"; for example, persons likely to become disabled or require expensive surgery. Consequently, a social insurance system will become financially unstable if the "good risks" are allowed to opt out. Moreover, some who opt out might eventually have to be rescued by taxpayers through welfare programs (Ball, 2000; Schulz & Binstock, 2006).

Consistent with the social goals of providing for the general welfare, maintaining dignity, and enhancing the stability of families and society, "social adequacy"—that benefits should meet the basic needs of the protected population—is the driving principle of social insurance. Absent a concern to provide widespread, adequate financial protection, there would be little reason for public social insurance (Hohaus, 1960). Protection against identified risks could be left to families and other private mechanisms (e.g., private savings, private insurance, IRAs). In such a case, many families would suffer, for such mechanisms do not provide universal and adequate protection.

Although less important than "social adequacy," "individual equity"—that the more one contributes the larger benefit returns should be—also influences the structure of social insurance programs. That is why social insurance benefits often bear some relationship to contributions made. For example, under Social Security, people who have worked consistently at higher wages, making larger payroll tax contributions into the program, receive larger monthly benefits. However, reflecting the adequacy principle, people who have worked for many years at low or moderate wages receive a benefit that is proportionately larger, relative to their payroll tax contributions.

The Social Security benefit formula protects against the risk of working long and hard for relatively low wages. Although people with higher earnings generally receive larger monthly benefits, Social Security's progressive benefit formula assures that benefits will replace a substantially larger portion of pre-retirement earnings for low- and moderate-income workers. The wage-indexing features of the Social Security benefit formula assure that Social Security retirement benefits will replace roughly constant amounts of pre-retirement earnings for people at different earnings levels. Low-income workers receive about 56% of their preretirement income when they become eligible, average-wage earners receive about 42% of their preretirement, and the highest wage earners receive about 27% (Ball, 1998; Cornman, Kingson & Butts, 2005; Kingson, Hirshorn & Cornman, 1986).

Of necessity, social insurance programs also reflect the concerns of taxpayers, economists, and politicians' for stable financing of the programs. In most social insurance programs, payroll tax contributions and other dedicated revenues flow to dedicated trust funds, earmarked to pay for benefits and program costs. Many safeguards assure stable financing. Legislative oversight, annual reports by program officials, and review by actuaries and independent panels of experts provide an early warning system for financing problems that will arise from time to time (Board of Trustees, 2008). The authority and taxing power of government as well as the self-interest of political leaders and the public to protect promised benefits—guarantees the continuity and financial integrity of social insurance programs.

Underlying the social insurance approach is the intergenerational compact. Princeton economist and Provost J. Douglas Brown (1898–1986), an architect of the old-age insurance provisions in the Social Security Act of 1935, spoke eloquently of an implied covenant in social insurance, arising from a deeply embedded sense of mutual responsibility in civilization. This covenant, he wrote, underlies "the fundamental obligation of the government and citizens of one time and the government and citizens of another time to maintain a contributory social insurance system" (Brown, 1977, p. 31–32).

Brown and other leading figures who guided Social Security through its first 50 years understood social insurance as:

- A practical means of enabling working persons to protect themselves and their families against financial risks that might otherwise be overwhelming;
- A program that would require monitoring and ongoing review to anticipate and adjust to changing economic and social conditions; and

- A trust between the American people and their government, held together by belief in the continuity of the nation's democratic processes and an understanding that it would be in the political interest of future congresses and presidencies to maintain the program's basic commitments.

Social insurance emerges from and reinforces the necessary interdependence among people, sectors, and generations. It balances individualism with an understanding that individuals thrive in the context of families and communities; that we, as a people have obligations to each other.

SOCIAL SECURITY AND THE INTERGENERATIONAL COMPACT

Social Security is an excellent example of how social insurance programs are expressions of and reinforcements of the concepts of interdependence and reciprocity. Social Security is the nation's most important intergenerational program, protecting persons of all ages and promoting the solidarity across generations that is integral to a well-functioning, progressing society. An embodiment of this interdependence, Social Security unites generations through its support of older Americans, severely disabled workers and their families, and family members surviving the death of a parent or spouse.

It is widely understood that Social Security is the basic building block for retirement income security for today's and tomorrow's retirees. About two-thirds of older Americans receive at least one half of their income from Social Security, and for one fifth of older Americans, it is their only source of income. The program is the only source of retirement income protection for 6 out of 10 private sector employees. Among the 50 million people receiving cash benefits each month, 38 million are retired or aged survivors (Social Security Administration, 2008).

It is also generally understood that the Social Security program, with its automatic cost-of-living-adjustments, assures that monthly benefits will maintain their purchasing power no matter how long a person lives, a critical feature given that many beneficiaries will live 20, 30, and even more years in retirement, disability, or survivorship.

Less well understood, Social Security is also the nation's major source of life insurance and long-term disability insurance for the great majority of the 163 million workers and their families covered by the program in

2007. As a result, nearly all of the nation's 73 million children under age 18 are protected against the death of a parent. The Social Security Administration estimates that without Social Security coverage, young working parents with two children younger than age 6 would, on average, need to purchase a $443,000 term life insurance policy to provide equivalent protection. The disability insurance for wage earners is valued at more than $414,000 for a family with two children younger than 6 years of age. These protections are the primary reason why benefits are received each month by 6.2 million disabled workers; 3.1 million children younger than age 18, 120,000 18-year-old students; 760,000 disabled children aged 18 and older; 210,000 non-aged disabled widows and widowers; and 340,000 younger spouses of disabled or deceased workers. (Cornman, Kingson & Butts, 2005; Social Security Administration, 2008).

Social Security is the largest and most substantial source of public cash benefits going to the roughly 2.4 million grandparent-headed households responsible for 4.5 million children younger than age 18. Another 2 million children, although not receiving benefits themselves, live with relatives who do. Indeed, about 36% of these households received Social Security benefits in 2000, averaging about $9,300 a year (Generations, United, 2005).

Interdependence and cross-generational exchanges provide the foundation for Social Security and other social insurance programs. Exchange relationships within families and society—the giving and receiving of care and resources over the course of the lives of family members—are reciprocal and change over time. Early in life, children and youth receive much more than they give—from families, teachers, and public institutions (e.g., schools). The balance shifts with movement into adulthood, with many giving care, for example, as parents or spouses, and also contributing to the economy and society as workers, taxpayers, and participants in their communities. As individuals age, they continue to give, though the need for assistance from families, friends, and society may increase for those experiencing serious functional disabilities (Kingson, Hirshorm & Cornman, 1986). Viewed at one point in time, it may look like adults are always giving. But viewed over time and with an appreciation of the interdependence of generations, it is clear that most people as they move through life both give and receive a great deal.

Similarly, at any one point in time, it may look as if today's younger working "generations" (cohorts) support through their tax payments older and younger "generations." But, again, when viewed over time, the reciprocity of giving and receiving and the need for generations to depend on each other for their well-being and advancement are apparent.

And finally, it is not well understood that the benefits of Social Security ripple through the family and the economy. By supporting the old, Social Security frees up middle aged family members to direct more financial resources (e.g., college tuition) on their children. By providing a floor of protection for nearly all Americans, Social Security strengthens and stabilized the national community, especially during recessions.

SOCIAL INSURANCE AND SOCIAL SECURITY VALUES IN AN "OWNERSHIP SOCIETY"

To return to where we started, the debate over the future of Social Security is about more than funding the program into the future.

Today's debate is deeply rooted in disputes surrounding the origins of Social Security, conflicts well symbolized by an exchange during a 1935 Senate Finance Committee hearing examining the merits of the proposed Social Security legislation (Altman & Kingson, 2008). Senator Thomas Gore, a Democrat from Oklahoma who had become increasingly critical of Roosevelt's policies, asks President Franklin Roosevelt's Secretary of Labor, Frances Perkins, "Isn't this socialism?" "Does the proposal involved in this legislation seek, in a sense, to substitute Social Security for the struggle for existence?" Disagreeing with the Senator's "Social Darwinistic" assumptions, the Secretary replies, "cooperation between individuals has accounted for as much civilization as any personal struggle. Most of us have tried to give a certain security to those who are dependent upon us from the more serious aspect of the struggle for existence... That is the purpose of civilization" (Alleviate the Hazards of Old, 1935).

At its core, today's debate is about whether the nation should move away from the vision enunciated by Roosevelt of using "the agencies of Government to provide sound and adequate protection against the vicissitudes of modern life" (Roosevelt, 1935)—embracing instead what President George W. Bush has called on "Ownership Society."

Proposals to carve private or personal accounts out of Social Security are consistent with one of the goals of an "Ownership Society," which is to tilt responsibility for handling risks from a broadly shared responsibility to individuals and their families. Indeed, some critics of this type of a society define the concept as individual ownership of risk.

Where the time-honored values of Social Security provide for civic cohesion, the Ownership Society is grounded in a narrowly conceived notion of "individualism"—each person for him/herself. It emphasizes individual responsibility, liberty and property, and reduced social responsibility, regardless of the impact on society as a whole or on disadvantaged persons in particular. By advocating individual control of health care, education and retirement savings, the proponents of the Ownership Society implicitly accept the fact that huge disparities in the access of low-income individuals, minorities, and women to comparable services would be an inevitable outcome (Cornman, Kingson, & Butts, 2005). Further, in addition to threatening the values informing Social Security and the traditional balance between interdependence and independence, Ownership Society proposals to privatize Social Security, in part or whole, would also undermine its basic purposes and benefits.

Privatization raises many questions and concerns about the key principles and values embodied in Social Security. Would inflation protections be maintained? Would, as has happened with Individual Retirement Accounts (IRAs), Congress eventually allow the holders of private accounts to raid their retirement savings for emergencies or down-payments on a first home, thereby undermining the goal of a secure retirement? Would the expenses associated with administering tens of millions of private accounts eat into the value of the nest egg that is accumulating? In an increasingly uncertain economic environment, will we be asking Americans to subject their basic life, disability, and retirement insurance protections to the vagaries of the stock market? Is it desirable to move Social Security, as private accounts would do, away from a system that seeks to assure a floor of protection for everyone by providing proportionately larger benefits to low and moderate income persons?

CONCLUSION

Wilbur Cohen—the first Social Security Administration employee, author of the Medicare legislation, and Secretary of Health, Education, and Welfare during the latter part of the Johnson administration—once quipped that "the economists" will kill Social Security. Cohen, of course, did not envision a cabal of the members of the "dismal science" "pulling the plug" one day on the nation's most successful and popular social policy. Nor was he unaware of the many important contributions of economists to the development of Social Security, Medicare, unemployment insurance, and other social insurance programs. But he was warning that too much reliance on technical details, with only limited appreciation of the social purposes and values at stake, could undermine the social insurance approach to economic security.

As Cohen, Robert Ball, and other social insurance pioneers understood (Berkowitz, 1995, 1997, 2004), Social Security, Medicare, Unemployment Insurance, and other social insurance policies are not just about taxes, benefits, financial projections, and government budgets. Social insurance programs give concrete expression to widely-held and time-honored American values and commitments. They are grounded in values of shared responsibility and concern for all members of society. They reflect an understanding of the social compact which suggests that, as citizens and human beings, we are "all in it together;" we all share certain risks and certain vulnerabilities, and we all have a stake in advancing practical mechanisms of self- and mutual support. They are based on the belief that government can and should uphold these values by providing practical, dignified, secure, and efficient means for hard-working Americans to protect their children, families, and themselves against risk to which all are subject (Cornman, Kingson & Butts, 2005).

When this is understood, it is clear that:

- The nation will not be well served by the tilting of the balance between fostering the interdependence of generations and individualism toward the latter;
- The benefit of putting more risks on families does not exceed the costs of that shift;
- This is not the moment in our history when the nation should make a drastic change in the principles of a time-tested approach that reduces the risks families face from the vicissitudes of life and strengthens the ties between generations.

The nation cannot afford to have social insurance policy discussions dominated by technical issues regarding structure, projected shortfalls, benefits, taxes, and administration. To do so, invites the type of disingenuous and dysfunctional policy claims so prevalent during the President George W. Bush years—that "the public good" is best served by the partial or full privatization of Social Security and Medicare.

The social insurance approach rests on an understanding that generations depend on each other; they are interdependent. It gives concrete expression to values supporting mutual aid and the obligation to care for our families, our neighbors, and ourselves. Consequently, the values at stake and moral choices embedded within social insurance policy discussions require explicit recognition and discussion.

Indeed, as social insurance policy discussion proceeds, it will be important to not lose sight of this moral dimension of the social insurance approach, which is a cornerstone of our society and its values.

DISCUSSION QUESTIONS

1. What is the relevance of societal values to our social insurance programs?
2. Describe the structure of social insurance programs.
3. Ownership Society proposals to privatize Social Security are based on what claims? What are the potential risks to Ownership Society principles?
4. You are asked to give a talk to a group of college students who resent the idea that their Social Security taxes might support others and not themselves in their retirement. Using concepts from Kingson, Cornman, and Torre-Norton's chapter, talk about why social insurance works this way. Provide examples of the interdependence of generations.

REFERENCES

Alleviate the Hazards of Old Age, Unemployment, Illness and Dependency: Hearings before the Committee on Finance, United States Senate, 74th Cong., 1(1935).

Altman, N. J. (2005). *The battle for Social Security: From FDR's vision to Bush's gamble.* Hoboken, New Jersey: John Wiley and Sons.

Altman, N. J., & Kingson, E. R. (2008, August 13). McCain's views on Social Security. *San Francisco Chronicle.* B7.

Ball, R. M. (1998). *Straight talk about Social Security: An analysis of the issues in the current debate.* New York: The Century Foundation Press.

Ball, R. M. (2000). *Insuring the essentials: Bob Ball on Social Security.* New York: The Century Foundation Press.

Ball, R. M. (2006, December). Meeting Social Security's long-range shortfall: A golden opportunity for the new Congress. Retrieved August 10, 2008, from http://robertmball.org/

Berkowitz, E. D. (1995). *Mr. Social Security: The life of Wilbur J. Cohen*. Lawrence, Kansas: University Press of Kansas.

Berkowitz, E. D. (1997). The historical development of Social Security in the United States. In E. R. Kingson, & J. H. Schulz, (Eds.), *Social Security in the 21st century*. New York: Oxford University Press.

Berkowitz, E. D. (2004). *Robert Ball and the politics of Social Security*. Madison, Wisconsin: University of Wisconsin Press.

Board of Trustees, Federal Old Age and Survivors Insurance and Disability Insurance Trust Funds. (2008). *2008 annual report of the trustees of the federal old-age and survivors insurance and disability insurance trust funds*. Washington, DC: U.S. Government Printing Office.

Brown, J. D. (1977). *Essays on Social Security*. Princeton, New Jersey: Princeton University Press.

Cornman, J. C., Kingson, E. R., & Butts, D. (2005, May/June). Should we be our neighbors' keeper? *Church and Society*, journal of the Presbyterian Church USA (*Special Issue on the Social Compact*), pp. 34–41.

Diamond, P. A., & Orszag, P. R. (2005). *Saving Social Security: A balanced approach*. Washington, DC: Brookings Institution Press.

Generations United (2005, September). The stake of children, youth and families in Social Security. Retrieved August 11, 2008, from http://www.gu.org/documents/A0/GUStakeChildrenSSFactSheet.pdf

Herd, P., & Kingson, E. R. (2005). Reframing Social Security: Cures worse than the disease. In R. B. Hudson (Ed.), *Aged based public policy in the 21st century* (pp. 183–204). Baltimore: Johns Hopkins University Press.

Hohaus, R. A. (1960). Equity, adequacy and related factors in old age security. In W. Haber, & W. J. Cohen (Eds.), *Social Security programs, problems and policies*. Homewood, Illinois: Richard D. Irwin, Inc.

Kingson, E. R., Hirshorn, B. A., & Cornman, J. C. (1986). *Ties that bind: The interdependence of generations*. Cabin John, Maryland: Seven Locks Press.

Kingson, E. R., & Schulz, J. H. (1997). Should Social Security be means-tested? In E. R. Kingson, & J. H. Schulz (Eds.), *Social Security in the 21st century*. New York: Oxford University Press.

Reno, V. P., & Lavery, J. (2005, February). Options to balance Social Security funds over the next 75 Years. *Brief* No. 18. Retrieved October 7, 2008, from http://www.nasi.org/usr_doc/SS_Brief_18.pdf

Roosevelt, F. D. (1935, August 15). Presidential Statement signing the Social Security Act.

Schulz, J. H., & Binstock, R. H. (2006). *Aging nation: The economics and politics of growing older in America*. Westport, CT: Praeger Publishers.

Social Security Administration (2008, August). OASDI monthly statistics, November 2007. Retrieved October 7, 2008, from http://www.ssa.gov/policy/docs/statcomps/oasdi_monthly/

Steuerle, C. E., & Bakija, J. M. (1994). *Retooling Social Security for the twenty-first century*. Washington, DC: Urban Institute Press.

White, J. (2001). *False alarm*. New York: The Century Foundation Press.

PART II

What's at Stake

Part II: What's at Stake

Introduction

ERICA SOLWAY

According to the U.S. Census Bureau (2008), the United States will continue to become older and more racially and ethnically diverse in the coming years. Today, roughly one third of the U.S. population are members of ethnic minority groups. It is estimated that more than half of the population will be from a minority group by 2050, making minorities the majority. Furthermore, by 2030, all baby boomers will be 65 years or older, and there will be more than double the number of people age 65 years and older in 2050 as there are today. Although there is expected to be only a small increase in the non-Hispanic white population, the Hispanic, black, Asian, American Indian and Alaskan Native, and Native Hawaiian and other Pacific Islander populations are expected to grow substantially in the next few decades (U.S. Census Bureau, 2008). Thus, while the U.S. population as a whole will become more diverse in the coming years, there will also be significant demographic changes to the older adult population or what Hayes-Bautista, Hsu, Perez, and Gamboa (2002) refer to as "the browning of the graying of America." Furthermore, it is important to note that there are more women age 65 and older in the United States than men of the same age, and women accounted for 56% of adult Social Security beneficiaries in 2007. Social Security comprised 90% or more of income for 20% of older beneficiary couples and 41% of the income for nonmarried beneficiaries (Social Security Administration, 2008).

The four chapters in the second section of the book illustrate what is at stake for women, minorities and, indeed, for all Americans, in the future of our social insurance programs. The authors point out that with privatization comes great risk and cost but that preservation of social insurance programs as public programs helps foster feelings of dignity, equality, and security and promotes social justice and social change.

Chapter 7 begins this section by providing a sociological perspective on citizenship as an important concept and framework for understanding the historical and contemporary politics of social insurance in the United States. The authors argue that social insurance programs reinforce a sense of citizenship and efforts aimed at privatization alter this sense by replacing an ethic of community with one of individualism and the guarantees of the State with the uncertainties of the free market. The authors suggest that whereas the early history of social insurance in the United States reflects a fairly continuous expansion of the boundaries of citizenship in terms of both what services the state deemed as social rights and who was given access to these rights, the last 3 decades can be mostly characterized in terms of containment and retraction of these boundaries. The authors assert that there are opportunities through the implementation of national health insurance coverage and the extension of services to several groups that would expand the boundaries of citizenship in the United States in an important move towards a more democratic and just society.

In chapter 8, Harrington Meyer discusses the ways in which universal old-age Social Security redistributes resources and thus helps reduce inequalities by gender as well as race, class, and marital status. Harrington Meyer notes that there are many reasons why older women rely on Social Security more than older men, including the fact that women earn significantly less in the labor force and perform more unpaid work in the home. This chapter notes that efforts to privatize Social Security would have an enormous impact on economic security for older women by increasing risk, concentrating responsibility, stripping protections, and likely reducing benefits while increasing economic insecurity and social inequalities. Harrington Meyer suggests that modest adjustments to the Social Security system can make the program more responsive to changing sociodemographic trends and strengthen the program's ability to provide economic security and reduce inequality.

In chapter 9, Wallace and Villa explore the consequences of reforms that would raise the minimum retirement age. The authors caution that reforms to our social insurance programs should take into consideration the potential harm to minority elders given the disparities in finances, health, and opportunities around education and employment that continue to exist for minority groups. For example, in terms of health, the authors note that African Americans are the most disadvantaged in terms of life expectancy in comparison to whites, and differences are most pronounced for women. In terms of wealth, although poverty rates for older adults in general have declined in recent decades, significant disparities remain for minority elders. Furthermore, high school graduation rates among ethnic minorities continue to lag behind those of white, and these differences in education result in differences in earning ability for individuals and families across the life course as well as higher rates of occupational injury and disability. Differences exist between various minority groups and also within minority groups and these differences should be taken into account when considering the needs of individuals and groups and the ways in which changes to social insurance may affect certain populations.

Finally, chapter 10 examines the ways various demographic changes demonstrate how the needs of elders of color and other vulnerable populations will continue to challenge the effectiveness of redistributive exchange policies and practices in our nation. The authors argue that our current service model can be characterized as "one size fits all." An example of this "one size fits all" perspective is that service programs continue to be inflexible with their eligibility practices. The authors suggest that this model is out of date given the diversity of the older adult population. The authors suggest that as we strive to achieve a more inclusive society and improve quality of life, it is important to adapt to the social needs, service needs, and preferences of our elders that reflect their individual backgrounds and culture.

In conclusion, this section describes what could be lost and what might be gained based on the future of our social insurance programs. Because health and financial inequalities are likely to increase if social insurance programs are privatized, there is also the possibility, according to Poole (2006), that "a reconstructed social welfare policy just might be one of our best future options for eradicating racial inequality from our midst" (p. 187). Our social insurance programs play a critical role in the lives of many people, and, thus, there is clearly a great deal at stake for women, for people from ethnic minority groups, and for our national sense of community and citizenship more broadly.

REFERENCES

Hayes-Bautista, D. E., Hsu, P., Perez, A., & Gamboa, C. (2002). The 'browning' of the graying of America: Diversity in the elderly population and policy implications. *Generations*, *26*(3), 15–24.

Poole, M. (2006). *The segregated origins of Social Security: African Americans and the welfare state*. Chapel Hill, NC: University of North Carolina Press.

Social Security Administration. (2008). Fast facts and figures about Social Security 2008. Retrieved September 9, 2008, from http://www.ssa.gov/policy/docs/chartbooks/fast_facts/2008/index.html

U.S. Census Bureau Newsroom. (2008, August 14). An older and more diverse nation by midcentury. Retrieved September 9, 2008 from http://www.census.gov/Press-Release/www/releases/archives/population/012496.html

7 One Nation, Interdependent: Exploring the Boundaries of Citizenship in the History of Social Security and Medicare

BRIAN R. GROSSMAN, ERICA SOLWAY, BROOKE A. HOLLISTER, CARROLL L. ESTES, AND LEAH ROGNE

This chapter provides a sociological perspective on the concept of citizenship related to the historical and contemporary politics of social insurance in the United States. We seek to illustrate the importance of citizenship as a framework through which to analyze the U.S. experience with social insurance. We argue that economic and health security across the life course are, in fact, key elements of citizenship, around which advocacy and education are worthwhile, if not required, activities. The chapter considers the ways in which social insurance programs reinforce a sense of citizenship and how current efforts toward privatization undermine this sense, replacing an ethic of community with one of individualism, and the guarantees of the State with the uncertainties of the "free" market.[1]

The chapter is comprised of three sections. We start with theoretical perspectives on citizenship. From here, we refract the well worn histories of both Social Security and Medicare through the prism of citizenship to identify the boundary-shifting processes that accompany the introduction of these policies. Then, we review the recent histories in which

[1] Our discussion of citizenship here is on the historical development of the broad concept of citizenship and its application to the case of social insurance. We are not considering citizenship in the narrow, exclusionary, xenophobic way it has been largely treated in the current public debates on immigration. Indeed, our intent is quite the opposite, as will be clear in this chapter.

the second Bush Administration aggressively advanced the concept of an "ownership society," passed the Medicare Modernization Act (MMA), and unsuccessfully attempted to privatize Social Security. We conclude with a discussion of the future opportunities for the continued expansion of citizenship in U.S. social insurance programs, identifying both a key service to be offered and multiple groups to which services need to be offered.

SOCIAL INSURANCE AND CITIZENSHIP: MAKING THE CONNECTION

> "Citizenship has been used to draw boundaries between those who are included as members of the community and entitled to respect, protection, and rights and those who are excluded and thus not entitled to recognition and rights" (Glenn, 1992, p. 1).

Before discussing the concept of citizenship, we examine the etymologic and historical notions of the word citizen. Dating back to the 12th century, the word was spelled *citisein* (in Anglo-French) and *citeaine* (in Old French) and has its roots in the older Latin term *civitas* and the Roman concept of *civitatus*. These French words roughly referred to those who lived in the city and by virtue of living in the city, were afforded rights (Random House, 2006; Turner, 1990). According to Harper (2001), it is not until the end of the 14th century that citizen takes on the broader meaning of the "inhabitant of a country."

Classical Notions of Citizenship

Our examination of the theoretical concept of citizenship begins with Marshall's (1949) theory of British citizenship that focuses on a dual process of "fusion" and "separation" (p. 73). Developing across 3 centuries, three distinct but overlapping forms of citizenship emerge—civil, political, and social. Simultaneously, the meaning of citizenship shifts from one of "I live in a city" to "this is my nation" (p. 73). With the increasing manifestation of each of these forms of citizenship rights, the "local" decreases in importance as the insurer of these rights as the "nation" becomes the arbiter of citizenship.

First, Marshall (1949) identifies the 18th century as the time in which civil rights were developed, primarily via the courts and resulting in a legal status of citizen that is similar to what we recognize today. In particular, he claimed the right to work as a key civil right, explaining that "By the end of the nineteenth century this principle of economic freedom was accepted as axiomatic" (p. 76). Marshall (1949) assigned the development of political rights to the 19th century, including increased access to the right to vote. In this century he described this right as secondary to civil rights. In his description of the 20th century, political rights shift from a byproduct of civil rights to a unique form of citizenship rights. Also in the 20th century, we come to social rights, those rights that are most relevant to the subject of this book, social insurance. Marshall's (1949) discussion of social rights includes the English Poor Law after the Act of 1834 and the rights of factory workers. However, it is public education, due to its free and compulsory nature, that Marshall identifies as the birth of social rights. It is based on these social rights that one may claim *social citizenship*, such that one may demand security from the state[2] in matters deemed social (e.g., education, health, income replacement).

Critical of Marshall's (1949) theory of citizenship for its singular focus on the development of British citizenship, Mann (1987) developed a more sophisticated, comparative analysis that identified five geohistorical approaches to the development of citizenship: (1) liberal, (2) reformist, (3) authoritarian monarchist, (4) fascist, and (5) authoritarian socialist. Appreciative of these efforts, but critical of the class focus in Mann's analysis, Turner (1990) instead offers an alternate model that highlights a double dichotomy between demands for citizenship from below and provision of citizenship from above, and between an emphasis on the public (political) sphere and a focus on the private (autonomous, economic) sphere. Turner (1990) develops a four-part typology of citizenship that includes revolutionary, passive democracy, liberal pluralism, and plebiscitary authoritarianism. He identifies the U.S. notion of citizenship with liberalism, correlating the U.S. history of (1) citizenship demands arising from below (revolution) and (2) the focus on private, individual rather than public, political space. Turner (1990) makes an interesting observation about the centrality of "localism" (p. 209) to U.S. citizenship and the impact this has on the development of a national welfare platform.

---

[2] The state is composed of major social political, and economic institutions including the legislative, executive, and judicial branches of government; the military and criminal justice systems; educational, health, and welfare institutions (Estes, 2001; O'Connor, 1973; Waitzkin, 1983). In the United States, we think of the state as the federal government, although there is also the local state and the 50 states, each of which have jurisdictions over many matters. In this chapter, when we use the term *the state*, we are referring to the nation-state, primarily the federal government and the multiple institutions associated with it.

Indeed, this tie between citizenship and localism may explain the country's policy commitment to the federally funded, state-governed welfare program that is Medicaid and the abysmal failure of the many attempts to legislate a national health program in the United States (Navarro, 1995). The intertwining of citizenship and localism is further reflected in the "states' rights" and new federalism arguments that undergird policies that foster the devolution of responsibility from the federal to the state and local levels of government, and from the government to the individual (Estes, 1979).

Citizenship and Social Policy: A Normative Approach

Citizenship is a relational category in which the individual and the state have entered into an asymmetric, consensual relationship, in which the individual is beholden to the state to fulfill certain responsibilities, and the state is accountable to the individual to ensure certain rights. The relationship between state and citizen is key. As Turner (1990) explains, "Any theory of citizenship must also produce a discussion of the state" (p. 193). In this case, the asymmetry of the relationship between the individual and the state stands as a reminder of the impunity with which the state has access to (and use of) violence to achieve its means (Weber, 1946). This does not imply that citizenship rights are not (and have not been) gained by struggles led by individuals with and against the state. As Turner (1990) explains, "it is important to put a particular emphasis on the notion of social struggles as the central motor of the drive for citizenship" (p. 193). At issue is the degree that these struggles may be both violent and effective on the part of the collectivity of individuals involved.

As part of the relationship between the citizen and the state, the individual is expected to fulfill many roles as a (pre)condition to "demanding" services, programs, and/or accountability from the state. We will refer to this as a normative perspective on citizenship in which there are expectations that must be fulfilled (both in the eyes of the state and the eyes of fellow citizens) in order to lay claim to citizenship.

In this section, we outline what we believe to be the five roles of citizenship in late capitalism and describe the responsibilities that accompany those roles. To claim services from the state, the individual citizen is expected to perform as (1) citizen as laborer, (2) citizen as mother, (3) citizen as soldier, (4) citizen as loyalist, and finally, (5) citizen as consumer. We will explore each of these five roles in turn before moving on to a discussion of citizenship as it relates to the history of social insurance in the United States.

Citizens as Laborer

We begin with *citizen as laborer* to emphasize the triarchic relationship among the citizen, the state, and the economy. Indeed, one cannot understand the status category of citizen without recognizing that the citizen is a key functional element in the economy. In practice, the citizen is expected to labor not only for her or his individual benefit but also for the benefit of her or his family, and for the continued operation of the economy. If people stop working, then the economy stops, period. In the United States, the call for citizens to labor to facilitate a thriving economy is buttressed by the desire for the United States to retain its dominant position in the global economy. In part, this is the impetus behind the focus on education, or what we view as *citizen as laborer-in-training* (rather than, for example, citizen as student, for student is not a status category for which people receive social rights). Citizen as laborer-in-training is represented in the modern day fear that the growing skilled labor force in countries like China, India, and Japan will allow their economies to outpace that of the United States. Additionally, it is this concept of citizen as laborer that guides both welfare and social insurance policy in the United States and fuels the suspicion of freeloaders and people "faking" the need for disability benefits (Stone, 1984).

Citizen as Mother

Although citizen as laborer may seem obvious, *citizen as mother* may seem less so. Clearly, citizen as mother is a gendered term. It is not about citizen as caregiver (as much of the feminist literature on social policy can attest, caregiver is not a status category that affords one full citizenship). Rather, citizen as mother is about the reproductive potential of the womb and the cultivation and actualization of that potential in the form of giving birth. Park (2002) describes the social consequences experienced by couples who are biologically able to reproduce but *choose* not to. She identifies pronatalism as a combination of social forces that drive the cultural expectation that women *will* reproduce and support the sociocultural ownership of women's bodies as reproductive units that must fulfill their (biological, religious, nationalistic) obligation to replenish and strengthen the population. The labor of childrearing is part of this as well, but the primary focus is on the physical act of giving birth (separate, of course, from physical acts of sexual pleasure and even the physical moments of coitus and conception, as increasingly demonstrated by the prowess of biomedical technoscience). However, giving birth does not fulfill one's duties as citizen as mother; to be successful as citizen as mother, the birth must be a biologically viable, healthy, socially malleable (disciplinable) child—one who can, in turn, become a model citizen.

The role of citizen as mother is central to any nationalistic endeavor for two reasons: (1) citizen as mother is (re)generative and results in multiple citizens emerging from one original, and (2) citizen as mother is both a (re)productive unit for the state and a socializing agent for the state, instilling the roles of citizen into citizens-to-be. Although U.S. policy reinforces cultural demands for women to fulfill the role of citizen as mother (and lifelong caregiver), social insurance programs provide little or no compensation for this vital (re)productive labor—despite evidence documenting the related financial and health consequences that accompany this undervalued status (Estes & Zulman, 2007).

Citizen as Soldier

When we discussed this list of citizenship roles, we intentionally listed citizen as soldier directly after citizen as mother. *Citizen as soldier* is central to the maintenance of the nationalistic project of the United States through military intervention. The role of citizen as mother is fulfilled when viable future citizen soldiers have been produced. Through both the reproductive and socializing activities of the role of *citizen as mother*, the citizens to be (because children do not have full citizenship status) that are produced have been woven into the fabric of nationalism. Citizens (and their bodies) are not only seeking discipline and willing to self-discipline (Foucault, 1979), but they are also willing to enact violence on behalf of the state as an act of nationalism and patriotism.

As a nation, the United States has historically used and continues to use violence (as evidenced by the nation's consistent military actions since World War II) as a mechanism to ensure global economic stability (Kagan, Schmitt, & Donnelly, 2000) and, as a consequence, maintain the economically dominant position of the United States in the global politico-economic order (Choudry, 2008; Klein, 2007; Mahajan, 2002; Meszaros, 2001). Additionally, these military endeavors have fueled a transglobal military industrial complex that disproportionately benefits the pockets of U.S.-based corporations providing white collar welfare to employees of big defense and infrastructure firms (Rothe, 2009).

In no small part, the military industrial complex is sustained with the bodies of citizen soldiers (and in particular the bodies of young people of color) (Statistical Information Analysis Division [Department of Defense], 2003). Although soldier generally refers to the formal institutions of the military, it could also refer to the less formal agents of the state including police officers, emergency workers, and firefighters. Citizen soldiers line up in defense of their country with the assumption that while in the line of duty and if injured in performing these duties, the state will provide them with some sort of income and health security. However, it appears that the Bush administration has eroded this confidence for those on the front lines (Preist & Hill, 2007). The paradox, here, is that while citizen soldiers are defending the *economic* and *military* security of their country, they are being denied the basic citizenship rights in the form of *social* security by the very same country for which they are fighting.

Citizen as Loyalist

Distinct from citizen as soldier, but related in the expectation of an internalized sense of duty and responsibility to maintaining the social (and economic and cultural) order, is *citizen as loyalist*. This role of the status category of citizen acts as a legitimizing concept for the ideology of xenophobia (exclusion of the stranger), which the very (local) notion of national citizenship is based. Additionally, citizen as loyalist has far-reaching implications and encompasses a broad variety of normative expectations, that if broken are means for varying degrees of degradation of citizenship status. Consequently, violating the role of citizen as loyalist demands sanctions such that the category of citizenship maintains both meaning and a position of privilege in comparison to that of "alien." On one extreme, there is the crime of apostasy, crimes against the state (including treason) that betray the role of citizen as loyalist. A particular affront to middle-class values, apostasy carries with it sanctions as extreme as execution, as illustrated in the case of Timothy McVeigh (Tittle & Paternoster, 2000). A less extreme example of the violation of citizen as loyalist would be a crime for which an individual becomes (literally) disenfranchised, having their right to cast a ballot revoked less for the actual crime that was committed and more for the symbolic threat to the social order that the crime represents. One could actually view the deprivation of educational opportunities that often accompanies imprisonment or denial of college financial aid for a drug offense as a further revocation of citizenship rights (in these cases, the social right to education).

Although it would be an unfair over-simplification, each of the four roles of the citizen status discussed above could be united under a more general categorization of citizen as producer. However, there are two reasons to follow this line of reasoning. First, it is impossible to explore the concept of citizenship in the United States without addressing the impact of capitalism on the status category and its accompanying roles. Second, and perhaps more importantly, we are able to draw a distinction between the other four roles of the citizenship status category and a fifth role, that of citizen as consumer.

Citizen as Consumer

The designation of the role of *citizen as consumer* recognizes the vital role of consumption for the maintenance of both national and global economies, and the financing of the state as well (Offe & Ronge, 1982). The citizen as consumer has been enlisted in a different campaign of domination than those in the other citizen roles. However, in a capitalist society, these campaigns intersect in myriad ways. The citizen as consumer role is integrally related to the ideology of individualism that underpins the market economy. O'Connor (1984), describes American individualism as "capital's most powerful weapon of ideological domination of labor in the USA" (p. 13–14) and notes that in the United States, individualism is equated with capitalism. Capitalism, then, clearly demands the citizen as consumer, whose consumption serves the interests of the capitalist class.

In her book, *Capitalism and Citizenship: An Impossible Partnership*, political theorist Kathryn Dean (2003) offers a critique of the individual responsibility project under capitalist social relations, highlighting its corrosive effects on democracy and citizenship.

> Individual autonomy has now become official policy, since, as governments attempt to 'roll back' the Welfare State, interpellations and practices are systematically designed to elicit individualized self-direction and maintenance. Autonomy is here conceptualized as atomism, as the self-interest of individuals who are in external relations with one another and with "society." This atomism is intensified by the unknowability of the world in which self-programmable workers find themselves. Standing readiness to

> change, and standing anxiety about the satisfaction of needs, together with the need for self-reliance without a sense of self are the characteristics of self-programmable workers. . . . the world remains an "alien power" standing over self-programmable workers as *individual* workers (Dean, 2003, p. 162).
>
> . . . self-reliance is demanded under threat of future impoverishment. The structurally irrelevant [workers/individuals] are just that: irrelevant. Their fate depends on the readiness of governments and their electorates to dole out ever more meager and grudgingly offered sustenance (Dean, 2003, p. 162).

This atomism is largely what Dean (2003) identifies as a major component of the "impossible partnership" between capitalism and citizenship. The impossibility of an amicable partnership between capitalism and citizenship resides in the distinction between democracy, which relies on inclusion of all members of society, and capitalism, which relies on exclusionary privileges bestowed from property and wealth. One byproduct of this partnership is that a form of individual rights (citizenship if you will) has even been conferred on corporations. In Klein v. Board of Tax Supervisors, 282 U.S. 19, the U.S. Supreme Court (1930) ruled that a corporation (later referred to as an artificial person) has many of the same rights and privileges in a court of law as an individual. This ruling was clarified that artificial persons are not "entitled to liberty protections under the 14th Amendment of the U.S. Constitution. An artificial person is, however, entitled to the constitutional protections of property and life, as well as equal protection" (M. Nelson, personal communication, August 25, 2008). In contrast with citizens, these artificial persons have access to vast resources (fiscal, political, and human capital) through which to claim and defend these constitutional protections. The consequence of this asymmetry is often the infringement of the rights of the citizen in favor of those of the corporation.

A major example of how the citizen as consumer is constructed resides in the commodification of old age through an individually based approach to service provision via a multitrillion dollar for-profit medical industrial complex and aging enterprise (Estes, 1979). These systems of service provision, directed by professional experts (sometimes referred to as agents of social control) have promoted the role of older citizens as consumer. The literature of market economists speaks about the benefits of market competition as being the creation of "choice" and efficiencies. This is the dominant rhetoric of privatizers. Despite much evidence to the contrary, there are major problems with both the concepts and reality of "real choice" and "efficiency" in private insurance and medical markets (Rice, 1997).

The atomism of the consumer citizen of which both O'Connor (1984) and Dean (2003) speak is a major product of the ideologies of individual responsibility under the capitalist state. That social contract has been built, in the case of Social Security, for more than 70 years upon the commitment of some set (albeit limited) of nation-state responsibilities to a willing community of citizens who have paid into a social insurance system in good faith, in return for an assurance of a minimum base of economic security in old age.

CITIZENSHIP AND THE HISTORY OF SOCIAL INSURANCE IN THE UNITED STATES

> We have tried to frame a law which will give some measure of protection to the average citizen and his family against the loss of a job and against a poverty-ridden old age. It is . . . a law that will take care of human needs and at the same time provide the United States with an economic structure of vastly greater soundness (Presidential Statement on Signing the Social Security Act, August 14, 1935, from Bernstein & Bernstein, 1988).

> If the guiding philosophy behind the traditional system of social insurance could be described as "We're all in it together", the philosophy behind the ownership society seems to be "You are on your own" (Obama, 2006, p. 178).

> Citizenship is one of the most coveted gifts that the U.S. government can bestow, and the most important immigration benefit that USCIS can grant (United States Citizenship and Immigration Services [USCIS], 2008, from www.uscis.gov).

An analysis of the history of social insurance programs in the United States from the 1930s to the beginning of the 1980s indicates a clear trend of continued expansion of the boundaries of citizenship. However, beginning with the Reagan presidency, this expansion was interrupted by attempts to contract these boundaries (Estes, 1991). In particular, there are two axes on which these expansions and contractions have taken place: (1) the breadth of categories of people who qualify as citizens (in the context of accessing entitlements) and (2) the range of services that compose social insurance programs (that may be claimed as entitlements by citizens). In this section, we use the history of Social Security and

Medicare to illustrate these processes of expansion of the boundaries of citizenship across both of these axes. Additionally, we discuss the more contemporary politics of the Reagan and the second Bush Administration as demonstrative of attempts to constrain and roll back the boundaries of citizenship in favor of the libertarian ideal of the atomized *Homo economus* free to roam the free market in search of profit maximization.

Social Insurance in the United States Before 1935

Workers' compensation is generally considered the first social insurance program in the United States with Wisconsin as the first state to adopt such a program in 1911. However, workers' compensation primarily operates as a state-level program.[3] Because this chapter is concerned with citizenship (at the national level), we will begin our analysis with the introduction of the Social Security old-age insurance program in 1935.

Prior to the introduction of a formal, nationwide Social Security program in 1935, laborers in the United States had no statutory guarantee or cultural expectation of economic security in old age, or in times of unemployment, occupational illness or impairment, or the death of a parent or partner beyond reliance on family and occasionally organized religion. However, some workers gained access to such security through membership in private fraternal organizations (many of which are still in existence today, such as the Kiwanis Club, the Odd Fellows, the Freemasons, and the Elks),based on employer-sponsored or military pensions, or via state old-age assistance programs (DeWitt, 2003).

Access to these benefits was inequitably distributed across the population and consequently, there were great differences between those who had access to benefits and those who did not (Social Security Administration, 2008a). The members of private fraternal- and employer-sponsored organizations (if available at all) were likely determined by varying social and occupational characteristics.

Additionally, there was great interstate variation in access to old-age assistance programs based on whether or not and when a state instituted such a program, whether or not it was optional for the counties to

[3] Even today, with the exception of the Federal Employees' Compensation Program, the Federal Employees' Occupational Illness Program, Longshore and Harbor Workers' Compensation Program, and Black Lung Benefits Program, which are handled by the United States Department of Labor's Office of Workers' Compensation Programs, workers' compensation is handled as a state-level risk and benefits pool (U.S. Department of Labor, n.d.).

participate in this program, and the generosity of the benefits offered.[4] These programs only provided income assistance if an individual *did not have* children or other relatives to financially support them. Furthermore, an individual's eligibility for such assistance could be revoked for any number of social reasons: deserting one's family, having been a beggar, or being incarcerated in a prison or asylum (Armstrong et al., 1935). Unlike Social Security, these state old-age assistance programs were not a universal guarantee of income assistance in old age.

The Expansion of Citizenship in U.S. Social Insurance Programs: 1935–1980

By contemporary standards, the pool of people originally granted access to Social Security benefits based on the Social Security Act of 1935 was quite restrictive. The program was introduced at a time when certain aspects of social and family life (e.g., single earner families with a male breadwinner) were deemed normative and fixed (Zones, Estes & Binney, 1987). The initial passage of Social Security, in true Progressive era fashion, attempted to redress some of the economic uncertainties associated with industrial capitalism; Social Security was a program in which industrial and commercial laborers paid in to the system and these same workers gained access to benefits upon retirement (Berkowitz & McQuaid, 1988). However, a number of classes of workers, including domestic and agricultural workers—occupations that were predominantly held by African Americans, were excluded from participation in the program (Achenbaum, 1986; Poole, 2006; Quadagno, 1994). One could argue that because only about 60% of workers were covered by the original legislation, Social Security had yet to actually become a *true* social insurance program, as it did not approximate universal coverage (McGill & Brown, 2005).

In 1939, before the first benefits were even paid out, the group of people who could contribute to and claim the benefits of Social Security

---

[4] Arizona and Alaska (then a territory) were the first to pass old-age assistance programs in 1915, but the Arizona law was later deemed unconstitutional. By 1928, there were only seven old-age assistance programs in the United States: Colorado, Kentucky, Maryland, Montana, Nevada, Wisconsin, and Alaska. By 1934, that number jumped to 30 (including 28 states and 2 territories), but approximately one quarter of these programs did not mandate counties to participate. Also in 1934, the average benefits ranged widely—from \$6.13 in Indiana to \$29.90 in Maryland, as did the number of pensioners being paid—with no one at all being paid in Kentucky and West Virginia, at one extreme, and 51,228 paid in New York, on the other extreme (Armstrong et al., 1935).

was expanded to include two new categories of beneficiaries. The first new category represents an expansion of citizenship in terms of who qualifies as a citizen: Spouses and children of the worker who had been previously unable to claim benefits upon worker retirement were granted access. The second new category illustrates the expansion of citizenship in terms of benefits available in social insurance programs: The same group of beneficiaries from the first category can now claim benefits *not only* upon worker retirement but also in the unfortunate instance of premature worker death. As originally passed in the Social Security Act of 1935, a worker's family was provided with a "lump-sum payment" (Berkowitz & McQuaid, 1988, p. 135) upon the death of a worker that was equal to that which the worker had paid into the system.

Both changes ushered in with the 1939 amendments represented a move away from the initial "contributory-contractual principle" (Berkowitz & McQuaid, 1988, p. 126) of Social Security to a family-oriented policy in which the laborer's continued financial responsibility to his or her family could be assumed by the federal government under extenuating circumstances. This change was reflective of the unique position of the federal government (as a public insurer) to consider, in the words of R. A. Hohaus, "adequacy" over "actuarial equity" (Berkowitz & McQuaid, 1988, p. 134). (For further discussion of the 1935 and 1939 versions of Social Security, see Chapter 20.)

The Social Security Act amendments of 1950 initiated a further expansion in the boundaries of citizenship, offering eligibility to agricultural workers and the self-employed. Ten million workers, who had previously been ineligible to contribute to the Social Security system, were added to the program (Cohen & Meyers, 1950). Their inclusion in the program represented a broadening concept of citizenship in that it provided access to state support for income security not only for factory workers but also for farmers and small business owners as well. From a political perspective, the 1950 amendments increased the popularity of the program because, with increased numbers of people paying into Social Security, there were more people who were eligible to receive benefits when needed.

In addition, the 1950 amendments acted to expand citizenship in terms of the services that people could expect. Until these amendments, Social Security beneficiaries were receiving the same amount of money each month as they did on the day they first collected benefits. For example, Ida May Fuller, the first person to receive Social Security retirement benefits, was still receiving the same $22.54 each month even 10 years after she retired (DeWitt, 2003). The 1950 amendments increased the amount of Social Security income to account for the inflation that had occurred since 1940 (Cohen & Meyers, 1950). This, too, helped to increase the popularity of the program. Not only were more people eligible for benefits, but the benefits themselves were more desirable than those provided through the competing systems of state old-age assistance programs.

Between 1954 and 1960, people with disabilities, too, were slowly integrated into the Social Security program and the boundaries of citizenship were expanded further. First, with the Social Security Amendments of 1954, workers who qualified as having a "permanent disability" were put on "disability freeze." The freeze was not the same as disability insurance, but it allowed workers to retain work credits until they retired and could access benefits. Second, with the Social Security Amendments of 1956, those workers older than age 50 who had a "permanent disability" were entitled to access their earned benefits. Although it had been discussed as early as the late 1930s, it was not until 1960 that a disability insurance program that covered all workers and their dependents was added to Social Security. With each of these sets of amendments, the notion of citizenship is expanded incrementally. Although still clearly tied to the notion of citizen as laborer, the recognition that the capacity to labor may become limited *and* that those who experience this "permanent" limitation deserve access to income security is a shift in American social insurance policy.

A related expansion of citizenship pertains to the age at which an individual is allowed to claim "early retirement," that is, the age at which the laborer is permitted to leave the labor force and still receive Social Security benefits, though they might be reduced. Women were granted the opportunity to retire at age 62 (with reduced Social Security benefits) in 1956. It was not until 1961, however, that men were afforded this same opportunity. Despite the discrepancy in when these entitlements were offered, together they represent a redefinition of citizenship in which the laborer is afforded the opportunity to withdraw from the labor force with a reasonable expectation of income security, albeit one that is reduced from their full benefit.

Until this point in U.S. history, social insurance was focused on providing income security. In 1965, with the passage of Medicare, social insurance expanded to include health security (in old age) as well.[5] From a citizenship perspective, Medicare was a departure from the slow process of including more people into existing services. Rather, Medicare expanded the benefits to which a select group of citizens (those ages 65 and older) have access. Additionally, Medicare represented the first successful step toward national health coverage in the United States, albeit for one group of citizens.

Prior to the passage of Medicare, there had been three unsuccessful attempts to legislate a national health program in the United States.[6] Advocates for national health insurance had learned from these earlier experiences and took a strategic approach with Medicare (Marmor, 1973). They proposed a program that (1) restricted coverage to the elderly who were "sicker, poorer, and less insured than other groups" (Oberlander, 2003 pp. 23, endnote 42), (2) utilized the existing administrative and political experience of Social Security, and (3) restricted the scope of mandatory services to hospitalization coverage[7] (Oberlander, 2003). After the passage of Medicare, President Lyndon Baines Johnson declared,

> No longer will older Americans be denied the healing miracle of modern medicine. No longer will illness crush and destroy the savings that they have so carefully put away over a lifetime so that they might enjoy dignity in their latter years. No longer will young families see their own incomes, and their own hopes eaten away simply because they are carrying out their deep moral obligations (Sundquist, 1968, p. 321).

President Johnson's description of Medicare as reversing the former "denial" of medical care to older people may be interpreted as a recognition that a part of the expectation of citizenship is access to health security. In this case, the expectation has only been extended to older people. Furthermore, Johnson frames Medicare as a program that provides direct services to older people, protecting not only the financial well-being of

---

[5] Medicaid, another important program, was also passed in 1965. However, since this program is means-tested it is not a social insurance program but rather a "welfare" program and will not be addressed in this chapter.

[6] National health insurance was removed from the original Social Security proposal to increase the feasibility of the bill's passage. Significant opposition from the AMA also led to the failure of subsequent attempts to pass national health insurance in 1943 (the Wagner-Murray-Dingell legislation) and later during the Truman administration.

[7] Medicare Part B, which was also introduced at this time, was voluntary. Eligible participants would enroll and pay a monthly premium for access to insurance for doctor's bills. When this benefit was offered, 90% of those who were eligible enrolled (O'Sullivan, 2008).

the older people themselves, but their family members as well. Through the expansion of the services to which citizens have access, Johnson is also reaffirming the intergenerational economic and social interdependence of family and society.

It is worth noting that although Medicare represented a victory toward national health insurance in the United States, health security for all Americans is not a citizenship right in the United States. However, the architects of Medicare were hoping to get a "foot in the door" that could be used to expand the health security program from one that guaranteed services to seniors to one that provided services to all Americans, thus expanding citizenship based on who was deemed eligible to claim services. As noted by Robert Ball, the former commissioner of the Social Security Administration, "we all saw insurance for the elderly as a fallback position . . . we expected Medicare to be the first step toward universal national health insurance . . . " (1995, pp. 62–63). Although the U.S. experience since 1965 may taint our interpretation of the optimism Ball expresses, it is important to recall that between 1954 and 1960, disability insurance followed a similar path (Berkowitz & McQuaid, 1988).

In 1972, there were two different expansions of citizenship in the context of U.S. social insurance programs, one was related to Social Security and the other to Medicare. Prior to 1972, increases in Social Security benefits needed to be approved by Congress on an "as needed" basis, as was the case with the first such benefit increase in 1950.[8] However, the Social Security Amendments of 1972 included a mechanism to provide automatic cost of living adjustments (COLAs) to benefits starting in 1975. The boundaries of citizenship in U.S. social insurance programs now included a new form of an existing service: Citizens could now expect income security not just in the form of a fixed income but in one that kept pace with the larger national economy.

Also in 1972, people with permanent disabilities and those with end stage renal disease (ESRD) gained eligibility to the health security offered by Medicare. In contrast with the change in the Social Security program, this new entitlement was about offering existing services to new groups of people. Those with ESRD had shifted into a new citizenship category by virtue of their diagnosis (a testament to their immediate need). But for people with permanent disabilities, the new benefit was conditional. The 1972 amendments required that people with permanent disabilities

---

[8] Similar increases were legislated by Congress such that Social Security benefits were readjusted in 1952, 1954, 1959, 1968, 1970, 1971, and 1972.

wait 2 years after beginning to receive Social Security disability benefits before they can receive Medicare.

Restricting Citizenship in United States Social Insurance Programs: 1980s to the Present

In many ways, the dual changes to Social Security and Medicare in 1972 represented the end of an era of gradual expansion of both the types of services that a citizen could expect from social insurance programs and the groups of people deemed eligible for these services. The initial optimism that Medicare would be the first step to health security for all Americans was quickly dashed as rising health care costs became the focus of policy interventions of the late 1970s and the 1980s. When looking at the history of Medicare from the 1980s to the present, one of the notable trends is that no new groups have been granted these benefits. Consequently, 1972 represents the last expansion of the groups who may claim citizenship in U.S. social insurance programs. In contrast to the era of expanding the boundaries of citizenship in U.S. social insurance programs described in the previous section, this second era (1980s to the present) could be characterized by active attempts to constrain the boundaries of citizenship in U.S. social insurance programs.

Predictions of economic shortfalls in Social Security were the impetus for the 1977 amendments. They included an increase in both the percentage of payroll tax contributions collected for Social Security and the maximum amount of wages on which Social Security was to be collected. Although these changes may be viewed as an increase in the "cost" of social citizenship, they also functioned to increase the degree of financial interdependence that accompanied such citizenship. In effect, people were contributing more to the "pay as you go" Social Security program to safeguard current and future benefit levels. Additionally, the 1977 amendments changed the way in which COLAs were calculated (Achenbaum,1986; DeWitt, 2003).

In 1980, concerns over the cost of providing services to people with disabilities ushered in amendments that introduced new eligibility reviews for people with disabilities. From a policy perspective, these reviews were more work than the staff assigned to conduct them could possibly complete. By 1983, the reviews were stopped and in 1984, the Disability Benefits Reform Act was passed (DeWitt, 2003).

In terms of citizenship, the introduction of these reviews represented an institutionalized attempt to restrict access to the category of "people with permanent disabilities." Deborah Stone (1984) explains that both the clinical definition of disability on which initial assessments for benefits are based and the use of doctors and other medical professionals as gatekeepers are meant to restrict the number of people who can initially gain access to services through this category. Further, the introduction of continuing disability reviews symbolized a new and sustained effort to continually "kick people off" of disability benefits.

The 1983 amendments to Social Security continued this period of restricting the boundaries of citizenship in social insurance, despite changes that extended services to those who were already eligible. For example, these amendments allowed those people receiving benefits as "disabled widows and widowers," "disabled surviving divorced spouses," and "surviving divorced spouses" to continue receiving benefits after they remarried, as long as it was after a certain age (50 if disabled, 60 if not).[9] In addition, these amendments permitted divorced spouses[10] to access benefits even if their ex-spouse had yet to retire or claim benefits (subject to the same reduction in benefits for early retirement as applied to other beneficiaries). Furthermore, benefits were increased for both "disabled widows and widowers" who were eligible for benefits before the age of 60 and those widows and widowers whose spouses died before qualifying for benefits at age 62 (Social Security Administration [SSA] Office of Legislation & Congressional Affairs, 1984).

As a whole, the 1983 amendments significantly redrew the boundaries of citizenship in social insurance programs by excluding people who would have been eligible under previous rules than they were in actually expanding the boundaries to include new groups of recipients. The 1983 amendments gradually increased the age of eligibility at which people could collect full Social Security benefits from 65 to 67 (depending on the year in which one was born). Additionally, although citizens could still access benefits at age 62, these amendments amplified the penalty for doing so at this "early age." In both cases, citizenship is restricted (SSA Office of Legislation & Congressional Affairs, 1984).

COLAs were also changed in 1983. This change represented a potential reduction in the degree of income security experienced by citizens

[9] For disabled widows and widowers and disabled surviving divorced spouses, benefits are retained if they remarry after age 50 (SSA, 2008b). For surviving spouses and surviving divorced spouses, benefits are retained if they remarry after age 60 (SSA, 2008c).

[10] As long as they were aged 62 years or older, had been married for a minimum of 10 years and divorced for a minimum of 2 years.

who qualified for benefits. Although the introduction of COLAs in the 1972 amendments had promised to increase the Social Security benefits of older Americans to keep pace with increases in the prices of goods and services in the economy, the 1983 amendments signaled that those citizens who qualified for income security, could expect COLAs to be less effective than before at helping their incomes retain "real value" (SSA Office of Legislation & Congressional Affairs, 1984).

The Medicare Catastrophic Coverage Act of 1988 offers a unique example of the rigid boundaries of citizenship in the context of social insurance. Signed into legislation in July 1988 and repealed just over a year later in November 1989, the act included the first major expansion of the services available to Medicare beneficiaries since the introduction of the program in 1965. Changes introduced by the Medicare Catastrophic Coverage Act of 1988 included (1) removing co-payments for hospital stays longer than 60 days in duration, (2) limiting the Medicare Part A deductible (to $560 annually), (3) introducing an annual maximum for the Medicare Part B deductible (to $1370), and (4) incrementally phasing in a prescription drug plan scheduled to start in January 1991. However, these new benefits were unlike previous service expansions.

The benefit increases were not funded by an across-the-board increase in the maximum amount of payroll income subject to tax. Instead, these services would have been primarily funded through a specific tax (labeled a "supplemental premium") that was restricted to those people who would be receiving benefits—that is older people, themselves. From a policy standpoint, this proved to be problematic for two reasons. First, only about 40% of older people would be required to pay this supplemental premium. The remaining older people would be exempt due to their lower income levels. Second, those paying the supplemental premium (those with higher incomes) were the group who were most likely to already have access to the benefits, especially an existing prescription drug plan (Rice, Desmond, & Gabel, 1990).

The Medicare Catastrophic Coverage Act continued the trend of restricting the boundaries of citizenship in social insurance that began in the 1980s. The Act did not expand existing services to a new group of people. Although it attempted to protect older adults from bankruptcy due to costs associated with catastrophic illness and to provide new services to an existing group of beneficiaries, the services were not generous enough (co-insurance instead of full coverage), did not address one of the major concerns of older people (long-term care insurance), and violated the social insurance principle of universality in financing (Himmelfarb, 2005; Holstein & Minkler, 1991). Furthermore, even when the Medicare Catastrophic Coverage Act attempted to provide new services, such as the prescription drug benefit, these services were restricted to those who did not already have access through other means. In some ways, the Medicare Catastrophic Coverage Act was a step away from social insurance and toward a means-tested program supported only by tax revenues from other older people. It is notable that the repeal of the act was in large part due to the dissatisfaction expressed by more affluent older people who would have been paying more of the taxes for it.

In 1996, President Bill Clinton signed the Contract with America Advancement Act that included a newly restricted definition of disability that affected both (then) current and future beneficiaries. For existing enrollees, alcoholism or drug addiction in and of themselves were no longer enough to qualify for disability benefits through either Social Security Disability Insurance or Supplemental Security Income (a means-tested program operated through the Social Security Administration). Consequently, on January 1, 1997, benefits were terminated for 220,000 people who had previously received SSDI or SSI (Social Security Administration, n.d.). With this act, disability as a category of citizenship had been restricted and the determination for who qualified for this category of citizenship had been altered for the future.

The next significant change to Medicare, the introduction of Medicare Plus Choice (Medicare Part C) as part of the Balanced Budget Act of 1997, may also be seen as a restriction of the boundaries of citizenship. In an effort to manage the cost of health care, Medicare beneficiaries were encouraged to sign up for health maintenance organizations (HMOs) to manage their care (O'Sullivan, 2008).[11] From a citizenship perspective, the mix of services (and the degree to which they are covered) offered through HMOs is highly variable, creating both instability and disparities in service coverage. Additionally, for many, entering an HMO means surrendering their current relationship with their long-time physicians in exchange for a new relationship with an HMO-approved doctor.

---

[11] HMOs, or their precursors, "prepaid group practice plans," had been part of the Medicare program from the beginning. However, it was not until the 1990s that enrollment in these programs really began to take off (from 3.7% of Medicare beneficiaries in 1990 to 13.5% in 1997). To more equitably distribute the benefits available through these programs, especially access to prescription drug plans, the Balanced Budget Act of 1997 offered payments that exceeded the local fee-for-service rate to private programs in certain areas of the country (Biles, Adrion, & Guterman, 2008).

Consequently, many Medicare beneficiaries have elected *not* to enter into Medicare Plus Choice plans but remain in traditional Medicare.

Changes arising from the Balanced Budget Act of 1997 made the provision of coverage through Medicare Plus Choice a less profitable option for health insurance companies resulting in both a reduction in benefits offered and the overall number of plans available in certain areas. Consequently, plans were both less desirable and less accessible to beneficiaries leading to an enrollment drop of almost 25% between 1999 and 2003 (Biles, Adrion, & Guterman, 2008). Enrollees whose plans reduced benefits or withdrew from the (local) market completely were greeted with an abbreviated and unstable citizenship experience.

In part, this reduction in Medicare HMO enrollees was the impetus behind the most recent attempts to redefine citizenship in the context of Medicare, the Medicare Modernization Act (MMA) of 2003. Among other things, the MMA introduced private insurance prescription drug coverage for Medicare enrollees. Coverage is provided either through stand-alone plans (Medicare Part D) or through Medicare Advantage (the reformulated Medicare Plus Choice HMO plans where now include prescription drug coverage).

To entice Medicare Advantage plans to enroll Medicare beneficiaries, these plans are reimbursed at rates that are more than 12% higher than traditional Medicare (Biles, Adrion, & Guterman, 2008). These "overpayments" represent a total cost of $33 billion between 2004 and 2008, money that could potentially be used in other ways to expand the boundaries of citizenship within Medicare. The promotion of HMOs and private prescription drug plans in Medicare has also created varying costs and cost structures for Medicare beneficiaries that are likely to reproduce basic class inequalities and to have negative effects on the low-income and disabled elderly (Geyman, 2006; Geyman, 2004; Oberlander, 1999; Biles, Nicholas, & Guterman, 2006).

Unlike the Medicare Catastrophic Coverage Act the MMA was not repealed despite its initial unpopularity (Himmelfarb, 2005). Like many other changes in policy since the 1970s, the MMA may at first seem to be a victory in terms of citizenship since a new service is being offered by the state to citizens. However, the market-first approach of the MMA—as characterized by the sole reliance on private industry in the prescription drug plan—is a negative tradeoff for the expansion of the boundaries of citizenship via the provision of greater health security. Indeed, money is siphoned away from citizens and toward corporations through the increased costs associated with billions of dollars of state subsidies for private prescription drug plans and Medicare Advantage plans that compete with traditional Medicare. In addition, the design of the MMA—prohibiting federal negotiation on drug costs and providing substantial state subsidies for private commercial insurance, management, administration, and provision of Medicare services—predictably does nothing to curb either the growth in Medicare costs or Medicare's contribution to the growth in overall healthcare costs.[12] This situation may be used to bolster the ideology that government-provided health care is inefficient and an unacceptable result of efforts to expand the benefits of citizenship. Overall, the passage of the MMA affords citizens access to prescription drugs through plans that are costly and favor corporate profits, resulting in a further infringement upon the ability of people to claim health security as a citizenship right delivered by the state in the guise of a new "expanded"service.

THE FUTURE OF CITIZENSHIP AND SOCIAL INSURANCE IN THE UNITED STATES

> The enactment of the Social Security Act marked a great advance in affording more equitable and effective protection to the people of this country against widespread and growing economic hazards. The successful operation of the Act is the best proof that it was soundly conceived. However, it would be unfortunate if we assumed that it was complete and final. Rather, we should be constantly seeking to perfect and strengthen it in the light of our accumulating experience and growing appreciation of social needs (President Roosevelt, in a Recommendation to Congress in 1938).

In this chapter, we have presented a sociological and historical analysis that has illustrated two very distinctive periods in the history of social insurance programs in the United States. In the first period, which spans from the 1930s through the late 1970s, citizenship in the context of social insurance expands in terms of the services guaranteed by the state and the people whom can gain access to these services. In contrast, the second period is characterized by a virtual stagnation in services

[12] It is instructive to address the rising costs of healthcare overall, rather than focusing solely on increasing Medicare costs. To place the blame on rising Medicare costs independent of larger health care costs runs the risk of reproducing ageism and places the problem squarely on the shoulders of older people rather than on the entire health care system.

offered and the active restriction of eligibility criteria for specific groups of people.

Social Security, as the U.S. social insurance program par excellence, was far from perfect when first introduced, since it did not provide universal coverage. Some people were not considered in the discussion of citizenship during the initiation of social insurance and at key times when changes were made. In particular, African Americans, by virtue of the occupational sectors that they inhabited, were systematically neglected from coverage under Social Security at its inception. As both Quadagno (1994) and Poole (2006) explain, the disadvantages experienced by black people, and specifically black women, as a result of this original exclusion have been perpetuated by Social Security policies. This includes the fact that African Americans receive less in lifetime benefits because of their lower life expectancy and the fact that black women's payroll taxes serve to subsidize the spousal benefit for nonworking married women, who are much more likely to be white. The history of racialized "work" in Social Security can be connected to the reproduction of inequality in an otherwise redistributive program (Poole, 2006). Proposals to address these experiences of inequality in the current Social Security system are addressed by Madonna Harrington Meyer and colleagues in chapter 8 of this volume.

Our analysis documents just how far the program has progressed (in the first historical period) and the ways in which it has regressed and/or stagnated (in the second). In this section, we identify the opportunities to continue the expansion of citizenship in the context of U.S. social insurance programs. In keeping with President Roosevelt's call to "perfect and strengthen" U.S. social insurance programs so that they may better address "social needs," we outline both what services are left for the state to offer and to whom exactly these services have yet to be offered. We identify a key service expansion that has not yet been implemented as a social insurance program in the United States—full national health coverage including long-term care services. Additionally, we identify *multiple* groups to which existing services need to be expanded to achieve the social insurance principle of universal coverage—single, unmarried individuals or those whose relationships are not recognized by the federal government; undocumented laborers; and the near old, those aged 55 to 64. Both the implementation of national health coverage and the inclusion of the groups listed above to those who already have access to social insurance programs would expand the boundaries of social citizenship in the United States in a dramatic step toward a more democratic and just society.

Expanding Services that People May Claim: Health Care and Long-Term Care

Single payer health care has been proposed and defeated numerous times in the history of American politics due to strong opposition from stakeholders and weak mobilization among advocates (Navarro, 1992; Navarro, 1995; Quadagno, 2004; Quadagno, 1988). The strongest advocates for single payer health care have been previously or currently disadvantaged groups of potential citizens (people with disabilities, women, minorities, people with low socioeconomic status). As stated previously, the United States is the only industrialized country without a national health insurance. More recent attempts to address the growing population of uninsured in the United States failed; the Bush administration's proposal for "health savings accounts" fizzled, and Clinton's broad plan for health-care changes fell flat (Fahrenthold, 2006, p. A01). However, several steps have been taken toward a single payer, universal health care system at the state level.

Since the enactment of Massachusetts' mandatory health insurance on June 30, 2006, 439,000 more people in Massachusetts have health insurance coverage; there has been a 37% decrease in total free care visits (from the now Health Safety Net) to hospitals and community health centers between October 1 and December 31, 2007, compared to between October 1 and December 31, 2006, meaning that low-income people are receiving more managed care that focuses on prevention and primary care rather than unmanaged care often through emergency room visits (Division of Health Care Financing and Policy, 2008).

After the passage of mandatory health insurance in Massachusetts, other states, including California, are attempting their own health care reforms. SB 840, the California Health Insurance Reliability Act (CHIRA) will "provide fiscally sound, affordable health insurance coverage to all Californians, provide every Californian with the right to choose his or her own physician and control health cost inflation (Health Access California, 2005). However, as Navarro (1992, 1995) argues, without a strong working class labor movement, attempts at reform are unlikely. In 2008, S.B. 840 was passed by the California legislature for the second time, despite the likelihood of a veto by Governor Schwarzenegger.

On the national level, HR 676 (United States National Health Insurance Act, 2005) would create a national single-payer insurance covering everyone for all medically necessary care (Medicare Rights Center, 2007). This would include physician, hospital, rehabilitation, diagnostic, long-term care, mental health, prescriptions, dental, vision, home health, and physical therapy (Political Affairs.net, 2005). The plan would improve care to everyone, even those who currently have insurance, and extend health care to the 45 million who are now uninsured. HR 676 would transform for-profit health institutions into non-profits, simplify administration through a single-payer system, and redistribute the savings through better care and extended coverage (Political Affairs.net, 2005).

The Presidential election of 2008 once again opens up a political window for national health insurance or substantial improvements therein. Candidate Obama would expand citizenship through mandatory insurance coverage for all U.S. children, with a goal of universal health coverage for all, building upon the health insurance infrastructure already in place including the Federal Employee Benefit Program. Candidate McCain would expand the private insurance market, giving all Americans modest vouchers to pay for that insurance while abolishing the present employer and employee tax subsidies for health insurance. Some experts estimate that this will drastically reduce the number of workers under modern employer-based health insurance, raising the number of uninsured by millions. As of this writing, we know only that the fate of social insurance programs of Social Security and Medicare and the possibility of national health insurance weight heavily in the balance depending on the November 2008 election (Collins, Nicholson, Rustgi, & Davis, 2008).

Expanding the People Who May Claim Services: Marital Status

As addressed by Walker (chapter 16) in his history of social insurance in Britain, social insurance programs have institutionalized values around family and labor that were, at the time of the programs' start, deemed static and universal. In light of changing labor force participation rates, divorce rates, rates of cohabitation, and the struggle for recognition of gay and lesbian relationships, marriage has become an increasingly weak and unequal mechanism for distributing benefits. For example, Tamborini & Whitman (2007) used the Survey of Income and Program Participation (SIPP) and found that in 2001, while three fourths of women aged 40 to 69 were eligible for Social Security benefits based on their marital histories, the cohort of women aged 40 to 49 were less likely to have married, were more likely to be divorced, and had shorter marriages prior to divorce than similarly aged women in 1985.

Furthermore, Harrington Meyer, Wolf, and Himes (2006) illustrate dramatic racial disparities in access to Social Security benefits based on marital status. The differences are greatest for African American women, and the gap is widening due to declining frequency and length of marriages for these women. Although marriage rates are expected to remain "nearly universal" (p. 241) for whites and Hispanics, it is projected that only 64% of black women born between 1960 and 1964 will ever marry (compared to 93% of whites). It is expected that only 50% of African American women born in the 1960s will reach retirement age having had a marriage that qualifies them for widows' or survivors' benefits. Thus, according to Harrington Meyer and colleagues (p. 255), the Social Security spouse and widow benefit as a "safety net is becoming increasingly irrelevant (p. 255)."

Expanding the People Who May Claim Services: Gay and Lesbian Cohabiting Couples

Another example of the inequities of distributing Social Security and Medicare benefits through marriage is the systematic exclusion of gays and lesbians from accessing spousal benefits. Under current law, same-sex spouses are not eligible for Social Security spousal benefits because they do not meet the gender specific definitions of "husband" and "wife" used in the Social Security Act. Although gay and lesbian couples can marry in the states of Massachusetts, California, and most recently, Connecticut,[13] the legalization of same-sex marriage at the state level has no validity for determining marriage at the federal level (Haltzel & Purcell, 2008). This has implications not only for Social Security but also for federal level tax benefits as well. (See chapters 18 and 19 for more on taxation issues related to Social Security.) Consequently, gays and lesbians, although able to access Social Security as individual laborers, are only entitled to partial citizenship once in a cohabiting relationship.

Moving away from a marriage-based model by decreasing the length of the marriage requirement, extending benefits to cohabitants, and establishing a higher minimum benefit would help increase financial equity

[13] It is worthwhile to note that although same-sex marriages have been legalized in these three states, since the introduction of the Defense of Marriage Act in 1996, 27 states have passed constitutional amendments that define marriage as between one man and one woman. Additionally, while same-sex couples can legally marry in the state of California as of the time this article was written, it is one of two states along with Florida that has a constitutional amendment on the November 2008 ballot (NCSL, 2008).

for retirees. Harrington Meyer and colleagues recommend that a "minimum benefit approach would create an income floor that is independent of martial or employment history and reduce inequality in old age" (p. 257).

Expanding the People Who May Claim Services: Undocumented Workers

Undocumented workers represent an interesting illustration of people who are afforded only partial citizenship in the context of social insurance programs. After the passage of the 1986 Immigration Reform and Control Act, employees were required to provide Social Security cards (even fake ones) to employers. In response, a number of undocumented workers have used fake Social Security numbers to secure employment and have consequently paid into the Social Security system. In 2004, this resulted in revenues equal to 10% of the Social Security surplus (Porter, 2005). An estimated 7 million undocumented workers in the United States are now providing the system with a subsidy of as much as $7 billion a year. SSA actuaries currently assume that about half of the illegal immigrants in the United States actually pay Social Security taxes although they are very unlikely to collect benefits (Porter, 2005). Although this group of laborers has not been recognized as official U.S. citizens (by the USCIS), they are incurring the *costs* of social citizenship by providing revenues for social insurance programs through income, Social Security, and Medicare payroll taxes. Additionally, undocumented workers help to sustain social insurance programs through the work of (re)producing children—children who will one day contribute through their own labor and income taxes. However, because their Social Security numbers are not valid, they are denied the *benefits* of social citizenship; that is they cannot make claims against the state to access services to which they contribute as part of their role as laborers.

Expanding the People Who May Claim Services: The Near-Old

Poor health is often experienced at earlier ages for people with low-income levels over the life course, including women, minority, and immigrant populations. Between one fifth and one third of persons aged 55 to 64 with low incomes have no health insurance (Plumb, Weitz, Hernandez,

Estes, & Goldberg, 2007). As a result, these individuals are likely to enter the Medicare system at age 65 in poorer health than other populations that had access to preretirement health insurance. Experts contend that disparities in health could be reduced and illness and the onset of disability could be prevented or delayed if the near old and others who are uninsured had access to health insurance. Beginning with President Bill Clinton, several policymakers have proposed the expansion of health insurance under Medicare to those aged 55 to 64 when more than 95% of older Americans are eligible for Medicare. With the deepening U.S. and global economic uncertainty, including the recent Wall Street meltdown, pressures are likely to intensify in support of expanding citizenship to mid-life person and newly unemployed workers between the ages of 55 and 64 who lose their health insurance. Despite the dire situation of millions, there will be major power struggles and pushback against any social insurance expansions as well as contests regarding the feasibility of continuing to support U.S. entitlement programs.

SUMMARY

In this chapter, we have outlined a descriptive model of citizenship that captures the five normative role expectations associated with U.S. social citizenship in late capitalism. The previous discussion highlights both the degree of citizenship one is afforded (based on certain eligibility criteria) and the services to which one granted citizenship can expect to have access (through an entitlement). Consequently, an individual or group can experience less-than-full citizenship or access to some state guaranteed services and not others. Furthermore, an individual or group can have full citizenship status but the state may not necessarily provide an entitlement to certain services.

We have traced the relevance of the concept of citizenship (and, in particular, social citizenship) through the history of social insurance programs in the United States. Although the early history of social insurance in the United States reflects a fairly continuous expansion of the boundaries of citizenship in terms of both what services the state deemed as social rights that needed to be met and who was given the right to access them, the past 3 decades can primarily be characterized in terms of containment and retraction. Looking to the future, it is clear that there are opportunities to engage in the renewed expansion of the boundaries of social citizenship so the people in the United States can truly know the meaning of income and health security, not only in old age but also across the entire life course. In the spirit of the architects of the original Social Security bill, such a change would foster a true sense of security from "cradle to grave."

DISCUSSION QUESTIONS

1. What are the five "normative" roles of citizenship in late capitalism identified by the authors?
2. What future expansions to the boundaries of citizenship are outlined by the authors?
3. Think about the boundaries of the categories of citizenship in social insurance programs in the United States. According to the authors, during what time period were these boundaries expanded? On what two axes did these boundaries expand? When were these boundaries beginning to contract?
4. When were people with disabilities first considered as part of the Social Security program? In what ways have the services for people with disabilities who qualify for Social Security expanded over time?
5. Use the information presented in the article to make a pictorial representation of the expanding boundaries of the category of citizenship described in this chapter. Begin with the groups of people who were included as beneficiaries in the original conceptualization of the Social Security program in the United States as articulated in the Social Security Act of 1935. Distinguish between those who were originally covered by the program and each boundary expansion between 1935 and 1972.

REFERENCES

Achenbaum, W. A. (1986). *Social Security: Visions and revisions.* New York: Cambridge University Press.

Armstrong, B. N., & Staff. (1935). *Old age security staff report.* Retrieved October 17, 2008, from http://www.ssa.gov/history/reports/ces/cesvoltwo.html

Ball, R. (1995). Perspectives on Medicare: What Medicare's architects had in mind. *Health Affairs, 14*(4) 62–63.

Bernstein, M. C., & Bernstein, J. B. (1988). *Social Security: The system that works.* New York: Basic Books.

Biles, B., Nicholas, L. H., & Guterman, S. (2006). Medicare beneficiary out of pocket costs: Are Medicare advantage plans a better deal? New York: The Commonwealth Fund.

Biles, B., Adrion, E. & Guterman, S. (2008). *The continuing costs of privatization: Extra payments to Medicare Advantage plans in 2008*. Retrieved October 17, 2008, from http://www.commonwealthfund.org/usr_doc/Biles_Medicareextra_1169_ib.pdf?section=4039

Choudry, A. (2008, August 22). Making a killing: The military-industrial complex and impacts on the Third World. *Toward Freedom*. Retrieved August 22, 2008, from http://towardfreedom.com/home/index.php?option=com_content&task=view&id=1386&Itemid=0

Cohen, W. J., & Myers, R. J. (1950). *Social Security Act amendments of 1950: A summary and legislative history*. Social Security Administration (SSA). Retrieved August 21, 2008, from http://www.ssa.gov/history/1950amend.html

Collins, S. R., Nicholson, J. L., Rustgi, S. D., & Davis, K. (2008). *The 2008 presidential candidates' health reform proposals: Choices for America*. Retrieved October 18, 2008, from http://www.commonwealthfund.org/usr_doc/Collins_presidentialcandhltreformprop_1179.pdf?section=4039

Dean, K. (2003). *Capitalism and democracy: The impossible partnership*. London: Routledge.

DeWitt, L. (2003). *Historical background and development of Social Security*. Retrieved December 12, 2007, from http://www.socialsecurity.gov/history/briefhistory3.html

Division of Health Care Financing and Policy. (2008). *Health care in Massachusetts last*. Retrieved August 2008, from http://www.mahealthconnector.org/portal/binary/com.epicentric.contentmanagement.servlet.ContentDeliveryServlet/Health%2520Care%2520Reform/Overview/key_indicators_0808.pdf

Estes, C. L. (1979). *The aging enterprise: A critical examination of programs and services for the aging*. San Francisco: Jossey-Bass.

Estes, C. L. (1991). The Reagan legacy: Privatization, the welfare state and aging in the 1990's. In J. Myles & J. S. Quadagno (Eds.), *States, labor markets and the future of old age policy* (pp. 59–83). Philadelphia: Temple University Press.

Estes, C. L. (2001). *Social policy and aging: A critical perspective*. Thousand Oaks: CA: Sage Publications.

Estes, C. L., & Zulman, D. M. (2007). Informalization in long-term caregiving: A gender lens. In C. Harrington & C. L. Estes (Eds.), *Health Policy* (pp. 142–151). Sudbury, MA: Jones and Bartlett.

Fahrenthold, D. A. (2006, April 5). Mass. Bill Requires Health Coverage: State Set to Use Auto Insurance As a Model. *Washington Post*, p. A01. Retrieved October 8, 2008, from http://www.washingtonpost.com/wp-dyn/content/article/2006/04/04/AR2006040401937.html

Foucault, M. (1979). *Discipline and punish*. New York: Vintage Books.

Geyman, J. P. (2004). Privatization of Medicare: Toward disentitlement and betrayal of a social contract. *International Journal of Health Services*, *34*(4), 573–594.

Glenn, E. N. (1992). Unequal freedom: How race and gender shaped American citizenship and labor. Cambridge, MA: Harvard University Press.

Gramsci, A. (1971). *Selections from the prison notebooks*. New York: International Publishers.

Haltzel, L., & Purcell, P. (2008, January 3). The effect of State-legalized same-sex marriage on Social Security benefits and pensions. CRS Report for Congress. Order Code RS21897.

Harper, D. (2001). Citizen. *Online Etymology Dictionary*. Retrieved August 15, 2008, from http://www.etymonline.com/index.php?search=citizen&searchmode=none

Harrington Meyer, M., Wolf, D., & Himes, C. (2006). Declining eligibility for Social Security spouse and widow benefits in the United States? *Research on Aging, 28*(2), 240–260.

Health Access California. (2005). SB840: The California Health Insurance Reliability Act (CHIRA). Retrieved October 8, 2008, from http://www.health-access.org/expanding/sb840.htm

Himelfarb, R. (2005). Echoes of catastrophic care? The passage of the Medicare prescription drug, improvement and modernization act and its implications for the future of Medicare. Paper presented at the annual meeting of the The Midwest Political Science Association, Palmer House Hilton, Chicago, Illinois. Retrieved October 8, 2008, from http://www.allacademic.com/meta/p86353_index.html

Holstein, M., & Minkler, M. (1991). The short life and painful death of the Medicare Catastrophic Coverage Act. In M. Minkler & C. L. Estes (Eds.), *Critical perspectives on aging: The political and moral economy of growing old* (pp. 189–206). Amityville, NY: Baywood.

Kagan, D., Schmitt, G., & Donnelly, T. (2000). *Rebuilding America's defenses: Strategy, forces and resources for a new century*. Washington, DC: The Project for the New Century.

Klein v. Board of Tax Supervisors, 282 U.S. 19 (1930).

Klein, N. (2007). *The shock doctrine: The rise of disaster capitalism*. New York: Metropolitan Books/Henry Holt.

Mahajan, R. (2002). *The new crusade: America's war on terrorism.* New York: Monthly Review Press.

Mann, M. (1987). Ruling class strategies and citizenship. *Sociology, 21*, 339–354.

Marmor, T. R. (1973). *The politics of Medicare*. Chicago: Aldine.

Marshall, T. H. (1949). Citizenship and social class. In T. H. Marshall (Ed.), *Class, citizenship, and social development*. Westport, CT: Greenwood Press.

McGill, D. M., & Brown, K. M. (2005). *Fundamentals of private pensions*. London: Oxford University Press.

Medicare Rights Center (2007, October 25) At last, a solution. Volume 7, Issue 42.

Meszaros, I. (2001). *Socialism or barbarism.* New York: Monthly Review Press.

National Counsel of State Legislatures (NCSL). (2008). *Same-sex marriages, civil unions, and domestic partnerships*. Retrieved October 18, 2008, from http://www.ncsl.org/programs/cyf/samesex.htm

Navarro V. (1992). *Why the United States does not have a national health program.* Amityville, NY: Baywood.

Navarro, V. (1995). Why Congress did not enact health care reform. *Journal of Health Politics, Policy and Law, 20*(2), 455–461.

Obama, B. (2006). *The audacity of hope: Thoughts on reclaiming the American dream.* New York: Crown Publishers.

Oberlander, J. (1999). Vouchers for Medicare: A critical reappraisal. In M. Minkler & C. L. Estes (Eds.), *Critical gerontology: Perspectives from political and moral economy* (pp. 203–220). Amityville, NY: Baywood.

Oberlander, J. (2003). *The political life of Medicare*. Chicago: University of Chicago Press.

O'Connor, J. (1973). *The fiscal crisis of the state*. New York: St. Martin's.

O'Connor, J. (1984). *Accumulation crisis*. New York: Basil Blackwell.

O'Sullivan, J. (2008). *Medicare Part D prescription drug benefit: A primer*. Washington, DC: Congressional Research Service.

Offe, C., & Ronge, V. (1982). Thesis on the theory of the state. In A. Giddens & D. Held (Eds.)*Classes, power, and conflict* (pp.249–256). Berkeley, CA: University of California Press.

Park, K. (2002). Stigma management among the voluntarily childless. *Sociological Perspectives*, *45*(1), 21–45.

Plumb, M., Weitz, T., Hernandez, M., Estes, C. L., & Goldberg, S. (2007). Improving care and assistance security for vulnerable older women in California. In *Women, Health and Aging: Building a Statewide Movement* (pp. 9–45) Los Angeles: The California Endowment.

Political Affairs.net. (2005). Health care: Nationwide hearings support hr 676′. Retrieved October 9, 2008, from http://www.politicalaffairs.net/article/articleview/1368/1/102/

Poole, M. (2006). *The segregated origins of Social Security: African Americans and the welfare state*. Chapel Hill, NC: University of North Carolina Press.

Porter, E. (2005, April 5). Illegal immigrants are bolstering Social Security with billions. *The New York Times*. Retrieved August 2008, from http://www.nytimes.com/2005/04/05/business/05immigration.html

Preist, D., & Hull, A. (2007, February 18). Soldiers face neglect, frustration at Army's top medical facility. *The Washington Post*, p. A01. Retrieved October 9, 2008, from http://www.washingtonpost.com/wpdyn/content/article/2007/02/17/AR2007021701172.html

Quadagno, J. S. (1988). *The transformation of old age security: Class and politics in the American welfare state*. Chicago: University of Chicago Press.

Quadagno, J. S. (1994). *The color of welfare: How racism undermined the war on poverty*. NY: Oxford University Press.

Quadagno, J. S. (2004). Why the United States has no national health insurance: Stakeholder mobilization against the welfare state, 1945–1996. *Journal of Health and Social Behavior 45*(Extra Issue), 25–44.

Random House. (2006). *Random House Webster's Unabridged Dictionary*. New York: Random House Reference.

Rice, T. (1997). Can markets give us the health system we want? *Journal of Health Policy, Politics, and Law*, 22(2): 383–426.

Rice, T., Desmond, K., & Gabel, J. (1990). The Medicare Catastrophic Coverage Act: A post- mortem. *Health Affairs* 9(3), 75–87. Retrieved October 9, 2008, from http://content.healthaffairs.org/cgi/reprint/9/3/75.pdf

Rothe, D. (2009). War profiteering: Iraq and Halliburton. In P. A. Adler & P. Adler (Eds.), *Constructions of deviance: Social power, context, and interaction* (pp. 433–445). Belmont, CA: Thomson Wadsworth.

Social Security Administration (n.d.). Detailed chronology: 1990s. Retrieved October 9, 2008, from http://www.ssa.gov/history/1990.html

Social Security Administration (SSA) (1938). FDR statements on Liberalizing the Old-Age Insurance System. Retrieved August 23, 2008, from, http://www.ssa.gov/history/fdrstmts.html#liberal

Social Security Administration (SSA). (2008a). Historical background and development of Social Security. Retrieved August 19, 2008 from, http://www.ssa.gov/history/briefhistory3.html

Social Security Administration. (SSA). (2008b). What you need to know when you get Social Security Disability Benefits (Publication No. 05-10153). Retrieved October 17, 2008, from http://www.ssa.gov/pubs/10153.pdf.

Social Security Administration (SSA). (2008c). Survivors Benefits (Publication No. 05-10084). Retrieved October 17, 2008, from http://www.socialsecurity.gov/pubs/10084.pdf.

SSA Office of Legislation & Congressional Affairs. (1984). Summary of P.L. 98-21 (H.R. 1900). Social Security Amendments of 1983. Retrieved October 15, 2008, from https://www.socialsecurity.gov/history/1983amend.html

Statistical Information Analysis Division (Department of Defense). (2003). Active duty military deaths – Race/ethnicity summary (as of March 15, 2003). Retrieved October 9, 2008, from http://siadapp.dmdc.osd.mil/personnel/CASUALTY/RACE-OMB-WC.pdf

Stone, D. (1984). *The Disabled State*. Philadelphia, PA: Temple University Press.

Sundquist, J. (1968). *Politics and Policy: The Eisenhower, Kennedy, and Johnson Years*. Washington, DC: Brookings Institution Press.

Tamborini, C. R., & Whitman, K. (2007). Women, marriage, and Social Security benefits revisited. *Social Security Bulletin*, *67*(4), 1–20.

Tittle, C. R., & Paternoster, R. (2000). *Social deviance and crime*. Los Angeles, CA: Roxbury.

Turner, B. (1990). Outline of a theory of citizenship. *Sociology 24*(2): 189–217.

Twine, F. (1994). *Citizenship and social rights: The interdependence of self and society*. Thousand Oaks, CA: Sage.

United States Citizenship and Immigration Services (USCIS). (2008). Citizenship. Retrieved October 9, 2008, from http://www.uscis.gov/portal/site/uscis/menuitem.eb1d4c2a3e5b9ac89243c6a7543f6d1a/?vgnextoid=96719c7755cb9010VgnVCM10000045f3d6a1RCRD&vgnextchannel=96719c7755cb9010VgnVCM10000045f3d6a1RCRD

United States Department of Labor (US DOL). (n.d.). Workers' Compensation. Retrieved October 17, 2008, from http://www.dol.gov/dol/topic/workcomp/index.htm

Waitzkin, H. (1983). *The second sickness: Contradictions of capitalist health care*. NY: The Free Press.

Weber, M. (1946). *From Max Weber*. Translated and edited by H. H. Gerth and C. Wright Mills. New York: Galaxy.

Zones, J. S., Estes, C. L., & Binney, E. A. (1978). Gender, public policy and the oldest old. *Ageing and Society*, *7*(Part 3), 275–302.

8 Why All Women (and Most Men) Should Support Universal Rather than Privatized Social Security

MADONNA HARRINGTON MEYER

Being an older woman is a very different experience than being an older man. For a variety of reasons that cut across all stages of the life course, older women rely on Social Security much more than older men do. As a result, they have a great deal more to lose if the United States privatizes the system.

After decades of being almost unthinkable, major revisions to the Social Security System have recently taken center stage. Since its inception in 1935, the history of Social Security has been one of broad-based political support. Between 70% and 90% of respondents in national polls favor universal old-age programs and think the United States should be doing more for the elderly (AARP 2005; Harrington Meyer & Herd, 2007). Long considered a sacred cow, few politicians threatened to restrict the program. Those who did would feel the sting as voters took to the polls (Harrington Meyer & Herd, 2007; Harrington Meyer, 2005; Estes, 2001; Binney & Estes, 1988).

By the 1980s, however, various criticisms of the program began to make headlines. Some critics suggested that benefits for the elderly—generally defined as those ages 65 and older—should be redirected toward the young because they had higher poverty rates and smaller income supports than the old (Binney & Estes, 1988; Estes, 2001; Friedman, 1994; Gilbert, 2002; Hacker, 2002). Others claimed that providing benefits for older baby boomers was too onerous for the smaller generations that followed them. Over time, the charge that the program was misguided became commonplace, even if not well supported by evidence (Ferara, 1980; Yergin & Stanislaw, 1998). Indeed, supporters of Social Security countered that those who were opposed to social spending for the elderly were also actively voting against social spending for children. Moreover, the sizable surplus would nearly cover expenditures for the aging baby boomers (Binney & Estes, 1988; Estes, 2001; Herd & Kingson, 2005).

Nonetheless, by 2004, President George Bush made the privatization of Social Security his top domestic priority. The main rationale given for privatizing Social Security was that the program would soon be fiscally unsustainable. Supporters of privatization prefer individual accounts that would maximize each person's choice and responsibility. The plan most often discussed would allow those younger than age 55 to divert as much as 4% of their 6.2% Social Security contribution to private accounts (Estes, 2001; Gilbert, 2002; Harrington Meyer & Herd, 2007; Herd & Kingson, 2005; President's Commission to Strengthen Social Security, 2001). Supporters of Social Security, however, argue that our current compulsory universal program is the most efficient and effective program for shoring up financial resources in old age. They point out that Social Security has a modest budgetary shortfall that is readily addressed and that privatization would introduce greater economic inequality and insecurity and a much greater budgetary shortfall (AARP, 2005; Estes, 2001; Gilbert, 2002; Hacker, 2002; Harrington Meyer & Herd, 2007).

This chapter explores why all women (and most men) should support universal Social Security over a privatized system. The reasons are wide ranging, but at their roots, they all point to one conclusion: Social Security is the most effective tool for reducing gender inequality in old age (Engelhardt & Gruber, 2004; Harrington Meyer & Herd, 2007; Korpi & Palme, 1998). It is worth noting that the Social Security debate is just one of many that are dominating the political landscape of the United States. At the core of these welfare state debates lays a question about whether the United States should implement welfare programs that are beneficial to the market or to families (Harrington Meyer & Herd, 2007). Privatizing Social Security would redirect enormous amounts of money to the stock market and to those who manage the market. It would also redirect risk from the state to older people and their families. By contrast, universal Social Security does little to benefit the market *per se*, but a great deal to insure financial security for older people and their families.

SOCIAL SECURITY: THE MOST IMPORTANT SOURCE OF INCOME FOR OLDER WOMEN

Throughout their lives, women average smaller and fewer income streams than men. Even though times have changed, women remain significantly less likely than men to be employed at all ages and significantly less likely to be working full time. Women's lower employment rates are linked in part to ongoing disproportionate responsibility for unpaid care work. The gendered division of labor is not as severe as it was in the 1960s and 1970s, but women continue to do about twice as much as men to care for children and frail older relatives (Bianchi, Robinson & Milkie, 2006; National Alliance for Caregiving & AARP, 2004). Only about 40% of women work full time, year round, and they receive wages that are only 77% of men's wages (Institute for Women's Policy Research, 2006; U.S. Bureau of Labor Statistics, 2006).

The combination of lesser wages with a greater responsibility for caring for children and frail older relatives means that women accumulate a great deal less in wages over their lives than men. Hartmann, Rose, and Lovell (2006) traced a cohort of college-educated women and men who were ages 25 to 29 in 1984. They found that by 1989, the women's average accumulated wages were $76,000 less than the men's wages. By 1999, the women were $273,000 behind the men. By 2004, the women were an astonishing $440,000 behind the men in cumulative wages. These lower wages translate into smaller savings, investments, private pensions, and public pensions.

By age 65 and older, the gap between men's and women's income is remarkable. Even though the poverty rate for all older people is below 10%, older women are nearly twice as likely to be poor. Currently, an older individual is considered poor if their annual income falls below about $10,000 (Social Security Administration [SSA], 2007). Older women are also twice as likely as older men to live alone. Older women are only one-half as likely to be married and twice as likely to live on their own, thus they enjoy neither the economics of scale of living together nor the possibility of two income streams. Moreover, their claims on private pensions are much smaller than men's. Older women are only about 60% as likely to receive a private pension, and when they do, that pension is only half as big as men's on average (Harrington Meyer & Herd, 2007; He, Sangupta, Velkoff, & Debaros, 2005; McDonnell 2005). Older women are equally as likely as older men to receive a Social Security benefit, but those benefits are, on average, just 75% of older men's (SSA, 2007).

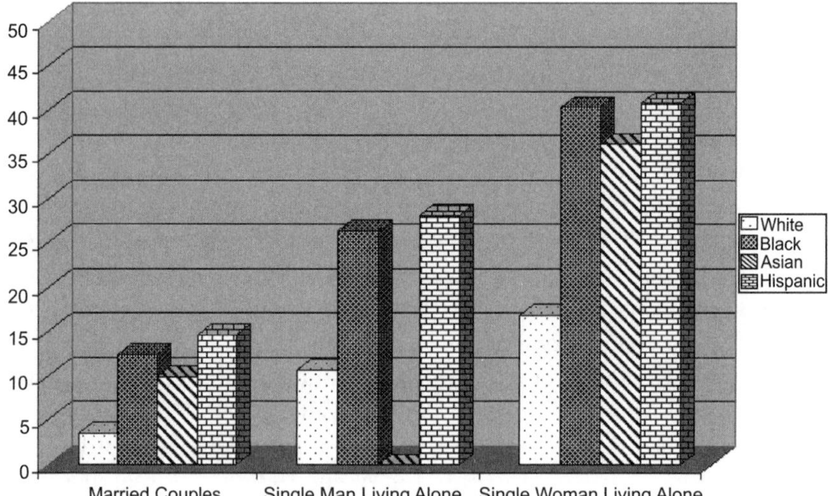

Figure 8.1 Source U.S Census Bureau 2005. Civilian noninstitutionalized persons. Reprinted with permission from Harrington Meyer and Herd 2007.

Variation between older women and men is substantial, but so is variation among women by race and marital status. Throughout their lives, black and Hispanic women tend to have less education, higher unemployment, lower wages, and greater responsibilities for care work for the young and the frail elderly (Harrington Meyer & Herd, 2007; He, et al, 2005; National Caregiving Alliance & AARP, 2004). By old age, the impact is clear. The U.S. Census reports that 10% of older white women are poor, compared to 16% of Asian, 22% of Hispanic, and 27% of black women. The differences are even more pronounced when we take marriage and living arrangements into account. As shown in Figure 8.1, 40% of single older black and Hispanic women who live alone are poor (U.S. Census Bureau, 2005).

Fewer market- and marriage-based resources make older women particularly dependent on Social Security. Indeed, fewer and smaller streams of old-age income means that Social Security benefits are much more important to older women than to older men. In general, Social Security comprises about 40% of income for all older people and 60% of income for all older women. Notably, Social Security contributes 100% of income for one in five older women (Porter, Larin & Primus, 1999; SSA, 2006). Because they live longer, women comprise 57% of Social Security beneficiaries. The program works effectively to help lift many out of poverty, and 60% of those lifted out of poverty by Social Security are older women.

Social Security is even more important for minority older people. Because of reduced access to private pensions and private savings, half of older Hispanics and African Americans rely on Social Security for 90% or more of their income (Torres-Gil, Greenstein, & Kamin, 2005; Wu, 2004). For black and Hispanic women, Social Security comprises almost 80% of their income. Some estimate that the overall poverty rate among women would be four times higher if they did not have Social Security income (Porter, Larin, & Primus, 1999).

Thus, efforts to privatize Social Security would have an enormous impact on economic security for older women. It is not clear exactly how privatization would shape women's retirement income because the welfare of older women has not been seriously addressed in most of the debates, but it is clear that privatization would increase risk for individual women and for older women as a group. And because it would eliminate some of the features that have benefited women, it is likely to reduce benefits for many. Any reduction in benefits would be problematic. Scholars estimate that even a 10% cut in Social Security benefits could lead to a 7% rise in poverty rates among the elderly, and older women would be especially hard hit by such cuts (Engelhardt & Gruber, 2004). In these next sections, I address several of the features of Social Security that have benefited women but would not likely be incorporated into a privatized system.

SOCIAL SECURITY REDIRECTS MONEY TO OLDER WOMEN

From its inception, the Social Security benefit formula has purposely provided a higher return on contributions by lower earners. On average, high-wage earners receive benefits that replace 28% of preretirement income, but low-wage earners receive benefits that replace 78% (Koitz, 1997; The Century Foundation, 1998). This redistributive benefit formula is particularly important for women, as on average they earn lower wages and are more likely than men to take time out of the labor force to care for children or frail older relatives. The redistributive benefit formula serves to reduce the size of the hit women take for lower and more disrupted earnings.

Privatized individual accounts would most likely not have mechanisms for redistribution from higher to lower earners. In fact, with privatization, the United States would likely shift from having a redistributive benefit formula to having no redistribution at all. Throughout their lives, people would contribute money to private accounts and their investments would fare however they fare. Some people would be able to save and invest a great deal of money and reap the rewards of very fortunate investment strategies. But at the other end of the continuum, many people would face the consequences of unfortunate investment strategies. There has been no discussion of implementing mechanisms that would shift money away from those who had either higher earnings or more successful investments toward those with lower earnings or less successful investments (Harrington Meyer & Herd, 2007). In fact, because they favor individualizing choice, risk, and responsibility, most supporters of privatized accounts would oppose such redistributive measures (Wray, 2005; Yergin & Stanislaw, 1998). Part of the initiative that drives privatization is the desire that as people age they would reap the results, however good or bad, of economic decisions made across their lifetimes.

SOCIAL SECURITY PROVIDES BENEFITS TO WIVES AND WIDOWS

Though the program was initially designed only to reward retired workers, Social Security legislation was changed early on to provide noncontributory benefits to wives and widows (Harrington Meyer, 1996). In 1939, wives and widows were given benefits equal to 50% and 75%, respectively, of their husbands'. Over time, the rules were made gender neutral so that benefits were available to husbands or wives. The rules were also relaxed so that those who had been married for at least 20 years could obtain benefits after a divorce. Eventually, the widow benefit was raised to 100%. And as divorce rates rose, the length of marriage requirement was decreased to 10 years (Harrington Meyer & Herd, 2007; SSA, 2006). Currently, 60% of older women receive benefits as wives and widows, rather than as workers, because the benefits they would receive as workers would be smaller. This is projected to be the case for the next several cohorts as they reach old age (Levine, Mitchell & Phillips, 2000; SSA 2006).

One of the most troubling aspects of discussions about privatizing Social Security is that supporters do not clarify what the impact of privatization would be for spouse and widow benefits. There is no indication of whether these benefits will shrink or ultimately disappear. Currently, spouse and widow benefits are funded by creaming off some of the funds and redirecting them to spouses. To put it differently, all workers could potentially receive higher retired worker benefits than they currently do, but instead the program channels some of the funds contributed through the FICA tax to cover spouses and widows. To date, there has been no discussion of implementing any mechanism that would divert funds from privatized accounts to make these noncontributory benefits available. What would happen to the financial outlook of women who have relied on these noncontributory benefits?

SOCIAL SECURITY PROVIDES ACTUARIAL ADVANTAGES FOR WOMEN

Women live, on average, 5 years longer than men, but Social Security does not reduce their benefits to offset this trend (Harrington Meyer & Herd, 2007). Life expectancy for all older women is now 80 years, compared to 75 years for men. Given that those who are currently old received full benefits at age 65, the gender difference in longevity might lead to a one-third reduction in women's benefits. But under Social Security, such actuarial distinctions have never been discussed, and this has been enormously beneficial to older women across the decades. Under a privatized Social Security system, however, the fact that women live longer could become problematic. Not only would women, on average, accrue significantly smaller amounts than men, but they would also need to pace their withdrawals to accommodate their longer lives. Women, more than men, would need to try to estimate how long they would live and try to adjust their monthly benefits to avoid running out of funds entirely before they die.

SOCIAL SECURITY IS A MORE EFFICIENT ADMINISTRATIVE SYSTEM

Currently, the SSA runs the single largest welfare program in the United States using less than 1% of the budget to cover all administrative costs. The Congressional Budget Office (Commonwealth Fund, 2004) calculates that if the United States switched to millions of privatized individual accounts and allowed account holders to make even a fraction of the decisions related to their investments, the administrative costs (which would then include stock broker and account manager salaries and expenses) would soar to between 5% and 30%. Deflecting that proportion of the funds to administrative measures would surely lead to either smaller benefits or larger taxes for all. And because many of the administrative fees charged to private account holders may be flat fees, they stand to take a much bigger bite out of the investments of lower income earners when compared to higher income earners. Although the administrative costs of Social Security are now paid for with a flat tax up to the tax ceiling, under a privatized system they would be paid for in a more regressive manner. Privatization would benefit many in the financial investment industry, as evidenced by the increase in lobbying groups from those sectors, but it would reduce financial security for most, particularly lower earners (Harrington Meyer & Herd, 2007; Herd & Kingson, 2005).

SOCIAL SECURITY SPREADS, RATHER THAN CONCENTRATES, RISKS

Under the Social Security system, everyone pays into and receives benefits from the same pool. Thus, any risks due to economic downturns or bad investment are spread across the entire older population. With privatized individual accounts, people face the outcomes of their economic fortunes and misfortunes on their own. Those with larger incomes can afford to put away more, take greater risks, and absorb unfortunate investment outcomes. Therefore, they are more likely to fare well in old age. But those with smaller incomes cannot afford to put much away, take higher risk strategies that might produce higher returns, or absorb losses (Harrington Meyer & Herd, 2007). Some families would be hard hit and it is not clear where they would turn for assistance.

SOCIAL SECURITY IS THE STRONGEST LEG OF THE "THREE-LEGGED STOOL"

For more than 60 years, old-age financial security in the United States has been addressed by a three-legged stool: Social Security, private pensions, and personal savings. In recent years, two of these legs have become much less stable. Private pensions, which historically have helped to determine who would and who would not be poor in old age, are the second largest income stream for older people. They are funded in part by government subsidies to corporations that total over $100 billion a year, but not everyone gets private pensions (Seldon & Gray, 2006). Among older people in the top earnings quartile, 63% have private pensions, and among those in the lowest earnings quartile, only 20% have private pensions (Employee Benefit Research Institute [EBRI], 2004).

Historically, most workers with private pensions were covered by defined benefit plans. Under these plans, employees received a benefit amount that went up with hours, salaries, and years of service. Recently, however, most companies have shifted to defined contribution plans. In fact, between 1979 and 2004, the population covered only by defined benefit plans dropped from 62% to 10%, while the population covered only by defined contribution plans rose from 16 to 63% (Harrington Meyer & Herd, 2007; EBRI, 2004). Defined contribution plans differ because they shift the responsibility and risks associated with private pension accumulation, and often much of the cost, from employers to employees. Because they are not as compulsory or as automatic, under defined contribution plans, employees are more readily able to opt out or reduce their contributions. They are also more readily able to withdraw money before retirement for expenses such as health costs, children's educations, or weddings. Women are significantly more likely than men to do both (Munnell & Sunden, 2004; Shuey & O'Rand, 2006). Because they concentrate rather than spread the risk of unfortunate investment strategies, defined contribution plans create shortfalls that are much harder for those with lower incomes to absorb. Finally, there is evidence that employers are contributing less to these plans, making employees even more responsible for their own pension accumulations (Munnell & Sunden, 2004; Shuey & O'Rand, 2006). What was once a very strong leg of the three-legged stool is now quite shaky, particularly for those with meager resources.

The personal savings leg is also looking shakier, especially for older women. It is difficult to explore gender differences in savings and assets among those who are married because they tend to be defined as household values. But among the growing share of older Americans who are not married, sharp gender differences are apparent. Single older men's assets are 30% higher than older women's assets (Levine, Mitchell, & Phillips, 2000). Among older women, one of the biggest determinants of private savings accumulation is whether women were single mothers (Harrington Meyer & Herd, 2007). Women ages 65 to 75 who were single mothers for at least 10 years report asset income equal to just one third of that for married mothers (Yamokoski & Keister, 2006). Across the board, savings in the United States are down (Zeller, 2007). In fact, in 2007, savings among families in the United States reached the lowest rates since the Great Depression. And savings and assets accumulation is especially low for those with lower incomes and higher demands on their income. Women, generally, and single mothers, in particular, average much lower assets in old age, and as a result, they are financially less secure.

Given that both private pensions and private savings are growing smaller and riskier, it seems particularly problematic to also be incorporating more risk into public pensions. But making Social Security more risky is precisely what privatization would do. And just as older women already come up short on the other two legs of the stool, experts expect that they would come up even shorter with a privatized social security system (Harrington Meyer & Herd, 2007).

SOCIAL SECURITY'S FISCAL SHORTFALLS ARE READILY ADDRESSED

Social Security is a pay-as-you-go system in which workers pay in through the FICA tax and the money is paid out to older beneficiaries. Aware that cohorts come in different sizes and aging baby boomers were going to draw out a great deal of benefits, the Social Security Administration purposely began accumulating a budget surplus decades ago. That surplus is now $2 trillion and rising at a rate of over $150 billion per year (SSA, 2007). As more and more of the baby boomers make claims, the surplus will begin to dwindle. By 2041, it is estimated that the surplus will be gone and the amount coming in from workers each month will cover 80% of the payouts.

While the modest budget shortfall that is predicted to appear in 35 years has been used as an excuse to dismantle Social Security, in fact, this shortfall is readily addressed (AARP, 2005; Harrington Meyer & Herd, 2007). One option is to temporarily raise the FICA tax by 1 to 2 %. That tax has not been raised since the mid 1980s and such a move would eliminate the fiscal shortfall that will occur during the aging of the baby boomers. Another option is to raise the cap on taxable earnings. Currently, earnings are taxed up to $102,000 per year (SSA, 2007). If that cap on taxable income was raised to $140,000, and then indexed to inflation, the increased revenues would cover a sizable share of the fiscal shortfall (AARP, 2005). Yet another option is to broaden the eligibility base to include the 30% of state and local government employees who are currently not participating in Social Security (Munnell, 2005). Any combination of these plans would reduce the shortfall and assure a seamless transition of the existing Social Security program through the aging of the baby boomers.

With privatization, the budgetary shortfall would be more substantial and more difficult to address. A switch to individual privatized accounts would be expected to shift the arrival of the shortfall forward from 2041 to 2017. And, because the Social Security Administration would have to simultaneously fund the old program and the new program for some time, privatization would amount to $1 to $2 trillion in new expenses (Diamond & Orszag, 2002; Harrington Meyer & Herd, 2007). Thus, not only would privatization increase inequality among the aged, it would also increase the tax burden on all Americans.

Despite all of the hyperbole, the real fiscal crisis with the current Social Security system is that the Federal government has borrowed nearly all of the trust fund for other purposes, repaying neither the interest nor the principle (Board of Trustees, 2008; SSA, 2007). Thus, the U.S. federal government owes the Social Security program nearly $2 trillion and must begin to repay that amount as baby boomers enroll in the program.

SOCIAL SECURITY'S OTHER SHORTCOMINGS ARE ALSO READILY ADDRESSED

Even Social Security's most steadfast supporters tend to think the program has shortcomings that should be addressed. For example, although Social Security does redistribute wages from higher to lower earners, it does not effectively offset time spent out of the labor force. All workers are allowed to drop the five lowest years of earnings, but many women spend more than 5 years out of the labor force or in lower paying jobs while they are performing unpaid care work (SSA, 2006). The corresponding reduction in benefits contributes to economic instability for those with primary responsibility for children and frail older adults. In general, Social Security benefits tend to be lowest for those juggling work and family—especially if they are not married long enough to be eligible for Social Security spouse and widow benefits. One solution would be to mimic policies that are already in place in some European countries by instituting care credits. The plan preferred in Harrington Meyer and Herd (2007) would be to eliminate the spouse benefit, and then introduce care credits that subsidize the worker benefit by giving credit for an amount equal to half of the medium wage for up to 5 years with one child and up to 9 years for more than one child. A person would not need to be a stay at home parent or married to benefit from this particular care credit; rather it would be beneficial to all who have lower wages due to child care.

Another shortcoming with Social Security is that noncontributory benefits are linked to marital status, and there is a growing race gap in marriage. Historically, black and white women were almost equally likely to meet the length of marriage requirement for spouse and widow benefits. Among women born in the 1920s, roughly 90% of white and black women were eligible for benefits based on marital status. But the ensuing retreat from marriage has been particularly notable among black women and by the time women born in the 1960s reach old age, 80% of white and Hispanic women, compared to only 50% of black women, will be eligible to receive benefits on the basis of their marital status (Harrington Meyer, Wolf & Himes, 2006). This means that older black women, who already have fewer economic resources and higher poverty rates, would be especially vulnerable in old age. One response to the growing inequality linked to race and marital status is to stop linking benefits to marital status and instead install a minimum benefit. The plan preferred in Harrington Meyer and Herd (2007) would be to create a minimum benefit equal to the poverty line, or about $10,000 per year. Coincidently, that minimum benefit would be nearly equal to the maximum spousal benefit, thus eliminating the need for that benefit altogether. And because it would bring Social Security beneficiaries up to the poverty line, it would nearly eliminate the need for Supplemental Security Income (SSI) for the aged, thereby offsetting some of the cost.

A related shortcoming is that Social Security does not acknowledge unmarried couples, whether gay or straight. Like many other nations, the United States has experienced an enormous increase in cohabitation among couples who do not plan to marry or whom are not allowed to marry. These couples are excluded from making claims for spouse or widow benefits. Expanding the eligibility requirements to allow cohabitators to make claims would help to shore up economic security in old age for couples who are not now legally recognized.

CONCLUSION

It is important that U.S. policy makers attend to these and other modest adjustments to the Social Security system, to make it more responsive to changing sociodemographic trends. Adjustments such as introducing care credits, generous minimum benefits, and recognition of cohabitating couples would strengthen the program's ability to shore up economic security in old age and reduce inequality linked to gender, race, class, and marital status. By contrast, privatization would strip away many of the protections provided by Social Security. And it would do so at a much higher cost. Rather than implement costly market-friendly policies that are sure to increase inequality, old-age policies should shore up effective family-friendly policies that will reduce old-age inequality (Harrington Meyer & Herd, 2007).

Even though older women rely more heavily on the program than older men, and older black and Hispanic women more than anyone else, the impact of privatization on older women has not been well explored. It appears, however, that under privatization, older women would lose many of the protective benefits afforded by redistributive benefit structures, spouse and widow benefits, the spreading of risk, and actuarial oversight. Moreover, the cost of administrative oversight for millions of individualized accounts would divert much of the resources. The strongest leg of the three-legged stool would become much shakier as, under privatization, financial insecurity linked to gender, race, class, and marital status would increase. For these reasons, all women, and any men who have a mother, daughter, sister, wife, or partner—or who themselves have lower wages or disrupted work histories—should support universal rather than privatized Social Security.

DISCUSSION QUESTIONS

1. Why might a woman receive benefits as a wife/widow even if she has a work history of her own?
2. Use Harrington Meyer's chapter to summarize both: (a) some of the ways that the current Social Security system benefits women, (b) some of the potential dangers that Social Security privatization potentially holds for women, and (c) some of the potential dangers that Social Security privatization potentially holds for all beneficiaries.
3. The title of this chapter references "all women (and most men)." In small groups, use the evidence provided in this article to discuss what the potential role of men could be in supporting universal Social Security. Think about how men might be involved in the push for the elimination of the spousal benefit and how this might impact heterosexual relationships (i.e., marriage) and the construction of the family in the United States.

REFERENCES

America Association for Retired People. (2005). *Public attitudes toward Social Security and private accounts*. Washington, DC: AARP Knowledge Management.

Bianchi, S. M., Robinson, J. P., & Milkie, M. A. (2006). *Changing rhythms of American family life*. New York: Russell Sage Foundation.

Binney, E. A., & Estes, C. L. (1988). The retreat of the State and its transfer of responsibility: The intergenerational war. *International Journal of Health Services, 18*(1), 83–96.

Board of Trustees. (2008). *The 2008 annual report of the board of trustees of the federal old- age and survivors insurance and federal disability insurance trust funds*. Washington, DC: U.S. Government Printing Office.

Century Foundation. (1998). *The basics: Social Security reform*. New York: The Century Foundation.

Commonwealth Fund. (2004). *Administrative costs of private accounts in Social Security*. Washington, DC: Congressional Budget Office.

Diamond, P. A., & Orszag, P. R. (2002). *Reducing benefits and subsidizing individual accounts: An analysis of the plans proposed by the President's commission to strengthen Social Security*. New York: Center of Budget and Policy Priorities and Century Foundation.

Employee Benefit Research Institute. (2004). Health insurance coverage of individuals ages, 55–64. *Notes, 25*(3), Figure 8:15.

Engelhardt, G. V., & Gruber, J. (2004, May). *Social Security and the evolution of elderly poverty*. (NBER Working Paper No. 10466). Cambridge, MA: National Bureau of Economic Research.

Estes, C. (Ed.). (2001). *Social policy and aging: A critical perspective*. Thousand Oaks, CA: Sage Publications.

Ferrara, P. J. (1980). *Social Security: The inherent contradiction. (Studies in Public Policy)*. San Francisco: Cato Institute.

Friedman, M. (1994). Comments on *The Road to Serfdom* by Friedrich Hayek. *Policy Review, 69*(14), 14–21.

Gilbert, N. (2002). *Transformation of the welfare state: The silent surrender of public responsibility*. New York: Oxford University Press.

Hacker, J. S. (2002). *The divided welfare state: The battle over public and private social benefits in the United States*. New York: Cambridge University Press.

Harrington Meyer, M. (1996). Making claims as workers or wives: The distribution of Social Security benefits. *American Sociological Review, 61*(3), 449–465.

Harrington Meyer, M. (2005). Decreasing welfare, increasing old age inequality: Whose responsibility is it? In R. Hudson (Ed.), *The new politics of old age policy*. Baltimore: Johns Hopkins University Press.

Harrington Meyer, M., & Herd, P. (2001). Aging and aging policy in the U.S. In J. R. Blau (Ed.), *The Blackwell companion to sociology* (pp. 375–388). Malden, UK: Blackwell Publishing.

Harrington Meyer, M., & Herd, P. (2007). *Market friendly or family friendly? The state and gender inequality in old age*. New York: Russell Sage.

Harrington Meyer, M., Wolf, D., & Himes, C. (2006). Declining eligibility for Social Security spouse and widow benefits in the United States? *Research on Aging, 28*(2), 240–260.

Hartmann, H., Rose, S. J., & Lovell, V. (2006). How much progress in closing the long-term earnings gap? In F. D. Blau, M. C. Brinton, & D. B. Grusky (Eds.), *The declining significance of gender?* (pp. 125–155). New York: Russell Sage Foundation.

Herd, P., & Kingson, E. R. (2005). Selling Social Security. In R. H. Hudson (Ed.), *The new politics of old age policy* (pp. 183–204). Baltimore: Johns Hopkins University Press.

He, W., Sangupta, M., Velkoff, V. A., & Debaros, K. A. (2005). 65+ in the United States. *Current Population Reports* (Special Studies Series P23, no. 209). Washington, DC: U.S. Census Bureau.

Institute for Women's Policy Research. (2006). Memo to John Roberts: The gender wage gap is real (IWPR #C362). Washington, DC: Institute for Women's Policy Research

Koitz, D. S. (1997). The entitlements debate. 97-39 EPW (Updated January 28, 1998). Washington, DC: Library of Congress, Congressional Research Service.

Korpi, W., & Palme, J. (1998). The paradox of distribution and strategies of equality: Welfare state institutions, inequality, and poverty in the western nations. *American Sociological Review*, *63*(5), 661–687.

Levine, P. B., Mitchell, O. S., & Phillips, J. W. R. 2000. Benefit of one's own: Older women's entitlement to Social Security retirement. *Social Security Bulletin*, *63*(2), 47–53.

McDonnell, K. (2005). Retirement annuity and employment-based pension income. *EBRI Notes*, *26*(2), 7–14.

Munnell, A. H. (2005). Mandatory Social Security coverage of state and local workers: A perennial hot button (Issue in Brief 32). Chestnut Hill, MA: Boston College, Center for Retirement Research.

Munnell, A. H., & Sundén, A. (2004). *Coming up short: The challenge of 401(k) plans*. Washington, DC: Brookings Institution Press.

National Alliance for Caregiving and AARP. (2004). *Caregiving in the U.S.* Washington, DC: Author.

Porter, K. H., Larin, K., & Primus, W. (1999). Social Security and poverty among the elderly: A national and state perspective. Washington, DC: Center on Budget and Policy Priorities.

President's Commission to Strengthen Social Security. (2001, December 21). *Strengthening Social Security and creating personal wealth for all Americans* (Final Report). Washington, DC: Author.

Shuey, K. M., & O'Rand, A. M. (2006). Changing demographics and new pension risks. *Research on Aging*, *28*(3), 317–340.

Social Security Administration. (2006). Annual statistical supplement 2005. Social Security Bulletin. Washington, DC: Author.

Social Security Administration. (2007). Annual statistical supplement 2006. Social Security Bulletin. Washington, DC: Author.

Torres-Gil, F., Greenstein, R., & Kamin, D. (2005). Hispanics' large stake in the Social Security debate. Washington, DC: Center on Budget and Policy Priorities.

U.S. Bureau of Labor Statistics. (2006, August 2). Usual weekly earnings of wage and salary workers: Second quarter 2006. Washington, DC: Author.

U.S. Census Bureau. (2005, September 16). Age-people (all races) by median income and sex: 1947 to 2001. *Historical Income Tables, People* (Table P-8). Washington, DC: Author.

Wray, L. R. (2005). *The ownership society: Social Security is only the beginning...* Public Policy Brief No. 82. Annandale-on-Hudson, NY: Levy Economics Institute of Bard College.

Wu, K. B. (2004). African Americans age 65 and older: Their sources of income (Fact Sheet 100). Washington, DC: AARP Public Policy Institute.

Yamokoski, A., & Keister, L. (2006). The wealth of single women: Marital status and parenthood in the asset accumulation of young baby boomers in the United States. *Feminist Economics*, *12*(1-2), 167–194.

Yergin, D., & Stanislaw, J. (1998). *The commanding heights: The battle between government and the marketplace that is remaking the modern world.* New York: Simon & Schuster.

Zeller, T., Jr. (2007, February 1). Savings rate at depression-era lows... Does it matter? *New York Times*.

9 Healthy, Wealthy, and Wise? Challenges to Income Security for Elders of Color

STEVEN P. WALLACE AND VALENTINE M. VILLA

INTRODUCTION

The public discourse around the future of Social Security and income security in old age is based on the image of the baby boom generation as healthy, wealthy, and wise. There is a public portrayal of the coming generation of retirees as being able to work well into their 60s and 70s. Boomers are seen as uniformly having good health and a long life expectancy, accumulated assets and other wealth that will supplement their retirement and make Social Security and other public programs less relevant, and high educational levels that gives them the capacity to plan for retirement and manage their extensive resources wisely so that income security is assured through their old age (Congressional Budget Office, 1999).

A monolithic view of the coming generation of elderly is unwise and underlies, in part, the justification for weakening social insurance programs and the social safety net for older adults. One proposal in this vein that this chapter will discuss is the proposal to raise the age for early Social Security benefits from age 62 to later, such as age 65 (Liebman, MacGuineas, & Samwick, 2005). Delaying the early retirement age is predicated on the assumption that there will be no adverse impact on the population because the next cohort of older persons will be in disproportionally good health, financially well off, and well educated.

Demographic data shows, however, that the baby boom population will be more racially and ethnically diverse than any previous generation, with 20% of boomers being members of a minority group (U.S. Census Bureau, 2006b). Angel and Angel (2006) argue that the current and expected increase in Latinos and African Americans among the ranks of the elderly translates into a growing number of individuals who are at risk of serious economic disadvantage. There are several factors that operate across the life course of minority populations that result in economic vulnerability in old age, including lower levels of human capital, less stable employment in low-wage jobs, low earnings for both husbands and wives, less accumulation of assets, and long-term sustained poverty (Whitfield, Angel, Burton, & Hayward, 2006; Angel, Jimenez, & Angel, 2007).

Social Security and other retirement income mechanisms are supposed to contribute to income adequacy in old age, but our measures of income adequacy for low-income older adults are flawed. The most common measure of adequacy is the "replacement rate," which is the percentage of preretirement income that the retiree obtains. The problem with this measure is that a full-time worker making minimum wage does not have a sufficient income to pay for basic expenses, so even a 100% replacement rate will not result in a decent standard of living in retirement.

Another measure that is often used to discuss income adequacy is the federal poverty line. This measure was based on consumption patterns in the 1950s of families that found that one third of their income was spent on food. The poverty line was then calculated as three times the Agriculture Department's stingiest food allowance. It did not take into account the different expenditure patterns of older adults or the variation in the costs of living by state. Even the author of the method conceded that the resulting poverty line was too low initially (Orshansky, 1993), and since its development, it has not be modified to account for the increased overall standard of living nor for the changing mix of costs. In particular, housing and medical care costs have taken a significantly larger share of the average expenditures of older adults in the past half century. Low-income older adults (those in the bottom quartile of earnings) now spend only 17% of their income on food, but 38% on housing and 14% on out-of-pocket health care costs (Social Security Administration [SSA], 2007a).

Because of these changes, basic income adequacy is best identified by a new measure, the Elder Economic Security Standard index, which varies by county and includes the actual needs for housing, health care, transportation, food, and miscellaneous expenses (see http://www.wowonline.org/ourprograms/eesi/eess.asp). In California, covering basic necessities requires an income of around 200% of the federal poverty line, on average (Wallace & Molina, 2008).

Understanding the potential impact that proposals such as raising the early retirement age hold for the baby boom population requires examining the health and socioeconomic status of the current preretiree population, people aged 50 to 61 years (the first large wave of the baby boom population). Although there are surely many individuals who fit the image of the healthy, wealthy, and wise older adults, there are many groups of older adults that do not and will not fit this optimistic and individualistic paradigm. In this chapter, we examine the health and economic status of racial and ethnic populations that constitute the current cohort of elders and preretirees and the impact that changes in the eligibility for early retirement benefits under Social Security will have on diverse populations.

ARE ALL OLDER ADULTS HEALTHY?

If all groups of older adults were equally healthy, then it might be logical to expect them to be able to work to older ages, but this is not the case for either the current generation of early retirement age adults nor for the coming generation—those aged 50 to 61.

African Americans in the preretirement ages are the most disadvantaged in life expectancy, with more than a 2-year shorter life expectancy at age 62 than whites (National Center for Health Statistics, 2007). During the preretirement ages of 62 to 64, both African Americans and Latinos face higher rates of disability that limits the amount and kind of work that they can do (Table 9.1). The disparity is most striking for women. About one quarter of white women aged 62 to 64 years report work limitations, but almost one half of African American women report work limitations in the same age bracket. Latinas fall in between, with about one-third reporting work limitations. The pattern is similar for men with modestly lower work disability rates for African American men than for women (Table 9.1). Among those with experience in the waged labor force, African Americans aged 62 to 64 years are most likely to report

Table 9.1

HEALTH PROBLEMS AFFECTING WORK, AGES 62–64

	HEALTH PROBLEM OR DISABILITY PREVENTS WORKING OR LIMITS KIND OR AMOUNT OF WORK		RETIRED OR LEFT JOB FOR HEALTH REASONS	
	Women (%)	Men (%)	Women (%)	Men (%)
African Americans	49.4	41.3	12.8	19.0
Latinos	32.0	32.6	11.3	14.8
Whites	25.3	26.4	9.2	11.3

Note. From "Current Population Survey, Annual Social and Economic Supplement, CPS Table Creator," by U.S. Census Bureau, 2007, Retrieved October 31, 2008, from http://www.census.gov/hhes/www/cpstc/cps_table_creator.html

not working due to health, with Latinos also more likely to leave work for health reasons than whites (Table 9.1).

Thus, many persons at early retirement age face health challenges to continued work, challenging the myth of the universally healthy aging population. And elders of color are the most likely to face those health challenges, making them particularly likely to be impacted by changing early retirement ages.

But isn't the next generation of workers healthier? Americans, overall, are living longer than ever before, and fewer older adults report physical disabilities (Federal Interagency Forum on Aging-Related Statistics, 2008). But data on the health of the baby boom cohort offers evidence of continued health vulnerabilities. Most (62%) of the population aged 50 and 64 years has at least one chronic condition such as diabetes, hypertension, arthritis, heat disease, or cancer (Collins, Davis, Schoen, Doty, & Kriss, 2006). By 2030, six of every 10 baby boomers will be living with more than one chronic condition. Moreover, obesity rates among baby boomers will increase, with one third of the population predicted as obese by 2030 (American Hospital Association, 2007). This is particularly troubling because of the link between obesity and several chronic conditions, most notably diabetes. The impact of these chronic diseases is greater for African Americans; for example, those with high blood pressure are more likely to have greater cardiovascular and renal damage than non-Latino whites (Clark & Gibson, 1997). Middle-aged black men also report a higher prevalence and incidence of many major chronic fatal diseases including hypertension, diabetes, and stroke (Hayward, Crimmins, Miles, & Yang, 2000). The pattern of poor health and chronicity is similar for Latinos as well, most notably the high prevalence of diabetes found among Latino populations. Latinos of all ages are two to five times more likely to have diabetes than the general population. The impact of diabetes is compounded by Latinos being more likely than non-Latino whites to be hospitalized for uncontrolled diabetes, as well as for diabetes with short- and long-term complications (AHRQ, 2008).

Thus, health disparities of both the current and coming generations of minority elders suggest that the African American and Latino populations will approach old age with disproportionately large numbers that have poor health status, making it difficult or impossible for them to work additional years before retirement.

ARE ALL OLDER ADULTS WEALTHY?

The socioeconomic status of the elderly in the aggregate has improved substantially in the past 40 years, with poverty rates among the elderly falling from 35.2% in 1959 to 9.4% in 2006 (Federal Interagency Forum on Aging-Related Statistics, 2008). But significant disparities between races and ethnicities remain in poverty rates, as well as in sources of income and levels of wealth.

The poverty rate for older African Americans and Latinos is about three times that of non-Latino whites (Table 9.2), and the poverty rate for older women is higher than that of men within every race (Federal Interagency Forum on Aging-Related Statistics, 2008). But, as explained earlier, the measure of poverty that we use is unrealistic and outdated. Large numbers of older adults have incomes just above the official poverty line; the proportion of all seniors living below 200% of the poverty line zooms to four times the proportion under the poverty line. And older adults from racial and ethnic minority groups are disproportionately in economically precarious positions. More than half of all older African Americans, American Indians and Alaska Natives (AIAN), and Latinos nationally have low incomes (below 200% of poverty). Although the economic situation of Asian elders overall is close to that of non-Latino whites, combining all Asian groups together obscures the bimodal distribution of outcomes. Some groups of Asian elders, such as second- and third-generation Japanese and Chinese elders, fare well overall, but others, including Indochinese refugees and Korean elders, have very low incomes (Park Tanjasiri, Wallace, & Shibata, 1995).

The economic situation of the next generation of older adults, those who are currently 50 to 61 years of age, is somewhat better. But those are adults who are theoretically at their peak earnings potential and typically are still in the labor force. Even with those advantages, one third of African Americans and Latinos aged 50 and 61 years have low incomes. Nonetheless, poverty rates for most minority groups are three times higher than for non-Latino whites, and the rate of those with low incomes is about twice that of those in poverty. This means that a substantial number of adults approaching old age, about one third of minority populations, are struggling to make ends meet and are likely to have no money left at the end of the month to put aside for retirement.

The foundation needed for economic security in retirement for the baby boomer generation is crumbling. Access to employer sponsored pensions and retiree benefits are decreasing across the working age population. Twenty-five years ago, 80% of large firms offered defined benefits where a worker was assured a predetermined pension for as long as they lived—today less than a third do so (Hacker, 2007). Less than half of the working age population have any private pension, and those who do primarily have a defined contribution-type plan like a 401(k), which carries returns that are neither predictable nor assured (Hacker, 2007). Minority elders have the worst pension coverage. In 2004, wage and salary workers had pension coverage rates of 63.9% for non-Latino whites, 59.0% for African Americans and only 38.4% for Latinos. Much of the difference in pension coverage between non-Latino whites and African Americans was a result of differences in their types of employment. But the large pension coverage gap with Latinos persisted even after controlling for a number of different employer characteristics, especially for immigrants (Copeland, 2005). The one third of minorities in their 50s who have low incomes have no discretionary resources to save or invest, and their low, insecure personal coverage compounds their lower incomes, leaving them with fewer resources in old age.

The low rates of pensions and savings for low-income workers leaves Social Security as the most critical source of retirement income for minority retirees who are between the ages of 62 and 64. When the head of household is in this early retirement age, just over half of both black and white households receive Social Security income, along with just under half of Latino and one third of Asian American households. The

Table 9.2

POVERTY AND LOW-INCOME (<200% POVERTY) RATES BY RACE/ETHNICITY, 2006

	NON-LATINO				
	WHITE (%)	AFRICAN AMERICAN (%)	AMERICAN INDIAN/ ALASKA NATIVE (%)	ASIAN AMERICAN (%)	LATINO (%)
Ages 65 and over, poverty rate	7.0	22.4	31.8	11.9	19.4
Ages 62–64, poverty rate	7.5	22.5	37.7	8.4	19.6
Ages 50–61, poverty rate	5.9	16.2	21.3	8.6	14.3
Ages 65 and over, low income (<200% poverty)	32.1	53.8	61.1	35.1	52.7
Ages 62–64, low income (<200% poverty)	22.0	45.8	49.3	32.0	43.6
Ages 50–61, low income (<200% poverty)	14.2	35.5	37.7	17.6	38.0

Note. From "Current Population Survey, Annual Social and Economic Supplement, CPS Table Creator," by U.S. Census Bureau, 2007, Retrieved October 31, 2008, from http://www.census.gov/hhes/www/cpstc/cps_table_creator.html

key differences by race and ethnicity are that minorities are less likely to have other sources of income and have lower total incomes. Among those receiving early retirement Social Security income, whites are about twice as likely to also have interest or dividend income as African Americans and Latinos (U.S. Census Bureau, 2006a). This reflects the fact that whites are more likely to enter retirement early with enough resources to supplement Social Security, and minority elders are more likely to have to rely entirely on Social Security for their entire income.

Racial differences in resources are especially evident for wealth. The median net worth of households headed by an older white person in 2005 was $226,900, but older black-headed households had assets of only $37,800. Most striking is that the wealth of older African American families has been relatively flat in constant dollars over the past 20 years, whereas the wealth of older whites has increased 80% (Federal Interagency Forum on Aging-Related Statistics, 2008). The result is an increase in both the relative and absolute racial disparity in wealth in older households. Data for household heads of all ages show that Latino families also have substantially lower assets than non-Latino whites. When home equity is excluded, the asset-gap ratio doubles, because African Americans and Latinos have a significantly lower proportion of liquid assets (stocks, savings) as well as a lower proportion of pension assets (401[k] plans, IRAs) (Orzechowski & Sepielli, 2003). This means that the more limited wealth of minority elders is concentrated in home equity, which is not easily accessed when needed for medical or other expenses.

Thus, although the income and assets of older adults has climbed over the years, the gap between whites and minority elders continues. A significant segment of minority elderly populations continues to struggle to meet basic expenses, and Social Security is the basic source of income for a large number of them.

ARE ALL OLDER ADULTS WISE?

Educational level is an important indicator of earnings ability as well as the knowledge and skills to structure adequate retirement savings. The latter is especially important for the coming generations of retirees who will have to rely predominately on defined contribution plans when they have pensions (such as 401(k) plans) rather than the traditional and more predictable defined benefit plans. Education is highly correlated with financial literacy related to retirement planning; both education and financial literacy are independently associated with enrolling in available 401(k) plans (Agnew, Szykman, Utkus, & Young, 2007).

Educational levels are rising with each succeeding generation, suggesting that future generations of older adults will be better able to plan adequately for retirement. Among the current generation of all older adults, 23.9% have not graduated from high school, but the rates are much worse for racial and ethnic minorities. Among current older adults, 42% of African Americans, 44.9% of American Indians and Alaska Natives (AIAN), and 57.8% of Latinos have not graduated from high school (U.S. Census Bureau, 2007).

The next generation of older adults, those currently aged 50 to 64 years, has a lower overall rate of no high school degrees, 12%. The rates for minority elderly continue to be worse than the overall rate, albeit improved at 17.6% for African Americans and 19.0% for AIAN. The 40.9% of Latinos aged 50 to 64 without a high school degree continues to be several times higher than the overall rate (U.S. Census Bureau, 2007).

Compounding the income disparities that future elders of color are likely to face, these educational patterns suggest they are likely to also face financial knowledge disparities that will further complicate relying on individuals to be entirely responsible for planning a reasonable retirement income.

The low quality of jobs held by many of the coming generation of older adults of color suggests that early retirement may be financially precarious but desirable from the perspective of job and life satisfaction. Although 44% of non-Latino whites aged 50 to 61 years hold management, business, and professional occupations, only 30% of blacks and 19% of Latinos are in those occupations (U.S. Census Bureau, 2006a). Those are the occupations with the best working conditions, making an extended work life least burdensome. On the other hand, Latinos aged 50 to 61 years are the most likely to be in the physically taxing and dangerous occupations of agriculture, construction, installation, transportation, and factory production (Wallace, Castañeda, Guendelman, Padilla-Frausto, & Felt, 2007), with African Americans also overrepresented in the latter two (U.S. Census Bureau, 2006a). These are occupations where older workers face particularly poor employment prospects and where the difficult working conditions necessitate retirement as soon as feasible. In addition, these blue collar and manual labor workers face a disproportionate risk of injury on the job, which can lead to unplanned retirement. Minority men, in particular, are more likely than non-Latino white men to have pathways to retirement that involve disability, unemployment, and part-time work. In other words, because of the type of work they do and the employment benefits provided, early retirement for whites is more often voluntary, whereas for minority workers, it is more often involuntary.

THE IMPACT OF RAISING THE MINIMUM RETIREMENT AGE ON MINORITY COMMUNITIES

With large economic and health disparities present in the coming generation of older adults, it is clear that a significant segment of the elder population will not be able to have a decent standard of living without Social Security starting at age 62. Both current policy and proposed changes to Social Security disproportionately harm this population.

As currently structured, those who retire at age 62 receive the same estimated lifetime benefits as those who retire at full retirement age. Because the lifetime amount is spread over more years, the monthly benefit is less for early retirees. As the full retirement age rises slowly to age 67, according to current law (to be fully implemented by 2022), those who retire early will receive an ever smaller monthly benefit. When full benefits were available at age 65, those retiring at age 62 received 80% of the full amount monthly. When the full retirement age is 67, they will receive 70% (Haverstick, Sapozhnikov, Triest, & Zhivan, 2007). Those with generous pensions, significant savings, and appreciated assets can offset the lower Social Security amounts if they voluntarily decide to retire early. Most minority elderly do not have those resources (Favreault, Mermin, Steuerle, & Murphy, 2007) and will, therefore, be adversely affected by the declining monthly payments. Similarly, proposals to push early retirement up to age 65 will disproportionately impact minority elders who are more likely to have to leave work for health reasons and have limited other resources.

There are several considerations that underlie Social Security and that should be reinforced when contemplating changes to the system. The first is adequacy. Even though Social Security was not intended as a sole source of income in retirement, it has become the only source for many. About one third of older adults rely on Social Security for basically all (90% or more) of their income. Social Security replaces a higher percentage of preretirement income for low-waged workers and their spouses than higher-waged workers at full retirement age—54% of earnings compared to 28% (Social Security Administration, 2007b). One solution to the challenge of falling retirement benefits that results from higher full retirement ages is to increase the replacement rate for the lowest-waged workers. Alternatively, full retirement age could be based on number of years worked rather than age, with early retirement a fixed number of years earlier. Because low-waged and manual laborers are more likely to enter the labor force at an earlier age than higher waged workers are, they would continue be eligible for benefits at an earlier age (Haverstick, Sapozhnikov, Triest, & Zhican, 2007). A third solution would be to reinstitute a minimum Social Security benefit that is high enough to assure a sufficient retirement income (Favreault, Mermin, Steuerle, & Murphy, 2007). The changes to Social Security suggested above have income adequacy as the most important policy goal. Fulfilling other goals, such as adequate financing, can then be met in ways that support adequacy in contrast to the current approaches that reduce adequacy as a means to improve financing. Any policy change that improves the adequacy of Social Security for the lowest wage workers will significantly improve the economic security of minority elders.

A second key consideration is equity (Sen, 2003; Estes & Wallace, 2006). The different preretirement income replacement rates noted above embody considerations of equity, where those with the greatest ability to shoulder a greater share of the financial responsibility than the poorest members of society. But policy recommendations are being based on the "average" older adult, with little consideration of the distributional consequences by income or race/ethnicity. As long as our society continues to be stratified by race and ethnicity in education, employment, and housing, it will be necessary to assure that policies do not disproportionately worsen the economic security of racial and ethnic minorities.

A final consideration that is key for Social Security reform is to not change the distribution of financial risk in the system. Currently, the investment risk and solvency risk is held by the government (Estes, 2001). This creates a collective risk so that individuals and their families are protected from the vagaries of the market, poor retirement planning, and unexpected life events, such as premature mortality. Moving early retirement to older ages serves to leave most of the risk of providing economic security to the individual during the early part of their 60s. Because Supplemental Security Income (SSI), a means-tested program for low-income elders, is not available until age 65, there is no social safety net to help those who have difficulty working because of physical or job market reasons and who are not disabled enough for Social Security disability.

As the aging of the baby boomers creates an increasingly diverse elderly population in the coming years, the challenges of maintaining an adequate income during the early retirement years of 62 to 65 will continue to be faced disproportionately in communities of color. Social Security serves as a foundation for the income of many in those communities, and moving delaying eligibility for early retirement will serve primarily to increase the economic precariousness of the aging families in those communities.

DISCUSSION QUESTIONS

1. Outline the disparities between white elders and minority elders in terms of health, income and wealth, and education. What are some differences *within* minority groups?
2. Some policy makers have proposed that the minimum age for receiving Social Security retirement benefits be raised because of increases in life expectancy. What evidence do the authors provide to show the negative consequences of this change for minority elders?
3. Wallace and Villa point out that education is correlated not only with income, but also with financial literacy. Considering the persistent lag in educational levels between whites and minority elders, how would an increasing emphasis on defined contribution retirement plans or reforms that would privatize Social Security differentially affect minority elders?
4. The authors suggest the principles of adequacy, equity, and shared risk that should be considered when looking at changes to the Social Security system. What kinds of changes to the system would you recommend that would uphold these basic principles, especially as they apply to issues related to minority elders?

REFERENCES

Agnew, J. R., Szykman, L., Utkus, S. P., & Young, J. A. (2007). Literacy, trust and 401(K) savings behavior (Working Paper). Chestnut Hill, MA: Center for Retirement Research at Boston College.

AHRQ. (2008). National healthcare disparities report. Rockville, MD: Agency for Healthcare Research and Quality.

American Hospital Association. (2007). When I'm 64: How boomers will change health care. Chicago: American Hospital Association.

Angel, J. L., & Angel, R. J. (2006). Minority group status and healthful aging: Social structure still matters. *American Journal of Public Health*, *96*, 1152–1159.

Angel, J. L., Jimenez, M. A., & Angel, R. J. (2007). The economic consequences of widowhood for older minority women. *The Gerontologist*, *47*(2), 224–234.

Clark, D. O., & Gibson, R. C. (1997). Race, age, chronic disease, and disability. In K. S. Markides & M. R. Miranda (Eds.), *Minorities, aging and health* (pp. 107–126). Thousand Oaks, CA: Sage.

Collins, S., Davis, K., Schoen, C., Doty, M. M., & Kriss, J. L. (2006). Health coverage for aging baby boomers: Findings from the commonwealth fund survey. New York: Commonwealth Fund.

Congressional Budget Office. (1999). Raising the earliest eligibility age for Social Security benefits. Washington, DC: Author.

Copeland, C. (2005). Employment-Based Retirement Plan Participation: Geographic Differences and Trends, 2004. EBRI Issue Brief No. 286. Washington, DC: Employee Benefit Research Institute. Retrieved November 11, 2008 from http://www.ebri.org/pdf/briefspdf/EBRI_IB_10-20051.pdf

Estes, C. L. (2001). Crisis, the welfare state, and aging. In C. L. Estes (Ed.), *Social policy and aging: A critical perspective* (pp. 95–117). Thousand Oaks, CA: Sage.

Estes, C. L., & Wallace, S. P. (2006). Older people. In B. S. Levy & V. W. Sidel (Eds.), *Social injustice and public health* (pp. 113–129). New York: Oxford University Press.

Favreault, M., Mermin, G. B. T., Steuerle, C. E., & Murphy, D. P. (2007, January 26). Minimum benefits in Social Security could reduce aged poverty (Brief No. 11). Washington, DC: The Urban Institute.

Federal Interagency Forum on Aging-Related Statistics. (2008). Older Americans 2008: Key indicators of well-being. Washington, DC: Government Printing Office. Retrieved October 13, 2008, from http://agingstats.gov/agingstatsdotnet/Main_Site/Data/Data_2008.aspx

Hacker, J. S. (2007). The great risk shift: Issues for aging and public policy. *Public Policy and Aging Report*, *17*(2), 1–7.

Haverstick, K., Sapozhnikov, M., Triest, R., & Zhivan, N. (2007, October). A new approach to raising Social Security's earliest eligibility age (Paper No. 08-4). Chestnut Hill, MA: Center for Retirement Research at Boston College.

Hayward, M., Crimmins, E. M., Miles, T. P., & Yang, Y. (2000). The significance of socioeconomic status in explaining the racial gap in chronic health conditions. *American Sociological Review*, *65*(6), 910–930.

Liebman, J., MacGuineas, M., & Samwick, A. (2005). Estimated financial effects of "a nonpartisan approach to reforming Social Security." Baltimore: Social Security Administration.

National Center for Health Statistics. (2007). United States life tables, 2003. Washington DC: U.S. Centers for Disease Control and Prevention. Retrieved October 13, 2008, from http://www.cdc.gov/nchs/datawh/statab/unpubd/mortabs/lewk3_10.htm

Orshansky, M. (1993). Measuring poverty. *Public Welfare*, *51*(1), 27–29.

Orzechowski, S., & Sepielli, P. (2003). Net worth and asset ownership of households: 1998 and 2000. *Current population reports, Series P70, Number 88*. Washington, DC: U.S. Census Bureau. Retrieved June 23, 2008, from http://www.census.gov/prod/2003pubs/p70-88.pdf

Park Tanjasiri, S., Wallace, S. P., & Shibata, K. (1995). Picture imperfect: Hidden problems among Asian Pacific islander elderly. *The Gerontologist*, *35*(6), 753–760.

Sen, A. (2003). *Inequality reexamined*. London: Oxford Scholarship Online.

Social Security Administration (2007a). Expenditures of the Aged Chartbook, Office of Research, Evaluation, and Statistics. Washington DC: Social Security Administration

Social Security Administration (2007b). Performance and Accountability Report, Fiscal Year 2007. Retrieved October 13, 2008, from http://www.socialsecurity.gov/finance/

U.S. Census Bureau. (2006a). Current Population Survey, 2006. Annual Social and Economic Supplement. Calculations by author. Retrieved October 31, 2008, http://www.bls.census.gov/cps_ftp.html#cpsmarch

U.S. Census Bureau (2006b). U.S. interim projections by age, sex, race, and Hispanic Origin. Washington DC: U.S. Census Bureau. Retrieved October 13, 2008, from http://www.census.gov/ipc/www/usinterimproj/

U.S. Census Bureau. (2007). Current population survey, annual social and economic supplement, CPS table creator. Retrieved October 31, 2008, from http://www.census.gov/hhes/www/cpstc/cps_table_creator.html

Wallace, S. P., Castañeda, X., Guendelman, S., Padilla-Frausto, D. I., & Felt, E. (2007). Immigration, health & work: The facts behind the myths. Berkeley, CA: Health Initiative of the Americas. Retrieved October 13, 2008, from http://www.healthpolicy.ucla.edu/pubs/publication.asp?pubID=236

Wallace, S. P., & Molina, L. C. (2008). Federal poverty guideline underestimates costs of living for older persons in California. Los Angeles, CA: UCLA Center for Health Policy Research. Retrieved October 13, 2008, from http://www.healthpolicy.ucla.edu/pubs/publication.asp?pubID=247

Whitfield, K., Angel, J., Burton, L., & Hayward, M. (2006). Diversity, disparities, and inequalities in aging: Implications for policy. *Public Policy and Aging Report*, *16*(3), 16–22.

10 Quality of Life for Communities of Color

E. PERCIL STANFORD, DONNA L. YEE, AND EDGAR E. RIVAS

Since the year 2000, proposals for privatization of public programs have called into question our country's commitment to the idea that everyone living here is on a shared journey as they age with the same destination of a comfortable retirement, adequate health care coverage, and financial security. This chapter will describe the landscape of social exchanges (e.g., transfer of public resources) that are the foundation of policies that impact all older persons and in particular, elders of color.

THE SOCIAL CONTRACT

As the global economy increasingly affects our everyday interactions, it is time to better understand how assumptions about social exchanges that underlie the social contract in the United States may vary, and how norms in other societies may strengthen our own responses to an increasingly diverse United States. For purposes of this discussion, we refer to the "social contract" as that agreement between community members and their leaders (Social Contract, 2008).

Various demographic factors point to how the needs of elders of color and other vulnerable populations will continue to challenge the effectiveness of redistributive exchange policies and practices in our nation, and thus affect the quality of life for all. In the year 2010, 13% of the population will be aged 65 years and older, whereas 2% will be aged 85 years and older. By the year 2050, those projections will increase to 21% and 5%, respectively. This indicates that the aging of the baby boomer cohort (born between 1946 and 1964) will almost double the number of individuals living into older age (U.S. Census Bureau, 2004).

In the year 2010, 14% of those aged 65 years and older will be elders of color; elders of color aged 85 and older will make up 11% of that total population. Projections for the year 2015 indicate that elders of color will make up 15% of those aged 65 and older and 12% aged 85 and older. Although these projections are for a more limited time period, they nonetheless point to the increasing diversity of this nation's aged and pose policy and practice challenges that affect the quality of life for elders of color (U.S. Census Bureau, 2004).

The social contract that exists in the United States is one in which the public sector (government) attempts to provide a safety net to protect its citizens from falling too far into poverty. None the less, many citizens believe that government provides too much assistance already. Some are of the opinion that government should not play a role in supporting individuals and that individuals should be totally self-reliant. However, absolute self-reliance is rarely possible, largely because communities are designed to be interdependent to improve the productivity and survival of every member. It can be argued that many children, elders, and individuals with disabilities are more interdependent and less totally self-reliant than others in the community. The proximity of more and less self-reliant and interdependent individuals influences the role of social exchanges that underlie a social contract, particularly in the use and claim on private and public resources.

The Heritage Foundation views the "American social contract" as a bargain between society and the individual, based more solidly on institutions that individuals value as integral parts of their lives, with the government aspect appropriately limited and sustainable and more just to future generations (Butler, 2007). Butler's position neatly places the social contract in the context of compassionate conservatism, that is:

> I call my philosophy and approach compassionate conservatism. It is compassionate to actively help our fellow citizens in need. It is conservative to insist on responsibility and results. And with this hopeful approach, we will make a real difference in people's lives. (President George W. Bush, Press Release, 2007)

Yet, policies extending from a philosophy of compassionate conservatism may appear to demonstrate conflicting ideals. For example, in his book, *Shredding the Social Contract: the Privatization of Medicare*, John Geyman (2006) offers an historical view of attempts over the past 30 years to privatize the Medicare program. Advocacy groups have argued that enactment of the Medicare Part D Program in 2003 was a step toward privatization, and Geyman offers stories about the problems that Medicare beneficiaries have encountered in privatized Medicare plans. He argues for a renewed commitment to the original vision of social insurance on which the program was based, which he equates to a social contract between the government and Medicare beneficiaries.

Similarly, in her analysis of the role of the social contract in the lives of African American elders, Anna Madison (1992) addresses the government's responsibility to provide long-term care to functionally impaired black elders. Functional impairment signifies living with three or more limitations in activities of daily living, such as transferring from a bed, bathing, feeding, dressing, and mobility. Madison posits a modern social contract theory that provides a way to understand the interdependent relationships among government, society, and the individual. Madison understands the notion of social justice as one that encompasses the redistribution of wealth, because all people do not have the same access to resources and opportunities. Her data suggest that although black elders are more likely to be at risk for needing long-term care, they are less likely to have the personal resources to pay for it, and thus are forced to forego needed care. Although there exists an acceptance that public assistance should be offered to functionally impaired elders who do not have the means for their own care, there is no agreement on the extent and nature of this assistance. Although the private sector only provides protection to African American and other elders who can afford such care, Madison concludes that they are dependent, therefore, on the federal government to guarantee their rights under the social contract.

Although these examples point to consensus about the definition and role of the social contract, there is less uniformity in the extent to which the contract should provide for the public good. Historically, our public policies have swung pendulum-like from providing for the public good (Social Security, Medicare, Older American Act, Low Income Home Energy Assistance Program, etc.) to retracting public assistance (welfare reform, unfunded and underfunded programs, privatization of public programs, etc.). Elders of color, many of whom depend on this assistance for their survival, are caught in the crossfire of ongoing struggles between politicians and corporations to define the appropriate balance in the social contract. It remains unclear as to whether these entitlements are forms of situational promises to share or exchange resources, or if they are institutional promises based on established norms that are a social contract.

MODELS OF REDISTRIBUTIVE EXCHANGE

Entitlements are legal obligations to provide funding for particular programs. Through the legislative process, Congress specifies eligibility criteria, which determine who qualifies to access these programs and who does not. Age and income status are two important examples of eligibility criteria as legislated by the Older Americans Act for its Senior Community Service Employment Program.

Gist (2007) defines our social welfare system as consisting of two categories of programs: (1) "entitlement" programs and (2) "tax expenditure" programs. Entitlement programs provide direct benefits to individual citizens through federal budget expenditures in the form of programs like Social Security, Medicare, and Medicaid. Although entitlement programs are those that are traditionally identified as constituting the welfare state, Gist expands this idea to include this second set of programs, tax expenditure programs. In these programs, individuals accrue financial benefits in the form of reduced taxes or tax-free income, such as employer-provided health insurance or tax deductions for mortgage interest payments. Gist finds that, in general, benefits from entitlement programs are distributed much more equally than those from tax expenditure programs. Even though entitlement programs broadly benefit the middle class, they are more closely targeted to those in need than are programs related to taxes. In his view, entitlement programs may better serve to honor the social contract that the Federal government has with low-income and middle class individuals.

However, entitlement program access can be restricted by the Congressional authorization and appropriation process. Authorizing legislation creates a law, which is then allocated funding for its implementation. Congress is responsible for allocating the federal budget dollars for programs, including all entitlements. A clear example of how Congressional inaction affects an entitlement program is in not reauthorizing the Indian Health Service (IHS), now 6 years overdue for reauthorization. As a result of this Congressional inaction, the funding and capacity of the IHS to fulfill its mission weakens with each passing year.

Earlier, we asked if a program for the good of the public is a form of the social contract or some form of voluntary exchange of resources. Exchange theory, in its simplest form, posits a reciprocal exchange of goods or services. In its more complex form, it posits a redistributive political exchange between haves and have-nots. Although we may rule out contemporary reciprocal exchanges across generations, because many elders are not in the position to exchange all needed goods or services for those they need to receive, reciprocal exchanges might be "credited" over a life span and across generations. Measures of equivalency of exchanges may be uneven and less reciprocal as family solidarity and social, economic, and political events cause uncertainty or failure to meet exchange obligations. These breakdowns raise questions about whether such reciprocal exchanges are reliable to meet the many needs of children, elders, or persons with disabilities in families.

Our social contract, as it is understood in modern industrialized societies today, is a form of redistributive exchange. Government collects taxes from everyone in society so that it can redistribute those taxes in the form of goods and services to those in need. Our social service and health care systems are partially based on redistributive exchange models as they are supported by taxes paid by all citizens, regardless of whether they will derive any benefit from them. Efforts to encourage citizens to believe that they will remain virile forever, reduce their risk for physical impairments and chronic conditions to nil, and live the middle-class dream of a government assistance-free retirement threaten to undermine the values of reciprocity on which the social contract is based. We run the risk of returning to a pre-industrial system of voluntary charitable contributions and norms of total self-reliance.

THE HISTORICAL CONTEXT

When Franklin D. Roosevelt signed the Social Security Act into law in 1935, it was a form of social insurance intended to keep older persons from falling into destitute poverty similar to that experienced during the Depression. Over time, the program has become a major source of retirement income for many individuals, although this was never meant to be the case. The misperception on the part of the public that Social Security is a retirement income plan is what leads to the debate over privatization of Social Security. Free-market proponents believe that the marketplace will provide for the best interests of the individual, and by extension, they see the payment of Social Security taxes as a redirection of the individual's income that could be better invested in the free market.

In 2005, President George W. Bush pushed Congress to study options for helping Social Security remain stronger financially in the long term. One option that he championed was partial privatization of the funds contributed by individuals. Unfortunately, the effort to privatize Social Security does little to assure that the individual "investor" has the knowledge base or capacity to make wise investment decisions or be protected from economic swings, thus setting the stage for possible destitution if the stock market trends up and down between bull and bear markets, as it invariably does over time. Elders of color, in particular, do not often have the resources for a successful retirement, because they are more likely to invest in education and home ownership. Therefore, they are particularly vulnerable and likely to suffer under these conditions in which the individual has responsibility for their own investment options.

One of the largest challenges confronting this country as the "face" of our aging society changes is with existing models for providing services to elders. Currently, policy dictates that our programs serve the greatest good, that is, that our programs are able to serve the widest range of average program constituents. When Medicare legislation was enacted in 1965, for example, all that was deemed necessary was access to doctors and hospitals for care. Over time, the program has expanded to add limited skilled nursing facility access, physician and nursing services, laboratory and diagnostic tests, influenza and pneumonia treatment, renal dialysis, vaccinations, limited ambulance transportation, outpatient medical treatments administered in a doctor's office, durable medical equipment, prescription drugs, and more. For a more thorough discussion of the Medicare program, please refer to the Web site for the Centers for Medicare and Medicaid Services (http://www.cms.hhs.gov/home/medicare.asp).

The Medicare program continues to change as economic and political pressures mount for the evolving health care needs of older people and other Medicare beneficiaries. Unfortunately, health care disparities—access and availability of culturally competent practitioners and care, research on the effect of different diseases and treatments on diverse populations—remain inadequately considered, as Medicare adapts to the changing health care environment.

Another example of a program that served the greater good but over time adjusted for the needs of elders of color is the Older Americans Act of 1965. When enacted as part of Lyndon Johnson's Great Society programs, it established eligibility for programs at age 60 and above. Later, the Act recognized that American Indian and Alaskan Native elders aged sooner, thus creating a Title VI program specific to their needs, thus incorporating the age 50+ years for eligibility in those tribes and villages, and taking sovereignty issues into consideration for funding and services. Later in the 1970s, when the program's network of aging services was found to be poorly serving elders of color, targeting language was added to the Act. This language, which read "those with the greatest social and economic needs," was meant to target the needs of elders of color and individuals living in rural communities.

TODAY'S CHALLENGES

What is missing from the updates of these Great Society programs of the 1960s and of many other public programs intended to address the needs of elders and their caregivers is that they do not address the increasingly diverse populations of elderly Americans. That is, federal programs in particular attempt to provide their limited resources to as many people as can be served, refusing to recognize that what may work for one group or community may not work with other population segments. Many senior centers, for example, may not recognize the native languages, food, or customs of all the communities they serve, and they may not feature ethnically or racially diverse staff. One size does not fit all in either clothes or service programs! Public health and social programs cannot continue to be enacted with eligibility guidelines that serve "everyone" targeted by that program, but in reality provides poor service to all of their constituents.

In the past, it was difficult to research program effectiveness with elders of color because there existed insufficient data about people of color. Thus, much of the earlier research on aging was assumed to be relevant and applicable for the majority of older persons, even though they overlooked or underestimated problems affecting elders in communities of color. Today, however, sophisticated data analysis techniques and the wealth of data available may inspire more culturally focused study models that will adequately answer questions about existing programs and their effectiveness for elders of color.

Similarly, policy makers and service providers alike must be reminded that all people of color, even when categorized by the Census as one major group, are not homogeneous and do not necessarily share the same needs or wants. Each major category of elders of color is comprised of subpopulations with distinct needs. For example, efforts to generalize study findings across Asian Pacific Islanders as a group can lead to interventions that serve neither recently arrived Hmong nor third-generation Japanese elders—ethnic groups with widely differing life span experiences and circumstances. Similarly, the needs of Dominicans in the Bronx, Mexican Americans in the Rio Grande Valley, and Spanish descendants living in northern New Mexico are all distinct—despite the fact that the Census classifies all of them as Hispanic/Latino.

Efforts to identify needed policy changes with regards to elders of color and efforts to assure the successful execution of such policies are in their infancy. Broader local discretion over the provision of Federal programs, such as Medicaid, Older Americans Act, or public health surveillance, requires practitioners in aging to work more diligently to assure that such programs adequately serve their local target populations.

Part of the challenge for both lawmakers and practitioners is for service systems to assess and correctly gauge the appropriate scale of the social exchange—the provision of services to those target groups stemming from the public's tax payments—across the target population groups. Even though elders may be living side by side and aging in place, they may well have distinct languages, religious traditions, and ethnic backgrounds, which dictate accommodations for service provision. For example, nutrition programs funded by the Older Americans Act increasingly use centralized kitchens to produce home-delivered meals for all clients in a geographic area. Menu choices do not accommodate most (if any) specific dietary restrictions and preferences (e.g., if an elder does not eat pork or beef, if an elder prefers rice to potatoes, if an elder is lactose intolerant). It is no surprise that some ethnic and religious groups decline to participate in such services, instead preferring to develop other programs to provide more appropriate services for their community members. Note, for example, the growth of Services & Advocacy for Gay, Lesbian, Bisexual, Transgender Elders (SAGE) program in New York City when lesbian, gay, bisexual, transgender elders were experiencing discrimination by paid caregivers in mainstream agencies. Similarly, the On Lok Program in San Francisco grew out of the needs of the Chinese and Italian communities in conjoining neighborhoods.

Another opportunity to better serve the needs of elders of color is for planners to consider incorporating the caregiving norms of each community in the development of program rules and administration. Are there norms, family caregiving patterns, and other factors that can inform why elders perceive certain programs as either acceptable or unacceptable? Yarry, Stevens, and McCallum (2007) found that clarifying the amount and types of care a spouse is providing, the caregiver's expectations of assistance from other family members, the actual extent of assistance provided by family members, and the family's comfort with the caregiving arrangement may help professionals avoid assumptions about the structure of the caregiving tasks within the family, especially in the context of ethnicity and culture. By more clearly understanding the strains that caregiving puts on families, however defined, with limited resources and with varied cultural norms, policy makers and planners can more realistically develop support systems, which meet the varied needs of their constituencies. Assuming that certain communities will simply "take care of their own" with no need for outside assistance is not an acceptable reason for abdicating responsibility for the social contract between a public jurisdiction and its constituency.

THE ROAD AHEAD

There is no refuting that contemporary American society is a more diverse mixture of global cultures than ever before. As we strive to achieve a more inclusive society, we need to adapt to the service needs and preferences of our elders, in response to their backgrounds and cultures. Our "one size fits all" service model is outdated and becoming increasingly irrelevant. Yet, current challenges such as downturns in the economy and backlash against immigrant communities make it even more difficult to uphold the social contract and continue to provide services to all members of our society. Meeting present and future service needs will take persistence and resources as well as explicit recognition of why such redistributive exchanges are part of the social contract. We will need to increase education efforts and cultural competency training not only for the direct support workforce, but also for policy makers, academics, and students alike in order to better comprehend the varied needs of constituents. As people of color move into increasingly responsible positions in policy development and in practice, they will have new opportunities to express their unique perspectives and backgrounds and apply their experiences as decision makers and caregivers. The development of their leadership is essential. One goal for a multicultural society, such as the one that presently exists in the United States, is for all of its members, not only people of color, to be encouraged to bring themselves fully "to the table" to broaden problem identification and problem solving. Fostering inclusiveness prevents people from losing their heritage—growing out of their differences—and encourages the sharing of our wisdom through time. The "American melting pot" is an historic cultural icon. A more useful icon today may be a "salad" with diverse flavors and fixings of many colors.

In this chapter, we have attempted to address how understanding the notion of a social contract as a redistributive exchange can positively affect this nation's multicultural elders. However, there are still many questions that remain unanswered. We now know that having everyone speak the same language does not foster an individual's quality of life. We no longer think of one primary family caregiver when we address "family" caregiving. We recognize that the traditional nuclear family is no longer the norm given the extent of single-parent homes, grandparents raising grandchildren, blended families, and nontraditional families from many backgrounds including lesbian, gay, bisexual, or transgender families. Perhaps we need to consider a new term to replace what has traditionally been called "family" with something like "a purposeful social support unit" or to what some refer to as their "chosen family?"

The recent MetLife Family Matters Study (2008) is a start at recognizing how blended and disconnected families across generations have increasing potential for sustained estrangement; long distances and changes in family membership and in individual commitments to support/sustain a sense of family will change patterns of support for older persons. Even the extent to which communities of faith and individuals with different abilities participate in providing care as a filial duty has a role in fulfilling the social contract. All of these factors affect the way social exchanges, which support and rely on a social contract for redistributive exchange at the societal level, affect the future quality of life for elders of color, all elders, and all of their caregivers.

DISCUSSION QUESTIONS

1. In what ways does social insurance impact communities of color?
2. Explain the demographic changes that are expected to take place in the older adult population in the next 5 to 10 years.
3. What are some ways in which service programs can be adapted to meet the needs of communities of color?
4. In what ways are social insurance programs an example of a social contract?

REFERENCES

Bush, G. W. (2007). Fact sheet: Compassionate conservatism. Washington, DC: White House Office of the Press Secretary.

Butler, S. M. (2007). *Restoring the American social contract.* Washington, DC: The American Heritage Foundation.

Centers for Medicare and Medicaid Services. (2008). Medicare. U.S. Department of Health and Human Services. Retrieved July 31, 2008, from http://www.cms.hhs.gov/home/medicare.asp

Geyman, J. (2006). Shredding the social contract: The privatization of Medicare. Monroe, ME: Common Courage Press.

Gist, J. (2007). Spending and tax entitlements. *Tax Notes, 115(2)*,145–154.

Madison, A. (1992). Social contract and the African American elderly. *Urban League Review, 15*(2), 21–28.

MetLife Mature Market Institute. (2008, February). *The MetLife family matters study: Examining the effect of varying family structures on retirement planning*. Westport, CT: MetLife Mature Market Institute.

Social Contract (2008). In *Merriam-Webster Online Dictionary*. Retrieved October 14, 2008, from http://www.merriam-webster.com/dictionary/social%20contract

U.S. Census Bureau. (2004, March). U.S. interim projections by age, sex, race, and hispanic origin. Retrieved October 14, 2008, from http://www.census.gov/ipc/www/usinterimproj/

Yarry, S. J., Stevens, E. K., & McCallum, T. J. (2007). Cultural influences on spousal caregiving. *Generations, 31*(3), 24–30.

PART III

The Ongoing Debates Over Social Insurance Programs

Part III: The Ongoing Debates Over Social Insurance Programs

Introduction

BROOKE A. HOLLISTER

Although debates about social insurance programs are nothing new in the United States, since 2004, debates about the sustainability and reform of Social Security and Medicare have been on the forefront of the political sphere. Although this attention and discussion of reforms brought many more people into the debate, the accuracy of information available to the public was frighteningly questionable. From the discrepancies between the Social Security Administration and the Congressional Budget Office projections of solvency, to the absurdity of projecting solvency past 10 years (how are war, fertility rates, changes to tax structures, economic growth, education, and disasters accounted for in these projections?), it was difficult even for experts on the topic to determine the facts. The authors contributing to this section were present and active in these recent debates. The following chapters focus on the debates over the current status and future structure of social insurance programs in the United States.

In chapter 11, Robert H. Binstock and James H. Schulz consider whether the threats to social insurance—and their potentially unfavorable consequences for older Americans—can be repelled. The chapter places U.S. social insurance in the context of changing eras in American political ideology. Binstock and Schulz then trace the political developments through which older Americans came to be portrayed as selfish citizens who cause and benefit from intergenerational inequities. Next, they delineate how depictions of the aging of baby boomers as a national crisis have become a foundation for policy threats to social insurance. Finally, Binstock and Schultz suggest strategies for repelling the threats to social insurance.

Expanding on Binstock and Schulz's explication of ideology, chapter 12, by Svihula and Estes, contends that current privatization efforts are (1) the result of an ideological social movement favoring privatization; and (2) institutionalized through various processes and structures. The authors use the theoretical frameworks of McAdam, Tarrow, and Tilly (2001) and Amenta (2006) to expand on their analyses of historical and legislative documents, databases, and Web sites. Through their analysis, the authors came to the conclusion that "the processes of ideological structuring and institutionalization follow decades of successful framing of the Social Security 'problem' and solutions around the market ideology and the wide propagation of these ideas by the media." However, as the antiprivatization movement continues to evolve and grow, Svihula and Estes believe that a reinstitutionalization of social insurance and the legitimacy of the state is possible.

In contrast to the ideologies of individualism fueling support for privatization, Martha Holstein addresses the moral values of dignity and gender equity in chapter 13. Holstein argues that "the best way to help assure the realization of dignity in old age is by a commitment to social solidarity and collective responsibility that unifies generations and different social and economic strata in our society." According to Holstein, social insurance programs achieve core values because they promote dignity and community rather than blame, humiliation, and shame promoted by means-tested programs. She argues that the bond created by Social Security and similar social insurance programs is morally honorable and a necessary condition for the flourishing of what she calls "the social citizen."

In chapter 14, Fay Lomax Cook and Meredith Czaplewski analyze polling data to assess the impact of ideology and discourse on the American public's views on Social Security and Medicare. Their analyses show that increasing proportions of Americans think Social Security is "in crisis." Even greater concern was expressed in polls about the financial outlook for Medicare. However, they find that support for privatization has gone down over time. Particularly, when reminded of the risks associated with investments in the stock market or transition costs, polls show that support for privatization is diminished. Not only is support for Social

Security and Medicare high for people of all ages, but people 18 to 29 years of age overwhelmingly support maintaining or increasing current spending levels on Social Security.

In chapter 15, Harry R. Moody discusses the paradox, noted by Cook and Czaplewski in the polls, of continuing widespread support for Social Security and Medicare, but declining confidence in the viability of the programs. He argues that the belief that a focus on generational equity is detrimental to public confidence in and support of social insurance programs is overstated. He argues that "there is no reason why politically progressive defenders of Social Security should refuse to recognize that issues of justice between generations are bound to arise when we transfer significant resources between age-groups and birth cohorts." Moody claims that the success of the 1983 amendments are due to the bipartisan efforts of the reform, shared burdens, incremental solutions, and the "rough justice" of "dedistributive" reform. It is through these successful reforms that Moody believes public confidence in these programs will be restored and an appreciation of social insurance renewed.

REFERENCES

Amenta, E. (2006). *When movements matter: The Townsend plan and the rise of social security*. New Jersey: Princeton University Press.

McAdam, D., Tarrow, S., & Tilly, C. (2001). *Dynamics of contention*. New York: Cambridge University Press.

11 Can Threats to Social Insurance in the United States Be Repelled?[1]

ROBERT H. BINSTOCK AND JAMES H. SCHULZ

During the first half of the 20th century, the problems and risks associated with old age in the United States were much more severe and widespread than they are today—especially the financial risks of inadequate income and the costs of health care. Before there was social insurance for income and health care, life in old age for the vast majority of elders was miserable and often dependent on the largesse of one's family and community.

Clearly, that has changed. During the second half of the 20th century, there was a spectacular revolution in the quality of life for elderly Americans, built on a foundation of the social insurance programs instituted during President Franklin Roosevelt's New Deal and President Lyndon Johnson's Great Society. Social Security and employer-sponsored pensions have substantially reduced the rate of poverty among older persons. Medicare, Medicaid, and employer-sponsored retiree health benefits have provided access to quality health services and long-term care for tens of millions of older persons. No wonder that the term "Golden Years" entered American culture in the 1970s and 1980s!

---

[1]Portions of this chapter are adapted from *Aging Nation: The Economics and Politics of Growing Older in America*, by James H. Schulz and Robert H. Binstock, copyright © 2006 by James H. Schulz and Robert H. Binstock, with permission of Greenwood Publishing Group, Inc., Westport, CT.

Now, the Golden Years are in danger of becoming tarnished. A great many pundits, politicians, policy analysts, insurance industry executives, mutual fund owners and managers, and some academics have become crisis mongers. We call them the "Merchants of Doom." They predict a catastrophic financial disaster in the country as a result of the aging of the baby boomers and their concomitant eligibility for social insurance benefits. As discussed in more detail later in this chapter, they use their crisis scenarios to set the stage for proposing radical changes in public policy, such as privatizing Social Security and limiting Medicare coverage. For some of the doomsayers, the agenda is primarily ideological—to shrink the role of government. For others, there are financial incentives—converting what are now public funds into private investment funds from which they and their firms and clients can benefit monetarily. Regardless of exaggeration and motive, the political agenda framed by the Merchants of Doom seriously threatens the social insurance programs that are vital to the financial well-being and health of most of today's and tomorrow's older persons.

This chapter considers whether the threats to social insurance—and their potentially unfavorable consequences for older Americans—can be repelled. It begins by placing U.S. social insurance in the contexts of changing eras in American political ideology. Then, it traces the political developments through which older Americans came to be portrayed as selfish citizens, who cause and benefit from intergenerational inequities. Next, it delineates how depictions of the aging of baby boomers as a national crisis have become a foundation for policy threats to social insurance. Finally, it sets forth suggested strategies for repelling the threats to social insurance.

SOCIAL INSURANCE IN THE CONTEXT OF CLASSICAL LIBERALISM

Why did it take until 1935 for the United States to establish Social Security as a policy? Consider that German Chancellor Otto von Bismarck's proposal for a German social insurance (or social security) scheme was established in 1889. During the next 25 years, his approach was adopted in one form or another in many European countries, for example, Denmark in 1891, Belgium in 1894, France in 1903, Britain in 1908, and Sweden in 1913 (Schulz & Binstock, 2008). But it was only in the midst of the

Great Depression of the 1930s that a U.S. Social Security retirement program was created by President Franklin Roosevelt, partly to reduce the number of older workers in the labor force so that younger unemployed workers would have less competition for jobs, as well as to provide income support in old age (Achenbaum, 1986). This long U.S. reluctance to adopt a Social Security program can be understood in the context of a pervasive liberal ideology in the United States that emphasized the primacy of individuals and the market and avoided (as much as possible) welfare provided by the state.

Danish sociologist Gøsta Esping-Andersen, in sorting out different national approaches to issues of social risk, has distinguished between two ideal types. One type is *Homo liberalismus* whose ideal is to pursue his personal welfare. "The well-being of others is their affair, not his. . . .His ethics tell him that a free lunch is amoral, that collectivism jeopardizes freedom, that individual liberty is a fragile good, easily sabotaged by sinister socialists or paternalistic institutions. *Homo liberalismus* prefers a welfare regime where those who can play the market do so, whereas those who cannot must merit charity" (Esping-Andersen, 1999, p. 171). In contrast is *Homo socialdemocraticus* who "is fully convinced that the more we invest in the public good, the better it will become. And this will trickle down to all, himself especially, in the form of a good life. Collective solutions are the best single assurance of a good, if perhaps dull, individual life" (Esping-Andersen, 1999, pp. 171–172). Esping-Andersen argues that the United States and Sweden are the closest living embodiments of the dreams, respectively, of *Homo liberalismus* and *Homo socialdemocraticus*.

Most students of American political life would agree with Esping-Andersen's characterization of the predominant political ideology in the United States. Indeed, in his classic and influential treatise on *The Liberal Tradition in America*, political theorist Louis Hartz (1955) argued that historically, U.S. political ideas, institutions, and behavior have uniquely reflected a virtually unanimous acceptance of the tenets of the English political philosopher John Locke, whose ideas were in harmony with the laissez-faire economics subsequently propounded by the Scotsman Adam Smith (1776 [2003]). In Lockean liberalism, the individual is much more important than the collective, and one of the few important functions of a limited state is to ensure that the wealth that individuals accumulate through the market is protected (Locke, 1690 [1924]). In this ideological context, it is easier to understand why it took the economic and political crisis of the Great Depression to make possible the adoption of Social Security in the United States, long after it had become commonplace as a policy in most European nations.

Aging and the Rise of Collective Concern

The dire collective and individual effects of the Great Depression, especially the manifest failures of the free market, made possible the acceptance (though not universal) of Franklin Roosevelt's New Deal programs to deal with market failures. The classical liberal ideology that characterized the American polity was temporarily submerged as a norm of activist government evolved from the New Deal, through World War II and beyond. Both Republican and Democratic presidents maintained this norm through 5 decades.

The ideological bulwark of individual responsibility was overcome with Social Security's establishment in 1935—a policy that singled out older Americans as a special group that needed to be, and worthy of being, collectively insured against the risks associated with old age. This new norm regarding older people, embodied in Social Security, was amplified in the years that followed. From the mid-1930s through the late 1970s, the construction of an old-age welfare state was facilitated by a compassionate ageism—the attribution of the same characteristics, status, and just deserts to a heterogeneous group of "the aged" that tended to be stereotyped as poor, frail, dependent, objects of discrimination, and above all "deserving" (cf. Kalish, 1979).

The stereotypes expressed through this ageism, unlike those of racism or sexism, were not wholly prejudicial to the well being of its objects, older people. During 5 decades, the American polity implemented the construct of compassionate ageism by creating many old-age government benefit programs, as well as by enacting laws against age discrimination. During the 1960s and 1970s, just about every issue or problem affecting some older persons that could be identified by advocates for the elderly became a governmental responsibility. Programs were enacted to provide older Americans with: health insurance (Medicare and Medicaid); nutritional, legal, supportive, and leisure services (Older Americans Act); housing; home repair; energy assistance; transportation; help in getting jobs; protection against being fired from jobs; public insurance for employer-sponsored pensions; special mental health programs; and on and on. By the late 1970s, if not earlier, American society had learned the catechism of compassionate ageism very well and had expressed it through a great many policies.

Aging and the Resurgence of Classical Liberalism

Then, after decades in which Social Security and the other old-age policies had become politically accepted as staples, the ideological pendulum swung away from collective concerns. Classical liberal ideology reemerged and flourished. This neoliberalism (popularly labeled as *conservatism*) once again emphasized the virtues of atomistic individualism and the virtues of free-market capitalism, while also stressing the evils of "big government," including government regulation and welfare programs (Pierson & Skocpol, 2007). This ideological context is important for understanding public political discourse and proposals for changing old-age policies today.

Neoliberalism emerged at the end of the 1970s and has persisted into the 21st century, spearheaded by the actions of a series of U.S. presidents. In the early 1980s, for instance, Ronald Reagan froze an annual cost-of-living adjustment in Social Security benefits, proposed (unsuccessfully) to make drastic cuts in the program's benefits, greatly tightened eligibility determination for federal disability insurance under Social Security, and deregulated a number of industries (such as the airlines). In the 1990s, William Clinton vowed to "end welfare as we know it" and "end big government," and he made progress on both fronts. The title of the welfare reform bill that Clinton signed into law expressed neoliberalism in clear terms. It was called The Personal Responsibility and Work Opportunity Reconciliation Act of 1996.

When George W. Bush took office in 2001, he had a long history of ideological distaste for the Social Security program and all government interventions. According to one of his professors at Harvard Business School in the mid-1970s, in his classroom Bush called Franklin Roosevelt a socialist, and specifically identified Social Security as one of several Roosevelt New Deal programs that he wanted to undo (Tsurumi, 2006). Bush spent the 8 years of his presidency promoting what he called "The Ownership Society," in which market forces (rather than government) are looked to for solutions to problems and individuals take on more responsibility for their welfare. In 2003, he successfully pushed for the passage of the Medicare Prescription Drug, Improvement, and Modernization Act (MMA) of 2003, which created a privately administered prescription drug program, Medicare's first means test, and a cap on Medicare expenditures. Then, in 2005, Bush tried hard (but unsuccessfully) to convert much of the Social Security program from social insurance into individual "privatized" accounts.

"GREEDY GEEZERS" AND INTERGENERATIONAL EQUITY

At the same time that classical liberalism was re-emerging, the compassionate stereotypes that had facilitated the building of an old-age welfare state underwent an extraordinary reversal. Older Americans began to be depicted by pernicious negative stereotypes. A key factor precipitating this reversal was that in the late 1970s journalists (e.g., Samuelson, 1978) and academicians (e.g., Hudson, 1978) discovered "the graying of the budget," a tremendous growth in federal funds spent on old-age benefits, which had made them comparable in size to spending for national defense. By 1982, an economist in the Office of Management and Budget had dramatized the comparison with the defense budget by reframing the classical trade-off metaphor of political economy from "guns versus butter" to "guns versus canes" (Torrey, 1982).

Another element in the reversal of the stereotypes of old age was the "discovery" of dramatic improvements in the aggregate status of older Americans, in large measure due to the impact of Social Security and Medicare. The success of these programs had improved the economic status of aged persons to the point where journalists and social commentators could—with only superficial accuracy (Quinn, 1987; Schulz, 2001)—describe older people, on average, as more prosperous than the rest of the population.

Whereas elderly persons had previously been stereotyped as poor and deserving, they now began to be portrayed as flourishing and a burden to society. As *Forbes* magazine succinctly and patronizingly expressed the new wisdom concerning "old folks": "The myth is that they're sunk in poverty. The reality is that they're living well. The trouble is there are too many of them—God bless 'em" (Flint, 1980, p. 51).

Throughout the 1980s and well into the 1990s, the new stereotypes, readily observed in popular culture, presented older people as prosperous, hedonistic, politically powerful, and selfish. A dominant theme in such accounts of older people was that their selfishness was ruining the nation. The epithet "greedy geezers" became a familiar adjective in journalistic accounts of federal budget politics (e.g., Salholz, 1990). And *Fortune* magazine went so far as to declaim that the "tyranny of America's old" was "one of the most crucial issues facing U.S. society" (Smith, 1992, p. 68).

In this climate of opinion, public discourse became increasingly hostile to governmental programs benefiting older people. Moreover, the aged emerged as a scapegoat for a wide-ranging list of other American problems. In the mid-1980s, for instance, when it was widely perceived (erroneously) that Japan had surpassed the United States as the dominant nation in the world economy, a former Secretary of Commerce suggested that a prerequisite for the United States to regain its stature as a first-class economic power was a sharp reduction in programs benefiting older Americans (Peterson, 1987).

Most of the problems for which older Americans were blamed were portrayed as issues of what was and still is called "intergenerational equity"—or, really, intergenerational *inequity*. A number of advocates for children blamed the political power of elderly Americans for the plight of youngsters who had inadequate nutrition, health care, education, and who also had insufficiently supportive family environments. One children's advocate even proposed that parents receive an "extra vote" for each of their children to combat older voters in an intergenerational conflict (Carballo, 1981). This construct of conflict between elders and children was given considerable respectability and momentum in 1984 when demographer Samuel H. Preston (1984), then President of the Population Association of America, erroneously argued that rising poverty among children was the direct result of rising benefits to older people.

Widespread concerns about spiraling American health care costs were also redirected, in part, from health care providers, suppliers, administrators, and insurers—the parties responsible for setting the prices of care—to elderly persons for whom health care is provided. A number of academicians and public figures, including politicians, expressed concern that health care expenditures on older persons would soon absorb an unlimited amount of our national resources. It was argued that the elderly were already crowding out health care for others as well as for a variety of additional worthy social causes (cf. Binstock & Post, 1991; Callahan, 1987).

These and other intergenerational concerns were highlighted by the efforts of an organization that called itself Americans for Generational Equity (AGE), founded in 1985 with backing from the corporate sector as well as from a handful of Congressmen who led it. According to its annual reports, most of AGE's funding came from insurance companies, health care corporations, banks, and other private sector businesses and organizations that are in financial competition with Medicare and Social Security (Quadagno, 1989). AGE's basic view was that the large aggregate of public transfers of income and other benefits to older persons is unfair, and that tomorrow's elderly baby boomers will be locked in conflict with younger generations with regard to the distribution of public resources. The AGE organization disseminated this viewpoint from its Washington office through press releases, media interviews, a quarterly entitled *Generational Journal*, a book by one of its staff members (Longman, 1987), and periodic conferences on such subjects as "Children at Risk: Who Will Support an Aging Society?" and "Medicare and the Baby Boom Generation."

Although the AGE organization eventually faded from the scene, by the end of the decade the themes of intergenerational inequity and conflict had been adopted by the media and academics as routine perspectives for describing many social policy issues (Cook, Marshall, Marshall, & Kaufman, 1994). It had also gained currency in elite sectors of American society and on Capitol Hill. For instance, the president of the prestigious American Association of Universities asserted in 1986, "[T]he shape of the domestic federal budget inescapably pits programs for the retired against every other social purpose dependent on federal funds" (Rosenzweig, 1990).

APOCALYPTIC DEMOGRAPHY AND THE MERCHANTS OF DOOM

As the aging of the baby boom drew near, the resurgence of classical liberalism, combined with the political transformation of older persons from needy objects of compassion to greedy geezers engaged in intergenerational combat, set the stage of public discourse for the entrance of what we called at the outset of this chapter the Merchants of Doom. We label them as *merchants* because of the common attribute of selling their concerns about the future in order to promote various interests—a particular ideological point of view and/or opportunistic selling of financial services products. We use the term *doom* to emphasize that their selling techniques are mainly exaggeration and fear. In addition to focusing on intergenerational equity, they have been tenaciously promoting the "crises" associated with population aging.

In 1986, the chairman and staff director for the Aging Society Project at the Carnegie Corporation of New York sought to alert policy makers and other readers to the problems that might be caused by what they termed *a demographic revolution.* Given the projected future population structure, they asked, "Would such [an aged] society, or anything approaching it, be viable?" (Pifer & Bronte, 1986, p. 5).

The alarming tenor of this question is typical of most writing on this topic, then and today. The literature on the impact of population aging is now quite large. First, there is the long-term decline in fertility rates, which means that the national *proportion* of older persons will continue to grow, reaching 20% by 2030. Second, there will be a large increase in the *absolute numbers* (basically a doubling) of older persons who will be eligible for old-age programs. And third, there is the substantial increase in average life expectancies at older ages, which means that persons eligible for old-age benefits will be receiving them for longer periods than in the past (National Center for Health Statistics, 2004). Today, a 67-year-old woman can expect to live, on average, over 18 years. So, when the youngest of the baby boomers has a 67th birthday in 2029, she may very well (given trends) collect Social Security benefits for over 2 decades, through the year 2050 or longer.

What are the consequences of these demographic changes? If one heeds the Merchants of Doom, the consequences are quite frightening, even menacing, for older people and society in general.

Bioethicist Daniel Callahan, concerned about health care expenditures for older people of today and tomorrow, wrote a widely read and influential book entitled *Setting Limits: Medical Goals in an Aging Society.* In it, he characterized the elderly population as "a new social threat" and a "demographic, economic, and medical avalanche . . . one that could ultimately (and perhaps already) do [sic] great harm" (Callahan, 1987, p. 20). Accordingly, he proposed old-age–based health care rationing—specifically, that Medicare reimbursement for lifesaving care be categorically denied to anyone aged in their late 70s or older. One might speculate as to why Callahan chose the unusual metaphor of an *avalanche* to describe the growing number of older persons. Our best guess is that he selected it because avalanches tend to bury whatever is in their paths. Perhaps his basic message is: Let's bury them before they bury us!

Economist Lester Thurow, former dean of MIT's school of management, has depicted aging boomers as a dominant bloc of voters whose self-interested pursuit of government benefits will pose a fundamental threat to our democracy:

> [N]o one knows how the growth of entitlements can be held in check in democratic societies. . . . Will democratic governments be able to cut benefits when the elderly are approaching a voting majority? Universal suffrage . . . is

going to meet the ultimate test in the elderly. If democratic governments cannot cut benefits that go to a majority of their voters, then they have no long-term future. . . . In the years ahead, class warfare is apt to be redefined as the young against the old, rather than the poor against the rich. (Thurow, 1996, p. 47)

Thurow's statement that "the elderly will be approaching a voting majority" is an excellent example of the misleading exaggerations proffered by the Merchants of Doom. In fact, even when all boomers are age 65 and older in 2030, they will still be only 27% of voting-age Americans (U.S. Census Bureau, 1998[2]). Moreover, to date, there is no evidence that older persons or boomers vote as a cohesive block (Binstock, in press).

Another opinion maker is Peter G. Peterson, a Wall Street financier. For years, he has written articles and books in which he argues that government obligations under social insurance entitlement programs must be drastically reduced. Yet, he warns that the political power of boomers may make these reforms difficult, if not impossible:

> Will global aging enthrone organized elders as an invincible political titan?. . . . Picture retiring boomers, with inflated economic expectations and inadequate nest eggs, voting down school budgets, cannibalizing the nation's infrastructure, and demanding ever-steeper hikes in payroll taxes. (Peterson, 1999, p. 209)

Peterson is so concerned about the impact of boomers on politics that he has established a foundation, funded by $1 billion of his personal assets, to carry forward his message. According to a report in the *New York Times* (Thomas, 2008, p. C4), he intends to foment intergenerational conflict, given that one of his specific objectives "is organizing a youthful equivalent to the powerful lobby group for seniors, AARP." To begin this effort he financed a media blitz in the summer of 2008, starting with a documentary film titled *I.O.U.S.A.*, which portrays long-run fiscal problems posed by Social Security and Medicare (Harwood, 2008).

Such doomsaying has not been confined to academics, financiers, journalists, and other commentators on public affairs. Politicians have also been among the Merchants of Doom. In 1993, President Clinton

[2]The most recent (2004) Census Bureau projections regarding the age distribution of American residents in 2030 does not break down information on 18- and 19-year-olds (who are old enough to vote) from the larger category of ages 5 to 19. Consequently, the 1998 projections, which do include a category that begins with age 18, are relied on for the total number of voting-age residents.

created a Bipartisan Commission on Entitlement and Tax Reform that included 22 members of Congress. Entitlement reform, of course, meant Social Security and Medicare reform. The Commission's report depicted continued government financing of Social Security and Medicare as an unsustainable economic burden for the nation (Bipartisan Commission on Entitlement and Tax Reform, 1994). Since then, many other national politicians have expressed similar concerns about the future of old-age social insurance programs.

President George W. Bush strongly entered the fray as a Merchant of Doom when he began his second term in 2005, in an attempt to carry out his long-held desire to dismantle social insurance. In a campaign without historical precedent, he personally undertook a speaking agenda, described by the White House as "60 stops in 60 days," to decry the status of the Social Security program. He repeatedly asserted that the program was imminently headed for disaster—that it soon would be "flat bust" (Bumiller, 2005) and that it was "headed toward bankruptcy" (e.g., Bush, 2005). He blatantly ignored the fact that a shortfall in benefits, then estimated to be around 26%, was not projected to begin until the 2040s—more than 3 decades hence. To undermine confidence in Social Security, Bush undertook a "photo-op" trip to an office building in Parkersburg, West Virginia, home of the U. S. Federal Bureau of Public Debt. There he ceremonially opened a file cabinet holding the U.S. Treasury bonds that have accrued as reserves in the Social Security trust fund and declared those U.S. bonds to be worthless; he described them as "just IOUs" and asserted that "there is no trust fund" (Vieth & Simon, 2005).

President Bush's primary solution to the Social Security problem was to partially dismantle the program. The president's favored approach was to divert some of the payroll taxes that are now dedicated to financing Social Security, and use them to set up private individual accounts that could be invested in the market to stimulate the private sector and, hopefully, earn high returns for investors. However, when confronted by experts who pointed out serious problems with his recommendations, President Bush admitted that what he was proposing would do nothing to solve a Social Security financing shortfall projected to occur decades hence.

FENDING OFF THE THREATS TO SOCIAL INSURANCE

The ingenious solution of the social insurance approach was (and still is) the national pooling of risks through insurance mechanisms, a solution that has produced meaningful financial security with dignity for most older Americans. Social Security keeps millions out of poverty and near poverty, and it provides a solid foundation on which it is possible to build a satisfactory financial situation in retirement with the addition of pensions and savings. Medicare finances health care for well over 90% of older persons in the country.

Despite the failure of President Bush's efforts to privatize Social Security, the threats to social insurance are very much alive, with the possibility of undermining America's successful approach to date for dealing with many major economic risks all of us confront as we grow older. Privatizing Social Security through individual accounts is still on the public policy agenda, buttressed by neoliberalism's emphasis on personal responsibility and the free market. Various measures for limiting Medicare expenditures on the health care needs of older persons are being actively investigated.

In our view, the crisis mongering by the Merchants of Doom has much to do with the persistence of these policy options. To be sure, the rapid aging of our population between now and 2030 presents substantial policy challenges. Yet, some historical perspective on declamations of so-called crises in the old-age policy arena reveals that they have been off the mark. Consider the following examples.

When Medicare was proposed (and finally enacted in 1965), leaders of the American Medical Association—a vigorous opponent of the legislation—made the ominous prediction that the program would quickly lead to "socialized medicine," causing a crisis in health care. No such thing happened. In the late 1970s and early 1980s, there was a so-called crisis in Social Security financing. Despite the extensive crisis rhetoric at the time, it turned out that the financing problem was not terribly difficult to solve (Estes, 1983). Still, another crisis was perceived in 1986 when Congress outlawed mandatory retirement at any age for almost all jobs. Many employers foresaw economic disaster. They predicted that business payrolls would be overwhelmed and production clogged by large numbers of very old, highly paid workers whose skills and energy had diminished with age. Once again, the fears turned out to be unfounded. Relatively few older persons chose to work longer (and most that did were highly productive).

Present shouts of "crisis" are not much different from the past, except perhaps for the massive uncertainty they are generating about the fate of Social Security and Medicare. By putting aside the rhetoric of crisis, it is relatively easy to see that the challenges of sustaining Social

Security can be met through relatively minor changes that do not require radical reform. For instance, the 2008 report issued by the trustees of the Social Security Trust Fund estimated that 22% of benefits could not be paid starting in 2041. This is a significant gap. Yet, the report also indicates that an increase of .85 of a percentage point in the payroll tax that finances Social Security—from both employer and employee—would fill the gap completely throughout the 75-year period for which such projections are made (Board of Trustees, 2008). Alternatively, a much smaller tax increase could be combined with a series of other minor changes, such as raising the annual ceiling on the payroll tax to generate more revenue from individuals with very high salaries, raising the "normal retirement age" in line with increases in life expectancy, slightly reducing the program's annual cost-of-living adjustment to benefits, and allocating all or some portion of the revenues from the estate tax to Social Security.

In the case of Medicare, the challenges are greater. The issue is not so much estimates of shortfalls from the Medicare Trust Fund, but rather the rapidly increasing costs of U.S. health care for people of all ages and its financing implications for the Medicare program. By 2036, the proportion of GDP spent on Medicare is projected to more than triple to about 8% of GDP (Medicare Payment Advisory Commission, 2006)—one twelfth of our national wealth, spent on one program. A number of studies have shown, however, that *population aging is a relatively minor factor in spiraling U.S. health care costs* (Reinhardt, 2003). Rather, the problem is expense factors in the overall system, in which costs rise much faster than the general rate of inflation. The major sources of rising costs per patient in the health care sector include a constant stream of new and costly technologies and procedures, high rates of utilization, huge private companies' administrative costs, and unnecessarily high comparative expenses and utilization in some regions and health centers as compared with others.

Consequently, efforts to contain Medicare costs—without limiting coverage for the health care of older patients—should in principle focus on reforming the health care system generally. But there are substantial political barriers to major, sweeping health care reforms because of the large financial stakes that the medical industrial complex has in current arrangements. Moreover, the larger health care arena is highly fragmented, so there is no entity "in charge" of it. In contrast, Medicare policies can be implemented more effectively because they can be centralized through concerted government policy actions. Consequently, attempts to contain health care costs are likely to continue focusing on limiting Medicare coverage.

REFRAMING THE ISSUES FOR AN AGING NATION

At the end of the day, sustaining social insurance in the United States will come down to two fundamental issues. Will there continue to be enough national wealth to fund Social Security and Medicare? And, will there be sufficient political will to do so? In our view, strengthening the requisite political will requires a reframing of the issues at stake in the social insurance arena.

In his book, *Don't Think of an Elephant: Know Your Values and Frame the Debate*, George Lakoff (2004) highlights principles for making effective political and policy arguments. Lakoff, a professor of cognitive science and linguistics at the University of California, Berkeley, illustrates the role of metaphors in framing issues, and the ongoing influence of rhetorical frameworks in the policy arena.

If the threats to the social insurance programs are to be repelled, who or what organization might undertake leadership in reframing old-age policy issues to counter the apocalyptic scenarios and radical policy options put forth by the Merchants of Doom? Among the potential candidates are many of the 53 organizations that belong to the Leadership Council of Aging Organizations (LCAO)—or the LCAO, itself—a coalition that defines itself as "dedicated to preserving and strengthening the well-being of America's older people" (Leadership Council of Aging Organizations, 2008). But, in our view, AARP (formerly the American Association of Retired Persons) is the best candidate for this leadership role. In the 21st century, it has become far more politically and financially powerful than any of its fellow old-age organizations, or all of them combined (Schulz & Binstock, 2008). Moreover, it has already begun the coalition building process. In conjunction with the Business Roundtable, the Service Employees International Union, and the National Federation of Independent Businesses, it has established "Divided We Fail," a campaign with the goal of ensuring "affordable quality health care and long-term financial security for everyone" (Divided We Fail, 2008).

Under the leadership of CEO William Novelli, a longtime public relations specialist, AARP is likely to continue drawing on its large resources and its standing as a massive membership organization of nearly 40 million older persons to play a visible and active policy role. Since Novelli took charge of the organization in early 2002, "positive social change" has become an explicitly avowed priority of the organization (AARP, 2003). Moreover, it appears that it is his intention to make the organization a major "player" in Washington politics, spending millions to influence public opinion.

In response to Democratic complaints that AARP had cooperated with the Republicans on the Medicare prescription drug legislation of 2003, he acknowledged that these actions had realigned AARP politically. Shortly after the legislation passed, he opined that, "AARP was taken for granted" by Democratic leaders in the past. He then observed that "the best thing we can do is not be aligned with either party" (Cook, 2003). This intent was demonstrated clearly in 2005 when his organization mounted a vigorous war of words and images in opposition to the Republican push for partially privatizing Social Security.

Perhaps the most effective issue-framing strategy to counter the Merchants of Doom and minimize conflict among generations would be for AARP to form a coalition with advocates for children (such as the Children's Defense Fund) and other key organizations concerned with the welfare of family members of all ages. Banding together its resources, the coalition should launch a sustained media campaign. The campaign should portray the aging of the baby boomers as *a challenge confronting boomers, their families, and society—rather than as a Social Security crisis and a Medicare crisis.*

The central focus of this coalition's campaign should be on *people rather than programs*. The key is to convey the consequences of radical policy changes in terms of what they would mean tomorrow for older people, the nature of family obligations and lifestyles, and the fabric of familiar social institutions that are integral to the daily life of Americans of all ages.

Such a campaign could be initially targeted to the 76 million baby boomers and be strong enough to compete with anti-aging marketing campaigns that tell this audience how to avoid growing old (Mehlman, Binstock, Juengst, Ponsaran, & Whitehouse, 2004). Its initial goal might be to convey to boomers (perhaps in a congratulatory fashion) that they will live for many, many years as older Americans. Perhaps a complementary aspect of this first "congratulatory" phase would be to effectively inform baby boomers about the existing array and financing of governmental benefits that reduce the risks of old age, making clear their roles and also their limitations.

A next element of the campaign would be to develop and convey scenarios that depict what life will be like for aged baby boomers *and their families* if nothing is done to maintain Social Security and Medicare in forms that sustain government supports at a level that is reasonably comparable to what older Americans experienced in the last 3 decades of the 20th century and the first years of the 21st century.

What will the budgets of elderly couples and aged widows be like in terms of how much they have to spend on food, shelter, clothing, utilities, transportation, medical care, and long-term care? For those who are less than wealthy, what limits might exist on their access to medical care—including high-cost, high-tech medical interventions—particularly at advanced old ages? How many older persons will have to be financially supported by their children, including the catastrophic expenses of acute health care and long-term care? Will American society witness, due to the necessity of family economics, the return of three- and, perhaps, four-generation households? Will the constant stream of emerging medical miracles be available to all of us, or only the very wealthy and "connected" in American society? Many such questions could be vividly posed.

The generation and promulgation of scenarios that answer these questions might be enough to help boomers and their families feel that a sufficient "crisis" looms in societal support for the basic needs of tomorrow's older people to warrant remedial, but not radical, policy action in the near-term future. If an issue as abstract, unfamiliar, and seemingly distant in consequences as Global Warming can reach public attention, then the challenges of population aging surely could, especially if the not-too-distant consequences are conveyed in terms of *daily lives for persons of all ages* rather than projected program deficits.

If the scenery for the play of daily life in our aging nation can be effectively painted for the American public, what else would be needed to mobilize popular support for maintaining the social insurance programs that have been so important? As implied above, the issues confronting older people are not now, and will not then, be hermetically sealed from the rest of society. Perhaps the way to gain widespread political support among all generations is to package policy options for our aging nation as *family policies* (see Harrington, 1999). In effect, this is what they are. We should not forget that the beneficiaries of the future will be all of us.

DISCUSSION QUESTIONS

1. Why do the authors suggest that the Golden Years are "in danger of being tarnished"?
2. Who are the Merchants of Doom? What do they believe and how do they spread these beliefs? What is their political agenda?
3. What are the authors' recommendations for repelling the threats to America's social insurance programs and reframing old-age policy?
4. What do the authors suggest as a way to gain widespread political support among all generations?

REFERENCES

AARP. (2003). *Annual report, 2002*. Retrieved March 27, 2004, from http://assets.aarp.org/www.aarp.org-articles/aboutaarp/annualreports2002-f.pdf

Achenbaum, W. A. (1986). *Social Security: Visions and revisions.* New York: Cambridge University Press.

Binstock, R.H. (In press). The boomers in politics: Impact and consequences. In R. B. Hudson (Ed.), *Boomer bust: Economic and political dynamics of the graying society*: Volume *I*: *Perspectives on the boomers.* Westport, CT: Praeger.

Binstock, R. H., & Post, S. G. (Eds.). (1991). *Too old for health care? Controversies in medicine, law, economics, and ethics*. Baltimore: Johns Hopkins University Press.

Bipartisan Commission on Entitlement and Tax Reform. (1994). *Commission findings.* Washington, DC: U.S. Government Printing Office.

Board of Trustees. (2008). *Annual report of the Board of Trustees of the federal Old-Age and Survivors Insurance and Federal Disability Insurance Trust Funds.* Washington, DC: Social Security Administration.

Bumiller, E. (2005, January 12). Bush presses his argument for Social Security change. *New York Times*, p. A18.

Bush, G.W. (2005, February 3). Transcript: President Bush's state of the union address. *New York Times*. Retrieved October 16, 2008, from http://www.nytimes.com/2005/02/03/politics/03btext.html?pagewanted-print&position=

Carballo, M. (1981, December 17). Extra votes for parents? *Boston Globe*, p. 35.

Callahan, D. (1987). *Setting limits: Medical goals in an aging society*. New York: Simon and Schuster.

Cook. D. (2003, December 11). The point man on AARP's controversial move. *Christian Science Monitor*. Retrieved December 29, 2003, from http://www.christiansciencemonitor.com/2003/12/11/p03s01-supo.hmtl

Cook, F. L., Marshall, V. M., Marshall, J. E., & Kaufman, J. E. (1994). The salience of intergenerational equity in Canada and the United States. In T. R. Marmor, T. M. Smeeding, & V. L. Greene (Eds.), *Economic security and intergenerational justice: A look at North America* (pp. 91–129). Washington, DC: Urban Institute Press.

Divided We Fail. (2008). *Get involved.* Retrieved July 25, 2008, from http://www.aarp.org/issues/dividedwe fail/get_involved

Esping-Andersen, G. (1999). *Social foundations of postindustrial economies*. New York: Oxford University Press.

Estes, C. L. (1983). Social Security: The social construction of a "crisis." *Milbank Memorial Fund Quarterly/Health and Society*, *61*, 445–461.

Flint, J. (1980, February, 18). The old folks. *Forbes*, pp. 51–56.

Harrington, M. (1999). *Care and equality: Inventing a new family politics*. New York: Alfred A. Knopf.

Hartz, L. (1955). *The liberal tradition in America*. New York: Harcourt Brace and Company.

Harwood, J. (2008, July 14). Spending $1 billion to restore fiscal sanity. *New York Times*, p. A15.

Hudson, R. B. (1978). The "graying" of the federal budget and its consequences for old age policy. *Gerontologist*, *18*, 428–440.

Kalish, R. A. (1979). The new ageism and the failure models: A polemic. *Gerontologist*, *19*, 398–407.

Lakoff, G. (2004). *Don't think of an elephant: Know your values and frame the debate—the essential guide for progressives.* White River Junction, VT: Chelsea Green Publishers.

Leadership Council of Aging Organizations. (2008). *Welcome to Leadership Council of Aging Organizations*. Retrieved October 16, 2008, from http://lcao.org

Locke, J. (1690 [1924]). *Of civil government, two treatises*. London: J.M. Dent & Sons, Ltd.

Longman, P. (1987). *Born to pay: The new politics of aging in America*. Boston: Houghton Mifflin.

Medicare Payment Advisory Commission. (2006). *Report to the Congress: Medicare payment policy*. Washington, DC: U.S. Government Printing Office.

Mehlman, M. J., Binstock, R. H., Juengst, E. T., Ponsaran, R. S., & Whitehouse, P. J. (2004). Anti-aging medicine: Can consumers be better protected? *The Gerontologist*, *44*, 304–310.

National Center for Health Statistics. (2004). *Health United States, 2004: With chartbook on trends in the health of Americans*. Hyattsville, MD, 2004. Retrieved September 28, 2005, from http://www.cdc.gov/nchs/data/hus/hus04trend.pdf

Peterson, P. G. (1987). The morning after. *Atlantic Monthly*, *260*(4), 43–49.

Peterson, P. G. (1999). *Gray dawn: How the coming age wave will transform America—and the world*. New York: Times Books.

Pierson, P., & Skocpol, T. (Eds.). (2007). *The transformation of American politics: Activist government and the rise of conservatism.* Princeton, NJ: Princeton University Press.

Pifer, A., & Bronte, L. (1986). Introduction: Squaring the pyramid. In A. Pifer & L. Bronte (Eds.), *Our aging society: Paradox and promise* (p. 5). New York: W. W. Norton.

Preston, S. H. (1984). Children and the elderly in the U.S. *Scientific American*, *51*(6), 44–49.

Quadagno, J. (1989). Generational equity and the politics of the welfare state. *Politics and Society*, *17*, 353–376.

Quinn, J. (1987). The economic status of the elderly: Beware the mean. *Review of Income and Wealth*, *33*(1), 63–82.

Reinhardt, U. E. (2003). Does the aging of the population really drive the demand for health care? *Health Affairs*, *22*(6), 27–39.

Rosenzweig, R. M. (1990). Address at the president's opening session, 43rd Annual Meeting of the Gerontological Society of America, Boston, MA (typewritten copy), November 16.

Salholz, E. (1990, October 29). Blaming the voters: Hapless budgeteers single out "greedy geezers." *Newsweek*, p. 36.

Samuelson, R. J. (1978). Aging America: Who will shoulder the growing burden? *National Journal*, *10*, 712–1717.

Schulz, J. H. (2001). *The economics of aging*. Westport, CT: Auburn House.

Schulz, J. H., & Binstock, R. H. (2008). *Aging nation: The economics and politics of growing older in America.* Baltimore: The Johns Hopkins University Press.

Smith, A. (1776 [2003]). *The wealth of nations*. New York: Bantam Classics.

Smith, L. (1992). The tyranny of America's old. *Fortune*, *125*(1), 68–72.

Thomas, L., Jr. (2008, February 15). Reconciling opposites: A crusade against cozy tax breaks, led by one who benefited. *New York Times*, pp. C1, C4.

Thurow, L. C. (1996, May 19). The birth of a revolutionary class. *New York Times Magazine*, pp. 46–47.

Torrey, B. B. (1982). Guns vs. canes: The fiscal implications of an aging population. *American Economics Association Papers and Proceedings*, 72, 309–313.

Tsurumi, Y. (2006, April 6). Hail to the robber baron? *The Harvard Crimson*, April 6. Retrieved on April 8, 2005, from http:///www.thecrimson.com/printerfriendly.aspx?ref=506836

U.S. Census Bureau. (1998). *Current population reports, series P2* (Middle Series Projections). Washington, DC: U. S. Government Printing Office.

Vieth, W., & Simon, R. (2005, April 6). President casts doubt on trust fund: Promoting his private account plan, Bush calls the Social Security bonds held for future beneficiaries "just IOUs sitting in a filing cabinet." *Los Angeles Times*. Retrieved October 16, 2008, from http://www.latimes.com/news/printedition/asection/la-na-bush6apr06,1,4700653,print.story

12 Social Security Privatization: The Institutionalization of an Ideological Movement[1]

JUDIE SVIHULA AND CARROLL L. ESTES

Social Security was enacted in 1935 amid political controversy (Domhoff, 1996). Until the passage of the Social Security Act amendments of 1950, Republicans, conservatives, and corporate leaders opposed the program, decrying it as burdensome to business, workers, and the state as well as an unfair liability on future generations. Yet, from 1950 through 1995, Congress and presidents generally agreed that the fundamental structure and principles of Social Security should be retained. Consensus politics continued through two periods of Republican majority control over the Democrats in Congress (1953 through 1955 and 1980 through 1986), but dissension began to mount when Republican majorities ruled both houses in 1994. We contend that (1) the dissension is the result of an ideological social movement favoring privatization and (2) this social movement has been institutionalized through various processes and structures. This chapter will review the history of the privatization movement.

[1]Parts of this chapter are adapted and revised from Svihula, J., & Estes, C. L. (2008). Social Security privatization: An ideologically structured movement. *Journal of Sociology and Social Welfare, XXXV*(1), 43–103.

DEFINITIONS AND THEORY

An ideology is any system of ideas, beliefs, values, and attitudes that justifies or legitimates dominant structural relationships or movements to change them (Jary & Jary, 1991; Johnson, 2000). Social movements are social processes wherein actors, linked by dense informal networks and sharing a distinct identity, are engaged in collective action against clearly identified opponents (della Porta & Diani, 2006; Diani & Bison, 2004). Based on their shared ideals, actors collectively resist or promote change in the political, economic, and/or cultural status quo.

Ideologically structured action is guided and shaped by ideological belief systems whereby adherents defend and attack current social relations and the social system (Zald, 2000). Actors with similar ideological commitments in different arenas shape their sense of friends and enemies, of alliance partners and opposition, and of right and wrong behavior and choices because of their shared commitments. Bureaucrats, legislators, jurists, and executives identify with movements and share ideologies with those we label activists and leaders.

Institutionalization is both "the process as well as the outcome of the process, in which social activities become regularized and routinized as stable, social-structural features" (Jary & Jary, 2000, p. 307). The institutionalization of a social movement encompasses both its process of formation and evolution as well as its outcomes, including the inculcation and adherence over time to value systems that become relatively stable and that both proscribe and constrain certain activities or behavior, such as the conceptualization and implementation of certain policy approaches. As cognitive scientist George Lakoff (2002) shows, the achievement of successful political inroads requires the binding of moral values with the political values (as in the linking of individual responsibility, the conservative version of "generational equity," and the market). Given the contemporary "speed of social change and . . . flexibility of social arrangements," sociologists increasingly "avoid treating institutions as if they were things, and . . . look more toward social processes—of institutionalization, de-institutionalization, and re-institutionalization—than to stable clusters of roles" (Turner, 2006, p. 301).

HISTORICAL AND LEGISLATIVE ANALYSIS

We used the theoretical frameworks of McAdam, Tarrow, and Tilly (2001) and Amenta (2006) to guide our study. To document the cumulative change in expressions of support for Social Security's social insurance ideals to privatization, we studied and selectively performed content analyses of historical and legislative documents, databases, and Web sites, including:

- Congressional and administrative documents
- Journal articles, reports
- Think tank Web sites
- Social Security Administration database
- Historical accounts on pension reform
- CQ Weekly online database
- Conferences on public pensions
- Eleven years of legislative hearings

POLITICAL SEEDS OF PRIVATIZATION

Although the seeds of dissention on Social Security's long-term financing appeared as early as 1977, it took the substantial efforts of conservatives to build the political momentum necessary to shift the institutional structures of government (Amenta, 2006; Domhoff, 1996; Light, 1995). President Roosevelt recognized the need for political action within the climate of the Great Depression and enacted Social Security in 1935 amid political controversy. Until the passage of the Social Security Act amendments of 1950, conservatives and corporate leaders opposed the program, decrying it as burdensome to business, workers, and the state, as well as an unfair liability on future generations.

In 1977, Congress directed the Social Security Commission to develop a system that would "best serve the Nation in the future." After extensive study, the Commission concluded that the Social Security system was sound in principle and the best of all alternatives for "stable income support, especially in times of economic adversity." Other alternatives would be "too costly or offer insufficient assurance" that workers' incomes would be there when they needed it. Until 2001, all presidents have backed the social insurance structure and principles of the Social Security Program. President Reagan stated, upon signing the 1983 amendments, the program "must be preserved." Subsequently, the first President G. H. W. Bush promised that the government would stand behind its social contract with its citizens (SSA, 1981, pp. 1–4, 20, 1996a).

The concept of privatization in Social Security debuted nationally when Pierre du Pont IV (R-Del.) called for private accounts during his

1988 presidential campaign (Birnbaum, 2005). Beginning in 1991, the Board of Trustees used new, more stringent tests of financial adequacy to test Social Security's solvency, resulting in estimates of insolvency over the long term (SSA, 1996b). Soon afterward, during President Clinton's first term, the Trustees recommended that the Advisory Council develop recommendations for restoring Social Security's long-range actuarial balance. Although the Technical Panel to the Council noted that privatization would require additional adjustments beyond what would be required to achieve system solvency, it concluded that private accounts deserved additional study.

NATIONAL ACTION

In the 1980s, market arguments began to proliferate in the U.S. government alongside pension privatization projects by conservative think tanks. Conservative think tanks united with the purpose of destroying Social Security (Ferrara, 1980). The Cato Institute (Cato) published an article, "Achieving a 'Leninist' Strategy," coauthored by affiliates of the Heritage Foundation, that called for "guerrilla warfare against both the current Social Security system and the coalition that supports it" by creating "a focused political coalition" to isolate and weaken its opponents (Butler & Germanis, 1983, pp. 547–556).

In the 1990s, recommendations for personal (private) accounts gained greater attention. Witnesses invited by the Republican-dominated Congress to federal hearings on Social Security reform expressed increasing support for privatization (Svihula & Estes, 2007). In January 1997, the Social Security Council recommended three different plans, two of which included private accounts. From 1998 forward, the Trustees have continually reported that the Trust Fund is not in long-term actuarial balance, placing greater emphasis, as time passed, on the importance of making changes to the program.

In his 2000 presidential campaign, Bush proposed a 2% diversion of the Social Security contributions of individuals to private accounts (SSA, 2001). By the time President Bush conducted his "60 cities in 60 days" campaign to privatize Social Security in 2005, he proposed allowing 4% of the 6.2% (almost two-thirds) of individual Social Security payroll contributions to be diverted into voluntary private accounts. Other privatization proponents have recommended the diversion to private accounts of 4% or essentially all of the individual's Social Security contributions in a phased-in transformation of the system. In 2001, members of the

President's Commission to Strengthen Social Security were appointed by Bush based on their acceptance of his injunction to include private accounts in their recommendations. Six of the members were affiliated with conservative think tanks, including three from Cato. In January 2005, the chairs of the House and Senate Republican Conferences developed a 103-page guide to educate Republicans on how to promote private accounts in Social Security (Pryce & Santorum, 2005). In 2006, 22 of the 26 reform proposals introduced to Congress included some form of personal carve-out accounts (SSA, 2006).

INTERNATIONAL ACTION

Although privatization efforts originated in the United States, the movement's first fruits were born internationally. The popularity of government spending as a means to improve the economy (known as Keynesian economics) declined with the stagflation and unemployment of the 1970s (Baker, 2007; Myles, 1984). The post-Keynesian political economy appears to have emboldened economists and others to promote market ideals. In the 1980s, Milton Friedman, a former Keynesian economist, lectured on the idea of free markets in his visits to Chile and elsewhere (Birnbaum, 2005; Commanding Heights, 2000). Shortly afterward, José Piñera, a Harvard economist trained by Friedman, masterminded the privatization of Chile's pension system (Pinera, n.d.).

President Reagan sent U.S. Treasury Secretary James Baker, III to promote market reforms at the annual meeting of the International Monetary Fund (IMF) and World Bank (WB) (Andrews, 2006; Boughton, 2001; Elahi, 1986; James, 1994; Williamson, 2000; World Bank, 2001). The U.S. government worked with the IMF and the WB in making market reforms, including pension privatization, a precondition of WB loans. Acting on advice she received from Pierre du Pont IV, who had received the acclaim of Milton Friedman, Prime Minister Thatcher privatized various government properties and programs including the country's public pension system. Beginning in 1994 with a publication titled *Averting the Old Age Crisis*, the WB has actively promoted privatization as a blueprint for pension reform worldwide.

PRIVATIZATION EFFORTS SINCE 2001

Since 2001, President George W. Bush has continually advanced private accounts via multiple venues (Center on Budget and Policy Priorities,

2006; House Committee on Oversight and Government Reform, 2007; Minority Staff Special Investigations Division Committee on Government Reform, 2005; Office of the Press Secretary, 2005; Schor, 2007; Wayne, 2006; Wayne & Tollefson, 2007). For example, a Department of the Treasury Office of Public Affairs Fact Sheet declares, "This Administration embraces the need for new ideas. The creation of personal accounts is critical to ensure Social Security's sustainability" (2004). Moreover, the Social Security Administration's (SSA) primary strategic goal of educating the public about the program was replaced in 2003 by a new objective to use public communication to "support reforms" to Social Security. Additionally, during two recent congressional recesses, Bush reappointed two public trustees—John Palmer and Thomas Saving, and appointed Andrew Biggs, Assistant Director of Cato's Project on Social Security Choice as associate commissioner of the SSA. Moreover, Bush has inserted estimated expenditures to fund Social Security private accounts in his proposed 2007, 2008, and 2009 national budgets.

BOARD OF TRUSTEES

Trustees have focused attention on what they label as a "crisis" of Social Security's solvency (long-term financing) and the urgency of reform (Baker, 2007; Estes, 2001; Light, 1995; Munnell, 2006; Wayne, 2005). Currently, four of the six Social Security trustees are political appointees of the president who are known to support private accounts. Recent Trustees' reports have had substantially more pessimistic assumptions than the nonpartisan Congressional Budget Office (CBO) resulting in as much as an 11 year earlier projected date of trust fund depletion by the Trustees when compared to the date projected by the CBO.

INTERNATIONAL AND NATIONAL DEVELOPMENTS

There have been recent developments in the market reform efforts (Sentido.tv Americas, 2006; SSA, 2007; Weisbrot, 2006; Young, 2007). In the international arena, the influence of the IMF in Latin America and middle-income countries has collapsed. Moreover, Chile is reforming its privatized system. Nationally, Democrats are staunchly against private accounts and Republicans are split on the reform option. Moreover, within the SSA, support for shifting the social insurance program to private accounts continues, and new and controversial actuarial techniques (e.g., infinite horizon budgeting) have been introduced that make the Social Security issue look worse.

Early in their campaigns, the 2008 U.S. presidential candidates were relatively quiet about Social Security, focusing more on health care (On the Issues, 2007). However, in November 2007, Republican candidate Fred Thompson, along with Democratic candidates Hillary Clinton and Barack Obama, began to debate the issue publicly. Thompson proposed personal accounts funded by additional individual payroll taxes that the government would match 2.5 to 1 through general revenues. Clinton said she anticipated ending the practice of borrowing from the Social Security trust fund and then appointing a bipartisan commission. Obama backed raising the income ceiling on payroll taxes. Thompson withdrew from the race; however, presidential hopeful John McCain was quoted in late 2007 as saying he did not support personal accounts that divert payroll taxes from Social Security (Sahadi, 2007). Instead, because he believed it more a political issue than an economic one, McCain supported reducing benefits rather than increasing taxes to shore up Social Security. Later, as the Republican nominee, McCain appeared to change his tone and suggested privatizing Social Security. Former Republican candidate Mike Huckabee had proposed either eliminating Social Security taxes entirely or allowing new retirees to opt for a lump sum payout.

In 2003, the SSA sponsored the Retirement Research Consortium (RRC) at $5 million or more per year through 2007 (SSA, 2007) to (1) conduct research and evaluation, (2) disseminate information on retirement research, and (3) train scholars and practitioners. The RRC has held events at which speakers and presenters have promoted personal accounts. At a conference in 2007, Andrew Biggs (the former lead on Cato's privatization work) and Sylvester Schieber were the two invited guest speakers. Sylvester Schieber, a partner with financial consulting firm Watson-Wyatt Worldwide, was appointed by President Bush to the Chairmanship of the Social Security Advisory Board.

One of the greatest objections to personal accounts has been the shift of risk from the government to the individual. Competitive economies pose risks to citizens. Social insurance programs, through universal coverage and risk sharing, provide security from individual risks. Social Security provides protection from individual risks such as the death of a parent in childhood, death of a spouse, loss of work wages due to disability, and outliving savings in retirement. At a 2006 RRC conference, five papers were presented on reducing the amount of individual risk associated with the introduction of private accounts into Social Security ("Reforming Social Security with Progressive Personal Accounts," "Reducing Social Security Personal Retirement Account Risk at the Individual Level," "Reducing the Risk of Investment-based Social Security Reform," "Changing Progressivity as a Means of Risk Protection in Investment-Based Social Security," and "Pricing Personal Account Benefit Guarantees: A Simplified Approach"). These papers sought to buffer against various problems created by privatization by attempting to anticipate and address the arguments of the opponents of Social Security privatization.

An accurate and unbiased public debate is overdue. Social Security is important to U.S. citizens; they support its social insurance values unequivocally, to the point of consenting to additional taxes to sustain the program (Cook, Barabas, & Page, 2002; Laurenti, 2000; PollingReport.com, 2009). Conversely, citizens do not favor the individual risk associated with personal accounts in Social Security. There is a great need for an accurate depiction of Social Security's status to be brought into national debate. As has been demonstrated in this chapter, market rationalists are prominent in the presidential administration, the Social Security Administration, the Department of Treasury, the Board of Trustees, and witnesses invited to congressional hearings on Social Security reform. Moreover, they have penetrated research institutions previously perceived as unbiased including Brookings and the Urban Institute. In the event of a conservative majority in Congress and/or the election of another conservative president in November 2008, it is possible that the legislative ambush similar to the Medicare Modernization Act of 2003 (MMA) will be replayed in Social Security. The MMA was a big step taken by conservatives to erode Medicare's social insurance structure. Conservatives, claiming to improve competition, have provided subsidies for private insurance companies and employers giving them incentive to remain in the market. At the same time, they prohibited Medicare from using its leverage to negotiate lower drug costs. Social Security reform options that contain private "carve out" accounts are a form of privatization that reduces the program's defined benefits.

Two international examples, Latin America and Chile illustrate the tensions and dynamics surrounding the privatization movement and the potential unwillingness of other nations to go along with the Bush Administration's proposal to privatize social insurance programs around the globe.

Latin America. Latin America has experienced an unprecedented long-term economic growth failure over the last quarter-century while implementing a number of market policies advocated by the IMF and WB (Sentido.tv Americas, 2006; Weisbrot, 2006). Recently, a number of countries rejected these policies and have elected governments with an explicit mandate to change course on economic policy. In 2007, the governments of Bolivia, Brazil, Ecuador, Paraguay, Uruguay, Venezuela, and Colombia decided to form a new "Banco del Sur" as an alternative to the IMF, WB, and allied institutions (Weisbrot, 2007).

Chile. As of 2004, several studies had concluded that a sizable majority of the Chilean workforce would not save enough to receive the minimum pension out of the private system, and they were not qualified for the safety net or public assistance programs. The results were confirmed by the WB (Sentido.tv Americas, 2006; Weisbrot, 2006). In 2007, Chile began to transform its private system into one with greater social insurance, beginning with free health care to individuals over 60 years of age and adding a national public safety net to the Social Security program.

INSTITUTIONALIZATION OF THE PRIVATIZATION MOVEMENT

The concept of *institution* refers to "arrangements involving large numbers of people whose behavior is guided by norms and roles." Institutionalization refers to "the process whereby the norms and roles expected in various situations are developed and learned," (Jary & Jary, 2000, p. 306). As noted earlier, institutionalization is both a process as well as the outcome of the process. As established in a prior study by the authors (Svihula & Estes, 2007), the ideology backing the Social Security privatization movement rests on the embrace of individual responsibility and the market as well as a rejection of collective responsibility and the state. Discrimination that becomes institutionalized (e.g., institutionalized sexism, racism, or ageism) may result from "the majority simply adhering unthinkingly to existing organizational and institutional . . . social norms" that are widely propagated (Marshall, 1996, pp. 250–251). In this and other ways, institutions "constrain or . . . determine the behaviour of specific social groups" (Marshall, 1996, p. 250).

We contend that the privatization movement is so well entrenched that it may be defined as institutionalized. This gives it a strength and solidity that braces it against the opposition, that is, those who seek to preserve and improve the existing Social Security defined benefit program. For the Social Security privatization movement, the institutionalization process, and the agents and structures that produce it are engaged in the continuing production and reproduction of crisis constructions around Social Security solvency and apocalyptic demography (Robertson, 1990), the unsustainability of entitlement costs by the state, and the inevitability of the privatization solution. These claims are promoted by a broad network of advocates in well-funded think tanks, private foundations, and representatives of the Bush Administration, such as Comptroller General David Walker and other conservative entities, and repeated in all forms of the media. The confluence of corporate, political, and religious interests asserting the morality of self-responsibility and the answer of the market have produced the desired "coherent political ideology" comprised of linked "categories of moral and political . . . reasoning about politics," through which voters learn a restricted framework of policy options (Lakoff, 2002 pp. 14–15). Channeled to a delimited view of a problem and solution, voters perceive no alternatives. Significantly, ideologies not only legitimate the dominance of particular structural interests (e.g., financial capital, antistatist sentiment), but also they generate societal consensus through their institutionalization (Gramsci, 1971; Estes, 1979).

In conclusion, the Social Security privatization movement has been institutionalized through political struggles over the morality and feasibility (affordability) of social insurance and the value (virtue or damnation) of collectively pooled risk versus individual responsibility. The forces of Social Security privatization had been nascent since its enacting legislation, but again roiled during the legislative battles leading to the passage of Medicare. The current re-invigoration of the privatization movement commenced in the 1980s, buoyed by President Reagan's election and conservative politics since (Svihula & Estes, 2008), and found fruition in the passage of the Medicare Modernization Act of 2003. The swelling number and influence of conservative think tanks and foundations have deepened and institutionalized the cultural and intellectual capital of the Right, supported by billions of dollars of private wealth accumulation. Perhaps the apex is the 2008 founding by Peter G. Peterson of a billion-dollar foundation to promote the ideas of fiscal responsibility and capitalism that is touting the unsustainability of three entitlements, Social security, Medicare, and Medicaid. Bryan Turner (2006) argues that detraditionalization and counter movements of reinstitutionalization may occur after one another. It appears that the privatization movement is a struggle for the detraditionalization of social insurance and Social Security. It certainly is a gambit aimed at the delegitimation of the bedrock social insurance safety net for older persons as well as younger disabled Americans. At the same time, there is an evolving, but less coherent and less developed resistance movement to Social Security privatization (Estes, 2008), which appears to be a struggle for the reinstitutionalization of social insurance and the legitimacy of the state as a protector of citizens and of the collective and communal values undergirding state policy.

The fledgling resistance movement against privatization was born of latent and fragmented civil servants, scholars, and progressives who were drawn into the struggles first emerging during Ronald Reagan's attacks on Social Security. These were followed by an explosion of media attention to demographic doomsayers, economists, think tanks, foundations, and corporations committed to rolling back the Welfare State and all forms of individual entitlements. Privatization proponents gained another foothold and significant state legitimacy through Cabinet and other federal appointments during the two-term Bush administration. The Medicare reforms of 2003 created another wake-up call, generating increased awareness of the consequences of privatization and encouraging coalitions of the concerned. The 2009 presidential elections and the divergent views on privatization of nominees, John McCain and Barack Obama, further thrust these issues into the limelight. One result is the growing formalization, visibility, and coordinated activities of entities opposing privatization. Indeed, they appear to have entered the early stages of a developing field of social movement organizations of privatization resistance (Estes, 2008; see McAdam, Tarrow, & Tilly, 2001; Zald, 2000). The privatization juggernaut surrounding Social Security and Medicare raises not only the social policy stakes, but also the potentially profound consequences for different sectors of the powerful and the powerless in the United States.

DISCUSSION QUESTIONS

1. What is a social movement?
2. The United States has exported the privatization perspective through entities like the World Bank and the International Monetary Fund. Which countries have moved toward privatization due to the encouragement/coercion of these entities?

3 The authors mention multiple examples of U.S. efforts to privatize previously public programs in other countries. Please identify one such example and explain the process through which privatization occurred. In the example you chose, what was the outcome of privatization?

4 The authors identify *the privatization of public programs* as an ideology. In your own words, describe ideology. Why is it important to identify ideologies? Explain what it means when the authors say that privatization is an ideology. What are the consequences of the ideology of privatization for the debate about Social Security in the United States?

5 The authors discussed the role of Presidential politics in the debate over Social Security privatization in the United States of America. In a paragraph, summarize the current President's position on Social Security (and whether or not she/he supports privatization). In a separate paragraph, write about how things *might have been different* if a different candidate were elected (or had been selected as the primary candidate).

REFERENCES

Amenta, E. (2006). *When movements matter: The Townsend plan & the rise of Social Security*. Princeton, NJ: Princeton University Press.

Andrews, E. (2006). *Pension reform and the development of pension systems: An evaluation of World Bank assistance*. Washington, DC: The World Bank Independent Evaluation Group.

Baker, D. (2007). *The United States since 1980*. New York: Cambridge University Press.

Birnbaum, J. (2005, February 22). Private-Account concept grew from obscure roots. *Washington Post*, p. A01.

Boughton, J. (2001). *Silent revolution: The International Monetary Fund 1979–1989*. Washington, DC: International Monetary Fund.

Butler, S., & Germanis, P. (1983). Achieving a "Leninist" strategy. *Cato Journal*, *3*(2), 547–556.

Center on Budget and Policy Priorities. (2006). *The President's budget: A preliminary analysis*. Retrieved October 20, 2008, from http://www.cbpp.org/2-6-06bud.htm

Commanding Heights. (2000). *Interview with Milton Friedman*. Retrieved October 20, 2008, from http://www.pbs.org/wgbh/commandingheights/shared/minitextlo/int_miltonfriedman.html

Cook, F., Barabas, J., & Page, B. (2002, Summer). Invoking public opinion: Policy elites and Social Security. *Public Opinion Quarterly*, *66*, 235–264.

della Porta, D., & Diani, M. (2006). *Social movements: An introduction*. Malden, MA: Blackwell.

Diani, M., & Bison, I. (2004). Organizations, coalitions, and movements. *Theory and Society*, *33*, 281–309.

Domhoff, G. W. (1996). *State autonomy or class dominance?: Case studies on policy making in America*. New York: Walter de Gruyter.

Elahi, M. (1986). The impact of financial institutions on the realization of human rights: Case study of the International Monetary Fund in Chile. *Boston College Third World Law Journal*, *6*, 143–160.

Estes, C. (1979). *The aging enterprise*. SF: Jossey Bass.

Estes, C. L. (2001). Crisis, the welfare state, and aging: Ideology and agency in the Social Security privatization debate. In C. L. Estes & Associates, *Social policy & aging: A critical perspective* (pp. 95–117). Thousand Oaks, CA: Sage.

Estes, C. L. (2008). A first generation critic comes of age: Reflections of a critical gerontologist. *Journal of Aging Studies*, *22*(2), 120–131.

Ferrara, P. (1980). *Social Security: The inherent contradiction*. Washington, DC: The Cato Institute.

Gramsci, A. (1971). *Selections from the Prison Notebooks* (Q. Hoare, & G. Nowell-Smith, Eds. and Trans.). London: Lawrence & Wishart

House Committee on Oversight and Government Reform. (2007). *Social Security reform costs* (No. GAO-07-621R). Washington, DC: Government Accountability Office. Retrieved October 20, 2008, from http://www.gao.gov/new.items/d07621r.pdf

James, E. (1994). *Averting the old age crisis: Policies to protect the old and promote growth*. Washington, DC: Oxford University Press.

Jary, D., & Jary, J. (Eds.). (1991). *HarperCollins dictionary of sociology*. New York: Harper Perennial.

Johnson, A. (2000). *The Blackwell dictionary of sociology* (2nd ed.). Malden, MA: Blackwell.

Lakoff, G. (2002). *Moral politics: How liberals and conservatives think* (2nd ed.). Chicago: University of Chicago Press.

Laurenti, J. (2000). *Public Priorities in the Allocation of the US Federal Budget*. NY: Global Policy Forum. Retrieved November 7, 2008, from http://www.globalpolicy.org/finance/tables/usspend.htm

Light, P. (1995). *Still artful work: The continuing politics of Social Security reform* (2nd ed.). New York: McGraw-Hill.

Marshall, G. (Ed.). (1996). *The concise Oxford dictionary of sociology*. New York: Oxford University Press.

McAdam, D., Tarrow, S., & Tilly, C. (2001). *Dynamics of contention*. Cambridge: Press Syndicate of The University of Cambridge.

Minority Staff Special Investigations Division Committee on Government Reform. (2005). *The politicization of the Social Security Administration*. Washington, DC: U.S. House of Representatives.

Munnell, A. (2006). Social Security's financial outlook: The 2006 update in perspective [Electronic Version]. *Issue Brief*, *46*. Retrieved November 3, 2008, from http://crr.bc.edu/briefs/social_securitys_financial_outlook_the_2006_update_in_perspective_2.html

Myles, J. (1984). *Old age in the welfare state: The political economy of public pensions*. Boston: Little, Brown and Co.

Office of the Press Secretary. (2005, January 11, 2006). *President participates in conversation on Social Security reform*, held at the Andrew W. Mellon Auditorium, Washington, DC.

Office of Public Affairs, U. S. D. o. t. T. (2004). *Fact sheet on 2004 Social Security & Medicare trustees' reports* (Fact Sheet JS-1252). Washington, DC: U.S. Department of the Treasury. Retrieved October 20, 2008, from http://www.treas.gov/press/releases/js1252.htm

On The Issues. (2007). *Social Security: Candidates' views*. Retrieved October 20, 2008, from http://www.ontheissues.org/Social_Security.htm#Headlines

Pinera, J. (n.d.). *The success of Chile's privatized Social Security*. Retrieved October 20, 2008, from http://www.cato.org/people/pinera.html

PollingReport.com. (2009). *Federal budget & taxes.* Retrieved November 7, 2008, from http://www.pollingreport.com/budget.htm

Pryce, D., & Santorum, R. (2005). *Saving Social Security: A guide to Social Security reform.* Washington, DC: House Republican Conference, Senate Republican Conference and Presentation Testing, Inc.

Robertson, A. (1990). The politics of Alzheimer's disease: A case study in apocalyptic demography. *International Journal of Health Services, 20*(3), 429–442.

Sahadi, J. (2007, November 29). The 3rd rail: Candidates take on Social Security. *CNN-Money.Com.* Retrieved Novemer 29, 2007, from http://money.cnn.com/2007/11/28/pf/taxes/campaign08_SocSec_proposals/?postversion=2007112815

Schor, E. (2007). Bush ties Democrats' hands with recess appointments [Electronic Version]. *TheHill.com.* Retrieved October 20, 2008, from http://thehill.com/index2.php?option=com_content_pdf=1=65272

Sentido.tv Americas. (2006). Bachelet takes office, Chile's first woman head of state. *Casavaria.com.* Retrieved November 3, 2008, from http://www.casavaria.com/sentido/global/americas/2006/06-0314-bachelet.html

Social Security Administration. (1981). *Social Security in America's future: Final report of the National Commission on Social Security, March 1981*. Washington, DC: Social Security Administration. Retrieved October 20, 2008, from http://www.ssa.gov/history/reports/80commission.html

Social Security Administration. (1996a). *1994–1996 Advisory Council on Social Security: Findings, recommendations and statements*. Washington, DC: Social Security Administration. Retrieved October 20, 2008, from http://www.ssa.gov/history/reports/adcouncil/report/findings.htm

Social Security Administration. (1996b). *1994–1996 Advisory Council on Social Security Technical Panel on assumptions and methods*. Washington, DC: Social Security Administration. Retrieved October 20, 2008, from http://www.ssa.gov/history/reports/adcouncil/report/tpa.htm

Social Security Administration. (2001). *The 2001 President's Commission to Strengthen Social Security, Charter*. Washington, DC: Social Security Administration. Retrieved October 20, 2008, from http://www.ssa.gov/history/reports/pcsss/charter.html

Social Security Administration. (2006). *Long-range solvency proposals*. Washington, DC: Social Security Administration. Retrieved October 20, 2008, from http://www.ssa.gov/OACT/solvency/list.html

Social Security Administration. (2007). *Partnerships: Retirement Research Consortium.* Retrieved September 21, 2007, from http://www.ssa.gov/policy/

Svihula, J., & Estes, C. L. (2007). Social Security politics: Ideology and reform. *Journal of Gerontology: Social Sciences*, *62B*(2), S79–S89.

Svihula, J. and Estes, C. L. (2008). Social Security privatization: An ideologically structured movement. *Journal of Sociology and Social Welfare*, *XXXV*(1), 43–103.

Turner, B. S. (Ed.): 2006. *The Cambridge dictionary of sociology*. New York: Cambridge University Press.

Wayne, A. (2005). Social Security overhaul supporters use trustees' report to push case. *CQ Weekly*, 793.

Wayne, A. (2006). Bush trustees reappointed. *CQ Weekly*, 1112.

Wayne, A., & Tollefson, J. (2007). Senate leaders decry Bush's use of recess appointments. *CQ Weekly*, 1126.

Weisbrot, M. (2006). *Latin America: The end of an era* [Electronic Version]. Center for Economic and Policy Research. Retrieved November 3, 2008, from http://www.cepr.net/documents/publications/end_of_era_2006_12.pdf

Weisbrot, M. (2007). A bank of their own: Latin America casting off Washington's shackles [Electronic Version]. *Alternet*. Retrieved October 20, 2008, from http://www.alternet.org/workplace/66529/?page=entire

Williamson, J. (2000). What should the World Bank think about the Washington Consensus? *The World Bank Research Observer*, *15*(2), 251–264.

World Bank. (2001). *Social protection sector strategy: From safety net to springboard*. Washington, DC: The World Bank.

Young, J. (2007). Following Social Security push, liberal coalition tackles Medicare Advantage. *TheHill.com.* Retrieved November 3, 2009, from http://thehill.com/business–lobby/following-social-security-push-liberal-coalition-tackles-medicare-advantage-2007-06-12.html

Zald, M. (2000). Ideologically structured action: An enlarged agenda for social movement research. *Mobilization*, *5*(1), 1–16.

13

A Normative Approach to Social Security: What Dignity Requires

MARTHA HOLSTEIN

Policy analysts often deny that policy and ethics share a central commitment—to make evaluative judgments of what is good or right in human conduct. Yet, policy is, after all, the expression of some common consensus, albeit generally tacit, of the values society chooses to incorporate into law. Although not all policy choices are about ethical values, if we think about the great policy debates that we are already facing in the 21st century, such as embryonic stem cell research, preemptive war, and access to health care, it is clear that ethical values repeatedly infiltrate policy analysis, policy making, and policy evaluation. They must. Even the popular cost-benefit analysis assumes the priority of one value—efficiency—and requires a determination of what goods will count as benefits.

Similarly, contemporary debates about Social Security are as much about values as about what ought to be done to keep the system from going "broke." Is the most important concern the individualistic one—return on investment, albeit often at high risk—or is it assuring a reliable, steady source of income through a collective commitment to older people, people with disabilities, and surviving family members no matter the contingent circumstances of their lives? Are we protecting the right of the autonomous person to act in his or her own self-interest, or are we acknowledging that because no individual is an island unto him or herself, we have obligations toward one another?

This chapter will address the moral values that I believe must be central to any system that so directly influences well-being for families and for individuals in later life. The values I support are dignity and gender equity, which must rest on a core commitment to social solidarity. These particular moral values have deep salience for women and other less privileged individuals. Contrary to the expectations of "third way" social welfare or the rhetoric of the "risk society," which assumes that primary responsible for well-being rests with individuals, families, and the market (Baars, 2006; Sevenhuijsen, 2000), few people or families are able to garner sufficient resources to manage their basic expenses in old age without a strong, reliable, and publicly guaranteed income floor that they cannot outlive. In the absence of this floor, dignity and the very possibility of autonomy are impossible. Economic insecurity damages self-respect and the possibility of living in valued ways. To assure this floor, a sustainable collective commitment to economic security and gender justice is necessary. The value-based analysis that I will undertake can elucidate the ethical choices at stake and the effects of alternative choices when policies are under development (prospectively), when changes are proposed, and when they are evaluated (retrospectively). It can also do more; it can defend the priority of certain moral values as central to a dignified old age.

If dignity in old age is thus central, as it is at other ages, I will argue that the best way to help assure its realization is by a commitment to social solidarity and collective responsibility that unifies generations and different social and economic strata in our society. It requires that all eligible individuals recognize that some intergenerational transfers, such as Social Security in which the taxes that working people pay help to finance benefits for the older generation, are a responsibility of citizenship. I would also hold that this commitment should serve, better than it does now, people who are poor or less well off, especially women.

Abandoning the universal, age-based features of Social Security for a means-tested or a privatized system (either in whole or in part) or reducing benefits, especially for the least well off, would threaten these critically important moral values and further jeopardize those individuals already disadvantaged by the current system. As a polity, we should not abandon the now historically sanctioned moral understandings that affirmed a collective responsibility for guaranteeing some portion of retirement income for all older people, regardless of their other sources of income. Maintaining Social Security as a universal age-based entitlement is the morally correct distributional scheme for the immediate and probably more distant future. This moral understanding requires only minimal renegotiation in anticipating the retirement of the baby boom generation.

SOCIAL SECURITY: HISTORICAL VALUE ASSUMPTIONS

Although the program that emerged in 1935 had a complex political history, it rested on implicit assumptions that reflected the social world occupied by the men who designed it—working men placed in economic jeopardy by the Depression most often through no fault of their own. In addition to moving them out of the work force, Social Security was seen as an earned prize rewarding men who followed the rules established by the genderized norms that dominated the 19th and early 20th centuries. The underlying social contract and the fact that everyone contributed to the system, its creators reasoned, would make it acceptable to those who scorned welfare as giving something for nothing. Social Security indirectly created another value that has long governed life in the industrialized nations.

By assuring some guaranteed income in retirement, Social Security supported the creation of a new life stage and became the central feature of what became the normative life course in the industrialized west (Kohli, 1991). This new normative life course, introduced in Germany in the last third of the 19th century, transformed age from a cultural category to an independent dimension of social structure. This transformation—resting on the greater certainty that one would reach old age, a certain normalization in the family cycle, the sharper age stratification of society with the advent of salaried labor, and the increasing focus on the individual and life as a designed product—has generated the perception that retirement is an entitlement, an earned right that comes after a sustained work life. That right is now under subtle attack and is one of the underlying but unarticulated tensions in the debate about the future of Social Security.

ACHIEVING CORE VALUES: SOCIAL INSURANCE VS. MEANS TESTING

I place dignity at the center of my assessment of public policies designed to provide an income floor. For Avashai Margalit (1996), an Israeli philosopher, dignity is "the feeling of respect people feel toward themselves as human beings." A decent society has institutions that "do not violate the dignity of the people in its orbit" (p. 51). For Canadian philosopher Charles Taylor (1989), dignity is the sense of "ourselves as commanding (attitudinal) respect" (p. 15). It shapes and, therefore, is prior to, our choices, desires, and interests and gives them a strong evaluative component. Our choices are thus related to our need to see ourselves as having dignity. This moral concern is not secondary to "either rational articulations of what an unencumbered human would choose or what utility calculations (e.g., cost–benefit analysis) suggest" (Taylor, 1989, p. 8). In a *Theory of Justice*, American philosopher John Rawls (1972) argues that most people, "would wish to avoid at almost any cost the social conditions that undermine their self–respect," which is "perhaps the most important of all the primary goods" (p. 440, p. 396). Robert Goodin (1982), an Australian philosopher, identifies what he calls moral primitives for which no further justification is needed; dignity is central. Dignity demands a minimum standard of decent treatment for every individual "not to be sacrificed for any less weighty considerations" (Goodin, 1982, p. 85). It is particularly important for older Americans when a sense of "otherness" (de Beauvoir, 1972) can overcome the belief that one is a person worthy of respect.

As Margalit (1996) points out, humiliation, which undermines dignity, "does not mean that one's rights have been violated, but rather that one is incapable of demanding them" (p. 36). The Social Security system, as constituted, gives us the simplest tools to assert our rights—our age, work history, and marital status—thereby supporting an elemental aspect of dignity. If we meet these criteria, we are guaranteed earned benefits. Compare this procedure to that required by Temporary Aid for Needy Families (TANF), which is provided on a categorical basis with specific provisions that recipients are expected to meet. Replacing traditional welfare programs, TANF carries the historic stigma associated with such programs. Stigma and proving one's deservingness cannot coexist with dignity. At no time in our history have means-tested programs recognized this fact. Although not usually phrased this way in the policy debate, the morally important distinction between social insurance and supplemental security income or TANF rests on this understanding of dignity and its centrality to human well-being.

The need to protect social insurance from the attacks of individuals who insist that we "cannot afford" entitlements rests on its further connection to what it takes to lead a human life—to do so requires a threshold of economic security. Not that long ago, the Director of the

Office of Management and Budget (OMB) was kown to have calmly stated that the country cannot afford the growing population of older people. Thus, substantial changes to entitlement programs were necessary. End of story. I detected no recognition from the speaker that this policy direction might affect real people who lacked his assurance of an adequate pension and the salary reserves that permitted saving. I use this example to suggest how the world as seen through the lens of privilege can ignore the human costs of its perspective. Individuals who see the world through this lens assume that their perspective is universal rather than partial; therefore, it requires no examination because it is putatively value-free, unfiltered. For people outside the privilege-power nexus, this partial perspective contributes to what feminists call oppression (Walker, 1998; Young, 1990). Oppression takes many forms, such as exploitation, marginalization, and exclusion. These characteristics are incompatible with dignity because they bar people from claiming their rights, render them relatively powerless, and deny them the chance to define their own needs (Fraser, 1987).

SOCIAL SOLIDARITY AND HUMAN INTERDEPENDENCE

In the case of old-age security, supporting dignity requires sustaining the muted American values of social solidarity and human interdependence. In an era that focuses almost exclusively on protecting individual autonomy, Social Security reminds us that each of us owes a debt to past generations. We would, quite literally, not exist "had not someone and some society taken responsibility for our welfare. . . . If we value our own life at all, then we must value and feel some obligation toward those who made that life possible" (Callahan, 1981, p. 77). Such ties are a "matter of moral intuition, social common sense, and obligatory notions of reciprocity, part of what once was called civil society" (Wolfe, 1989, p. 101). They also reflect emerging feminist views about relational autonomy, the social embeddedness of the self, and the inevitability of unchosen obligations (MacKenzie & Stoljar, 2000; Baier, 1994).

Ties of social obligation and reciprocity are ways to assure that, for example, we raise the next generation of children to understand the meaning of justice or to know what a promise means (Baier, 1994; Elshtain, 1995). Social Security thus recognizes that we are, throughout our lives, inevitably and importantly connected to others and that we would not have grown to be adults without the help of previous generations

(Wolfe, 1989). Social solidarity is a "necessary condition for the flourishing of the subjective life"; a human being understood holistically is more socially committed, socially shaped, and socially nourished than much recent ethical thinking would have us believe (Anjos, 1994, p. 139).

In contemporary American society, with its prevailing emphasis on atomistic individualism, there are few public expressions of social solidarity and interdependence. Yet, many of our deepest moral sentiments, supported by research in moral psychology and other domains, reinforce the importance of the social. Without visible expressions of community, we lack the social glue that binds individuals into a society. Yet, we rarely acknowledge the social goals of Social Security, and so, we do not stimulate informed discussion about the losses that might occur if those goals withered. Social Security, though framed in terms of a contract, more accurately embodies what are generally deeply held notions of reciprocity. Although relations of social obligation and reciprocity are not always freely chosen, they are required for the continuity of a just society (Baier, 1994). The fact that each of us pays in to the system and then anticipates receiving benefits through a tacit relationship with generations to follow reinforces the important moral concern with reciprocity. This aspect deserves more attention than it has received. Such bonds are not merely incidental, they are morally honorable and necessary.

Recent suggestions to privatize Social Security, although subject to criticism on many grounds, would fundamentally challenge the intergenerational compact that the existing system embodies. The moral understanding that has long seemed to be in place is that society has obligations to its members if they have, throughout their lives, honored their commitments. Social Security reflects that obligation. Amitai Etzioni (2005) points out that "to deny or to significantly dilute these commitments evokes the same sense of unfairness and injustice we experience upon hearing that an insurance company has canceled its policies when its policyholders became sick or when they retroactively and unilaterally change the terms of the policy" (p. 39).

Although cloaked in individualistic language, Social Security represented a collective effort, which Martin Kohli (1991) described as "morally bounded claims and expectations" (p. 276), which join one generation to another in a formally enacted system of transfer. In this way, Social Security also created what Kohli labeled a "social citizen." Social citizenship implies social obligation; by virtue of having met certain criteria in the past, one has claims on common social resources. Each subsequent generation has similar claims. An intergenerational compact, tacit or otherwise, must exist for this claim to be practically realized. This social citizen had "legitimate claims to continuity throughout the life course" (Kohli, 1991, p. 286). The operative word here is continuity.

Such claims, when combined with Social Security provisions that support adequacy (in contrast to equity), illuminate efforts to incorporate two conceptions of justice: The meritocratic, that is, rights earned by the hard work that all had the opportunity to pursue, and protection of the most vulnerable among the aged population. Indirectly, by giving the individual the foundation, though hardly adequate, to live his or her life in rough continuity with the past, the system nurtured individual autonomy. Such cash transfers support dignity (Margalit, 1996). In this way, the response of the United States to the perceived situation of its older members has blended different—and conflictive—normative assumptions that reflect alternative approaches to meeting norms of reciprocity as collectively understood in given times and places.

Social Security permits the sharing of risks at a time in life when risk is potentially imminent. By providing some help to younger generations in terms of financing their parents' retirement, it helps to assure the stability of generations over time. One need only recall the "family economies" of the late 19th and early 20th centuries (Haber & Gratton, 1994) to understand the potentially bruising results that future generations would experience from increased family responsibility. The Depression simply re-emphasized what most middle-class and working class families already knew—the family economy could not withstand endless pressures (Haber & Gratton, 1994). Today, with the average incomes of younger adults lower than they were 30 years ago (Herbert, 2007), they would be especially hard-pressed to provide financial assistance to parents or grandparents. For the older generation, Social Security lessens fears about being a burden on their children and, for some, facilitates continued contributions to successor generations. In this way, it encourages the ongoing recognition and practice of reciprocal and interdependent relationships while mitigating the troubling aspects of asymmetrical relationships that develop, as parents need more from their children.

Thus, Social Security contributes to maintaining ties of interdependency and solidarity. The normative life course, which Social Security helped to create and sustain, frees up a number of individuals, often in relatively good health, to contribute to society in ways often unavailable to younger working parents of families. We might, of course, achieve the same ends if benefits were needs–based, but it would be less likely for two reasons. First, the sense of security that comes with assured age–based entitlements is liberating and can encourage the person to pursue socially constructive interests. Second, there is always the risk that means testing can, for example, insist on work requirements for the healthy without concern for the number or quality of jobs available. In this way, the possibilities of contributing to the social good through alternative activities would be reduced while also exacerbating income inequalities between the healthy and those with health problems.

With these values paramount, Social Security does not place the older people, people with disabilities, and surviving widows and children in a position of subordination to legislators and bureaucrats who make decisions about other social welfare policies. As noted above, claiming their rights is nondemeaning, because it does not require such subordination to power. These collective commitments have reduced poverty among older people, one of the great achievements of the past half century. In apt phrasing, Schultz and Binstock (2006) warn us that without such strong commitments, the "Golden Years" can easily become the "Tarnished Years" (p. 7). We must each be able to rely on the moral sense and commitment of future, unknown strangers to keep public commitments in place and to acknowledge what is contrary to the individualism that is so pervasive in American society, that we live in an interdependent world where our successes and failures are "never entirely our own" (Robertson, 1997, p. 446).

GENDER EQUITY

Women's economic status is a harsh reminder and indictment of the neoliberal assumption that the market, the individual, and the family can be responsible for old-age security. It is particularly ironic because, as I write these words, the market is gyrating and losses are dramatic. But even in the absence of this continued erosion of savings, how will people who have raised two or three children on less than $50,000 a year (and that is considerably above the poverty line) be able to save the approximately 17% to 25% of their income from the time that they are 21 years of age that is necessary to assure some modicum of ease in old age (Polivka & Longino, 2006)? To be near poor means one is always at risk for losing one's home or not being able to afford rent in a decent neighborhood, being unable to afford medical care despite Medicare, or reducing their food budget, and having no resources for any leisure time activities. These bare statistics hide great suffering and mock the rhetoric of a dignified old age (Holstein, unpub., 2007).

Our ability to make ends meet and to weather the vicissitudes of life in old age are laid down by midlife are largely structural in origin. We have less control over the genderized labor market and normative family expectations than we might wish to have. As a result, advantages and disadvantages accumulate over time (Crystal & Shea, 1990; O'Rand, 1996; Dannefer; 2003). Today, we must also add neoliberal ideology to the factors that make escaping structural constraints all the more difficult. For people who were never well-served by the market, today's market crises can only make it worse and enlarge the number of people harmed by market failure.

Furthermore, as other chapters in this book detail more fully, the normative life course that Social Security helped establish did not speak to women's experiences. Their responsibilities for the health and well-being of children, grandchildren, elderly parents, and spouses meant their work experiences differed from those of men. Although women may treasure these responsibilities (and maybe also resent them or feel a combination of pride in accomplishment and resentment simultaneously), they are essentially unchosen and directly connected to Social Security. Both anticipated and unanticipated interruptions of work affect Social Security benefit levels. The more dropout years she has, the lower her benefit level will be when she retires. This penalty might not matter for the woman who stays married to the same, higher-earning man for her entire married life, but this pattern is becoming more and more uncommon in a society where divorce affects one out of every two marriages. Even the much praised and prized Family and Medical Leave Act of 1993 does not consider the long-term implications of taking time away from paid work. To achieve gender equity will require a rethinking of social insurance more generally.

CONTEMPORARY CHALLENGES TO SOCIAL INSURANCE

Although Social Security has changed over the years, contemporary challenges are different—they are highly politicized and ideological. The crisis mentality, which permits, indeed encourages, actions that might not be countenanced without the aura of crises, can also be understood as a renegotiation of the moral understandings that have formed certain patterns of responsibilities and accountabilities to the elderly over the past 50 years. Although few politicians would attack the program openly, indirect attacks and attacks from the "facts" are common. The indirect attacks started in the early 1980s, couched in the terms of "intergenerational equity." The accusations were bold and seemingly based on the incontrovertible evidence that the old were no longer the poorest segment of American society. Yet, there is no compelling evidence that entitlement programs for the old hold hostage—both literally and figuratively—current and future generations of children (Williamson, McNamara, & Howling, 2003). As an opening wedge in the war against the old, however, the arguments fed into the strengthening conservative ideology, whose grip on the country has withstood multiple failures of business and public policies. Yet, despite downward trends, poverty rates among America's older population are still the highest among the rich nations (Smeeding & Sullivan, 1998, cited in Myles & Quadagno, 1999). Few are wealthy or even near wealthy; for example, three quarters of Medicare recipients have incomes under $25,000 a year.

Purposefully seeking to divide the old from the young in this way will serve neither group. Entitlement programs are important for both young and old and can be accurately described as family policies (Schultz & Binstock, 2006). For those older people with substantial disposable incomes, the fairest way to "recoup" excess income is to tax all higher-income people at a more progressive rate. The income tax, which is sensitive to individual fluctuations in income, also protects older people who may experience a sudden and substantial reduction in their incomes because of catastrophic illness or the costs of long-term care. Indeed, if we move to the needs–based programming that "generational equity" supporters advocate, the most likely political scenario is that all will lose (see below for a further discussion of means testing). While in a different political environment that might not happen, in the United States today, the prevailing attitude of lawmakers suggests losses for all if efforts are made to dissolve the boxes of age-segregated policies (Hudson, 2007). Ironically, the success of Social Security, the savings, investment, the work habits of a Depression–era generation, and the thriving post–World War II economy have come to haunt this generation of older people.

Most dramatic have been the proposals to privatize the system in whole or in part and means testing in some way. Privatization, couched in terms of "saving" Social Security while also improving individual returns, is part of a larger agenda to undermine collective responsibility for economic well-being in old age (Holstein, unpub.). Further, the neoliberal position denies the structural origins of social inequality, holding instead that individuals are free to make decisions about their own lives, especially savings and investment decisions. Even if they had the resources to make such decisions, privatization can do little for the most vulnerable who do not have very much to put into private accounts, who have no history of investing, and who, when they do invest, do so cautiously (Hardy, 2000). Nor does it recognize the difficulties faced in old age by those who were unable to 'compete effectively during the relatively few years in which capital must be earned and partially invested for the future" (Baars, 2006, p. 31).

Less radical are changes that would delay the age at which an individual could collect full benefits and reduce overall benefits. These proposed changes rest on the premise that Americans are healthier than they once were and that the retirement of the baby boom generation can overload the system's financial stability. Discussion of these proposed reforms tend to ignore the ill health of many older Americans and the inability or the unwillingness of American business to support the continued working life of their older employees. Delaying the age at which a person may collect full benefits serves the wage system even as it responds to the better health of some of today's older people. By making retirement less attractive and less possible for many people, especially women, such changes in Social Security move a previously exempt class of workers into the competitive job market. Because women tend to have fewer alternative sources of income than men do, they will experience the strongest pressure to continue working at whatever jobs are available. This move does not then support gender equity.

The elevation of individual responsibility (with little concern for the larger economic or social context in which people have grown to old age) and increasing disregard for common concerns over, or at least parallel to, individual ones dominate the political agenda. This insistence on contextualism acknowledges that we can achieve important human ends differently and that historical and political location shape and shade the available moral options that forward those ends. As such, I favor a critical theory perspective that grounds normative reflection in a specific historical and social context (Young, 1990, p. 5). To understand (and judge) morality adequately, we must be able to envision the effects of its enactment in the lived world. We must also be concerned with how people, affected by these social and political practices, understand them. Thus, the state ought to guarantee those conditions under which its citizens can actually make choices that support their version of the good life.

In this environment in which there are few guarantees that programs for the most needy will not be subject to a wide range of political ends, including a balanced budget or tax reduction, means-tested programs are not a good response. Means testing would require older people, at a time when they may already have lost much of what is valued in American society, to "prove" that they are worthy of receiving benefits to gatekeepers of resources. They would have to do so in the face of many competing priorities for public resources in a period of tough parsimony, or what some have called "tough love."

There are also significant racial and gender dimensions to consider. Those who will be in the competitive pool are far more likely to be women, and especially women of color. This in itself presents another significant problem of justice. In the late 19th century, English researcher Charles Booth conducted an extensive study of poverty. He found that "there is no parallel in feeling between the taking of a sum of money to which a man is legally entitled and the suing in *forma pauperis* for a benefit that might be granted or postponed or withheld, and the granting of which must, in the public interest, be protected by preliminary suspicion and searching inquiry" (quoted in Goodin, 1985, pp. 37–38). This contrast—between a benefit to which one is legally entitled and one of which one must "sue" on the basis of poverty—continues to hold today. Older people willingly accept benefits based on social insurance but they often apply for means-tested benefits, such as Medicaid, reluctantly, especially if it means opening one's finances to public scrutiny as the "price" of becoming eligible for benefits.

Moreover, we could not assure that future political leaders would not hold lower–income older people "accountable" for their low incomes. Blame, not unfamiliar on the American political landscape, is inherently antithetical to dignity and solidarity. Means testing cannot guarantee that individuals have claims that cannot be denied; thus, means testing cannot support the dignity that comes with claiming what one deserves by right. Means testing further weakens the already eroded sense of a commonality among Americans of vastly different backgrounds. It is unlikely that it could support the two moral values this essay holds as central (dignity and gender equity). Needs are notoriously shifty concepts; so too are expectations placed on recipients of publicly granted benefits. In contrast, benefits offered as age–based entitlements do not require explicitly determined needs that others have the power to define (Elshtain, 1995). The tax system provides the most equitable vehicle to moderate even this outcome. Moreover, "it is arguable that more poor elderly have been helped by the relative invulnerability of age–based programs than would have been helped had programs been more narrowly targeted to the poor" (Daniels, 1988, p. 10). It is better, therefore, that some get more than they need than for many to be left with an uncertain future when they have scarce opportunity to improve their situation.

It is also beneficial to remember that losses often accumulate in old age. New images of "successful" or "productive" aging cannot foreclose this reality for large numbers of older people. Death of a spouse or a child, illness, and disability give the older person few chances to recoup. Savings are quickly consumed and emotional reserves exhausted. Yet, it would be at this very time that the older person would have to prove worthy of public support if programs were means tested. Simultaneously, when individuals are at their weakest, the needs for social solidarity are the strongest. Needs–based programs cannot respond to this requirement.

Perhaps even more importantly, there are some values that "constitute moral progress over particular alternatives," because they support human welfare (Kekes, 1993, pp. 160, 214). Attributing primary moral importance to dignity and the social solidarity required to support it, affirms that there are valued moral "goods" that are superior to economic or market values and that cannot be sacrificed without compelling reasons. In this present period public, universal, age–based policies are an important means to support dignity in old age. Simultaneously, they are reminders that we are indebted to the past, owe to the future, and have responsibilities for the more vulnerable amongst us. They also offer the greatest possibility for creating reforms that are sensitive to women's lives. This position does not mean that any policy modifications are unacceptable (they would be acceptable as long as they upheld the core values defined above). In particular, the system can eliminate the worst of its regressive features by general fund financing and a more progressive income tax. However, for now, these options do not even appear to be near, let alone on, the table.

CONCLUSION

Social Security, despite recent efforts to derail and discredit it, is extremely popular. It is also inadequate, in part, because it reinforces the polarization of wealth that occurs throughout one's lifetime and fails to account for changes in family structure (i.e., divorce, single parent households). Yet, at the very least it tilts toward adequacy. Public resistance to privatization schemes suggests that most people believe its goals are both important and reasonably well met. In this country, we seem to have a fairly consistent belief that poverty (and ill health) in old age are sources of threat that deserve a response (adapted from Baier, 1985). (These needs are equally pressing at younger ages, but so far, we have failed to respond adequately.)

Once the goals of Social Security are extended to include the moral values of dignity and gender equity supported by the elevation of social solidarity over individual autonomy, an argument based on alternative framings, such as the utilitarian criteria of efficiency and effectiveness, becomes difficult to support. Such arguments rarely include these non-quantifiable moral values. Without addressing the wide–ranging critique of such thinking (Williams & Sen, 1982), it is still safe to say that it ignores much of what moral psychology has learned about what humans value and how these values support qualitative distinctions of worth (Taylor, 1989). Arguments based solely on utilitarian criteria cannot sustain a broad democratic ethos in which ties of relationships are central and where the notion of citizenship means active participation in the good of the community. Efficiency/effectiveness arguments thus obscure important social values. Efficiency is but one among many values that ought to count in deciding how to respond to human need. Yet, it has played a particularly strong role in policy formulation. Seemingly quantifiable, "it purges moral analysis of all of its difficult—and essential characteristics." That is, its singularity means that choices among competing ethical values do not even appear as problematic (Amy, 1984, p. 587). This position evades the complexities of democratic decision making and the core demands of citizenship.

Although Social Security alone cannot support a wavering democratic ethos, it serves as a reminder that ties of social obligation (even if not specifically chosen) and mutual interdependence are part of what it means to be human. Moreover, they contribute to the provision of social goods that most of us view as primary. Of course, one might suggest that, because these goods are so highly valued, they should be made available to all Americans. And if our social accounting considered all social welfare costs rather than just the direct costs, we might discover the resources necessary to provide these goods more broadly. However, given the unlikeliness of such a scenario, it makes no sense to take away from the old what would be desirable for all to have.

DISCUSSION QUESTIONS

1. According to Holstein, what is the key criticism of plans to privatize Social Security?
2. For what reason is Holstein critical of the use of efficiency/effectiveness (cost-benefit analysis) as the only tool for policy analysis and evaluation?
3. What is interdependence? In what ways does Social Security recognize and reflect interdependence? What is reciprocity? In what ways does Social Security require and support reciprocity?
4. Holstein argues that dignity and gender equity are important values through which to analyze the current Social Security system and future policy options. Using the Internet, newspapers, and magazines, but *not* academic journals, locate at least two examples of approaches to Social Security that are based in either or both of these values. Your examples may be as small as a paragraph in a larger news article or a one-page ad in a magazine.
5. In a small group, select a current policy debate and identify the multiple values used to evaluate the policy and to justify changes to it. At least one person must focus on the use of efficiency/effectiveness as a value through which the policy is discussed. Other possible values include dignity, gender equity, human/civil rights, environmental sustainability, nonmalfeasance, or others that you identify. Create a poster that identifies the multiple values circulating in this policy debate, and which groups of people are employing which values to make their case.

References

Amy, D. J. (1984). Why policy analysis and ethics are incompatible. *Journal of Policy Analysis and Management*, 3, 573–591.

Anjos, M. (1994). Bioethics in a liberationist key. In E. Dubose, R. Hamel, & L. O'Connell (Eds.), *A matter of principles? Ferment in U.S. bioethics* (p. 139). Valley Forge, PA: Trinity Press International.

Baars, J. (2006). Beyond neomodernism, antimodernism, and postmodernism: Basic categories for contemporary critical gerontology. In J. Baars, D. Dannefer, C. Phillipson, & A. Walker (Eds.), *Aging, globalization, and inequality: The new critical gerontology* (pp. 17–42). Amityville, NY: Bayview Publishing Co.

Baier, A. (1985). *Postures of the mind.* Minneapolis, MN: University of Minnesota Press.

Baier, A. (1994). *Moral prejudices: Essays on ethics*. Cambridge: Harvard University Press.

Callahan, D. (1981). What obligations do we have to future generations? In E. Partridge (Ed.), *Responsibilities to future generations: Environmental ethics* (p. 77). Buffalo, NY: Prometheus 1988.

Crystal, S., & Shea, D. (1990). Cumulative advantage, cumulative disadvantage, and inequality among elderly people. *The Gerontologist, 30*(4), 437–443.

Daniels, N. (1988). *Am I my parent's keeper?* New York: Oxford University Press.

Dannefer, D. (2003). Cumulative advantage/disadvantage and the life course: Cross-fertilizing age and social science theory. *Journal of Gerontology: Social Sciences, 58B*(6), S327–S337.

De Beauvoir, S. (1972). *The coming of age*. New York: Putnam.

Elshtain, J. B. (1995). *Democracy on trial*. New York: Basic Books.

Etzioni, A. (2005). End game: What the elderly have earned. *American Scholar*, Spring, pp. 32-40.

Fraser, N. (1987). Women, welfare, and the politics of needs interpretation. *Hypatia, 2*, 103–121.

Goodin, R. (1982). *Political theory and public policy*. Chicago: University of Chicago Press.

Goodin, R. (1985). Self—reliance versus the welfare state. *Journal of Social Policy, 14*, 25–47.

Haber, C., & Gratton, B. (1994). *Old age and the search for security*. Bloomington and Indianapolis, IN: University of Indiana Press.

Hardy, M. (2000). Commentary: Control, choice and collective concerns: Challenges of individualized social policy. In W. Schaie & J. Hendricks (Eds.), *The evolution of the aging self: The societal impact of the aging process* (pp. 251–268). New York: Springer.

Herbert, B. (2007, October 6). Send in the clowns. *New York Times*, p. A27.

Holstein, M. (2007). *Economic (in)security across generations: Background, analysis, and policy recommendations, a white paper.* Unpublished manuscript.

Hudson, R. (2007). The political paradoxes of thinking outside the life-cycke boxes. In R. Pruchno & M. Smyer (Eds.), *Challenges of an aging society: Ethical dilemmas, political issues* (pp. 268–284). Baltimore: Johns Hopkins University Press.

Kekes, J. (1993). *The morality of pluralism.* Princeton, NJ: Princeton University Press

Kohli, M. (1991). Retirement and the moral economy: An historical interpretation of the German case. In M. Minkler & C. Estes (Eds.), *Critical perspectives on aging: The political and moral economy of growing old* (pp. 273–292). Amityville, NY: Baywood Publishing Co.

MacKenzie, C., & Stoljar, N. (2000). *Relational autonomy: Feminist perspectives on autonomy, agency, and the social self.* New York: Oxford University Press.

Margalit, A. (1996). *The decent society.* Cambridge: Harvard University Press.

Myles, J., & Quadagno, J. (1999). Envisioning a third way: The welfare state in the twenty-first century. *Contemporary Sociology, 29*(1), 156–167.

O'Rand, A. (1996). The precious and the precocious: Understanding cumulative disadvantage and cumulative advantage over the life course. *The Gerontologist, 36*(2), 230–238.

Polivka, L., & Longino, C. (2006). The emerging postmodern culture of aging and retirement security. In J. Baars, D. Dannefer, C. Phillipson, & A. Walker (Eds.), *Aging, globalization, and inequality: The new critical gerontology* (pp. 183–204). Amityville, NY: Baywood Publishing Co., Inc.

Rawls, J. (1972). *A theory of justice*. Cambridge: Harvard University Press.
Robertson, A. (1997). Beyond apocalyptic demography: Towards a moral economy of interdependency. *Ageing and Society*, *17*(4), 425–446.
Schultz, J., & Binstock, R. (2006). *Aging nation: The economics and politics of growing older in America.* New York: Praeger.
Sevenhuijsen, S. (2000). Caring in the third way: The relations between obligation, responsibility and care in third way discourse. *Critical Social Policy*, *20*(5), 5–37.
Smeeding, T. M., & Sullivan, D. H. (1998). Generations and the distribution of economic well-being: A cross-national view (Luxembourg Income Study, Working Paper Series, No. 173). As cited in J. Myles & J. Quadagno. *Envisioning a third way: The welfare state in the twenty-first century*.
Taylor, C. (1989). *Sources of the self.* Cambridge, MA: Harvard University Press.
Walker, M. U. (1998). *Moral understandings: A feminist study in ethics.* London: Routledge.
Williams, B., & Sen, A. (1982). *Utilitarianism and beyond*. Cambridge, England: Cambridge University Press.
Williamson, J. B., McNamara, T. K., & Howling, S. A. (2003). Generational equity, generational interdependence, and the framing of the debate over social security reform. *Journal of Sociology and Social Welfare*, *30*(3), 3–14.
Wolfe, A. (1989). *Whose keeper? Social science and moral obligation.* Berkeley: University of California Press.
Young, I. M. (1990). *Gender and the politics of difference.* Princeton, NJ: Princeton University Press.

14

Public Opinion and Social Insurance: The American Experience

FAY LOMAX COOK AND MEREDITH B. CZAPLEWSKI

Generations of Americans have come to think of Social Security and Medicare as part of the lexicon of the American experience—programs to which they have contributed and on which they or their parents or grandparents rely. Since their enactment—Social Security in 1935 and Medicare in 1965—both programs have grown incrementally in response to changing needs and changing times. Both programs have experienced enormous public support in the past (Cook & Barrett, 1992; Page & Simmons, 2000), but in recent years, critics have harshly criticized Social Security and Medicare and called them into question as bad investments, financially unsustainable, and ready for major reform (Kotlikoff & Burns, 2004; Peterson, 2004). Proponents have argued just as strongly that Social Security and Medicare remain excellent investments and financially sustainable with reasonable adjustments and incremental reforms (Marmor & Mashaw, 2006; Baker & Weisbrot, 1999).

At the policy elite level, the discussion about Social Security and Medicare has gone from a *politics of consensus* in which there was widespread support and relatively few publicly expressed differences of opinion to what might be called a *politics of dissensus,* where disagreement is heated and a tremendous amount of political rhetoric is being espoused about the state of the programs (Oberlander, 2003; Cook, 2005). Where does the public stand?

With rhetoric flying about the "crises" surrounding the programs, political commentators, interest group spokespersons, and policy makers often invoke what they claim are the views of the public to make the points they want to make. The problem is that the claims they make are often wrong (Cook, Barabas, & Page, 2002). At a time when the debates about Social Security and Medicare are likely to continue and when various reform proposals are being forwarded, it is useful to step back and assess where public views of the two programs stand and what reforms, if any, the public favors. That is the purpose of this chapter.

Public support for Social Security and Medicare are often said to rest on two pillars of public opinion: (1) a belief in the purpose of the programs and a commitment to them and (2) a belief that the programs are affordable public expenditures (Marttila, 2005; Cook & Barrett, 1992). Given the claims about the "bankruptcy" that the programs face as well as the debates about the programs that have played out in the mass media, to what extent has there been an erosion in these two sets of beliefs? Proponents of reform often rest their arguments for change on the charge that the public is losing confidence in the programs and that the lowered confidence will produce an erosion in public support, reflecting a loss of belief in the purpose of the programs. Furthermore, the claims of bankruptcy that buttress reform proponents' demands for change could well undermine the public's belief that Social Security and Medicare are affordable public expenditures. Using a wide range of public opinion polls, this chapter examines the extent to which the public actually holds both sets of beliefs in the purpose of the programs and in the viability of each as public expenditures.

Public opinion toward Social Security and Medicare needs to receive careful evaluation. Particular attention should be paid to survey items that were worded in identical or similar ways over a long period of time. As survey researchers know, poll results are very sensitive to how questions are worded because even slightly different wording can sometimes result in different responses. Examining identically or similarly worded questions from several surveys over time allows real trends and patterns in public opinion to be identified. In this chapter, we present a review of dozens of separate public opinion survey items. The review demonstrates that members of the public remain highly committed to the two programs, but have concerns about the programs' financial situations.

FROM THE POLITICS OF CONSENSUS TO THE POLITICS OF DISSENSUS

Until the mid-1990s, the politics of both Social Security and Medicare were marked by relative consensus with, for the most part, deliberative, bipartisan support of incremental policy changes (Cook, 2005; Oberlander, 2003). For Social Security, the Republican Congressional landslide in 1994 brought with it attacks on Social Security as unaffordable and an unwise financial investment. Since then, critics have claimed that the way to "save" Social Security is to partially privatize it by allowing people to invest some or all of their Social Security payroll taxes in the stock market, while defenders have often argued that the program is "sacrosanct" and that any tinkering would be destructive (Marmor & Mashaw, 2006).

The most recent Social Security debate began during the second term of the Clinton administration and came to a head during the second term of the Bush administration when President Bush made reforming Social Security the major item on his domestic policy agenda. In his 2005 State of the Union address, he called the Social Security system "unsustainable," "in crisis," and "bankrupt" (Bush, 2005). He advocated incorporating within Social Security a system of personal retirement accounts into which workers would invest a certain percentage of their payroll Social Security contributions (4% was proposed by his Commission). President Bush's proposal to partially privatize Social Security stalled in Congress in 2005 and 2006, but in 2008, each of the initial six Republican presidential candidates said they supported private accounts. The initial eight Democratic presidential contenders offered a variety of incremental policy changes, such as higher payroll taxes on higher wage earners and raising the age of eligibility (AssistGuide Information Services, 2007). Clearly, the debate will continue to be marked by divisions between the leadership in the Republican and Democratic parties.

Similar to Social Security, until the mid-1990s, Medicare politics was marked by consensus, with deliberative bipartisan support of major policy reforms and implicit acceptance of the idea that Medicare should be operated as a universal government program (Oberlander, 2003). However, this consensus fell apart abruptly in 1994, as elites became ideologically differentiated over the understanding of the program's philosophy. This division occurred primarily along the view of whether medical care should be considered a market good or a medically determined need (Oliver, Lee, & Lipton, 2004). While there was common acceptance among elites in the 1990s that the Medicare program needed adjustment (Marmor, 2000), advocates for health care reform were ever more dividing into "marketist" and "medicalist" camps (Glied, 1997). Earlier politics of Medicare focused on technical issues concerning the most efficient ways to pay for the program while accepting the program's existing structure, but new political battles were overwhelmingly fought over the fundamental purpose of Medicare and the role of markets in social insurance provision (Oberlander, 2003).

Oberlander suggests three main factors that combined to shift Medicare politics to a state of dissensus. First, projections of a "trust fund crisis" became salient after reports in 1995 stated that Medicare would be solvent for only 7 more years. Second, the Republican Party's "Contract with America" emphasized large spending cuts to balance the budget. Third, the nature of health care systems was undergoing a change, with "managed care" plans becoming the dominant form of insurance (Oberlander, 2003). This politics of dissensus continued into the new century, making Medicare reform a hot topic in political debate.

Public opinion must be seen within the context of the dissensus created by the political debate about the future of Social Security and Medicare. Has the dissensus at the elite level caused overall public support to weaken? Or has public support splintered such that what was once "one public" has become "many publics" with divisions by partisanship, ideology, and age? As noted in the three sections that follow, the recent literature on such divides among the public causes us to think it is important to examine support for Social Security and Medicare along these lines.

Partisanship: Republicans versus Democrats

American politics in the past few decades has grown increasingly polarized, as parties, once thought in decline, have undergone a resurgence (Fiorina, 2002). Though researchers differ over whether the behavior of elites or the mass electorate first drove the increasing polarization (Jacobson, 2000; Layman, Carsey, & Horowitz, 2006), the realization is that politics at the beginning of the 21st century is party politics and that the public has grown more polarized in their party preferences.

This increasing polarization has resulted in a public for which party identification is a very real force on their voting behavior and on the construction of policy preferences. Using data from the National Election Studies (NES) survey, Bartels (2000) finds that the proportion of respondents who claim to be "strong party identifiers" has increased significantly since 1976. Furthermore, this identification has had a real effect on electoral behavior with levels of party voting higher than they have been in the recent years (Hetherington, 2001). Such dynamics were strongly felt in the 2004 presidential election that saw turnout levels among partisan voters higher than the average for elections between 1972 and 2000, strong partisan differences in responses to almost every polling question regarding which party would better handle policy issues of the day, and a nearly 80% difference in presidential approval between Republicans and Democrats (Jacobson, 2005).

The effect of increasing partisan polarization is not only an electoral phenomenon expressed at the ballot box. More importantly for our purposes, partisanship has increasingly differentiated policy preferences. Individuals are dramatically more likely to perceive differences between the parties on many issues since the 1970s, and the difference between the policy positions of Democrats and Republicans on seven out of eight issues[1] was higher in the 1990s than in the 1980s and 1970s (Brewer, 2005). Additionally, the average correlation between policy positions and party ID on every one of these issues has increased from 1972 to 2004 (Abramowitz & Saunders, 2005). Furthermore, research has found that party identification influences beliefs on equal opportunity, self-reliance, and limited government in the social welfare domain across all levels of political sophistication (Goren, 2004). To what extent are these partisan differences seen in support for Social Security and Medicare?

Ideology: Liberals versus Conservatives

Although political scientists have found that the mass public is unlikely to exhibit ideological consistency in their belief systems (Campbell, Converse, Miller, & Stokes, 1960; Converse, 1964; Zaller, 1992), there is evidence that suggests that individuals will use ideology as an aid in constructing their preferences. Self-placements on ideological continuums can help predict policy preferences (Jacoby, 1991), and when ideology is defined as a "symbolic predisposition" (or a stable, affective position), it is a strong predictor of individuals' attitudes (Sears, 1993). Research has shown that ideology plays an important role in the formation of attitudes, not only on *individual* policy issues (Jacoby, 1994; Sears,

---

[1] These issues came from the National Election Study and included health care, support for guaranteed jobs, civil rights, government insured school integration, aid to African Americans, role of women in society, school prayer, and abortion.

Huddy, & Schaffer, 1986; Lau, Brown, & Sears, 1978) but also across distinctly different policy domains (Jenkins-Smith, Mitchell, & Herron, 2004).

There is also evidence that ideological thinking may be on the rise. As Jost (2006) proclaims, those scholars who declared the end of ideology may have done so too quickly. Instead, politics has become much more ideological than it had been when scholars were discrediting the role of ideology in the construction of individual preferences. Using NES data, Jost finds that three fourths of respondents since 1996 placed themselves on bipolar liberalism/conservative scale with a reasonable degree of accuracy, stability, and coherence. Additionally, self-identification of liberalism or conservatism had a correlation of over .90 with voting decisions (Jost, 2006).

The question for this chapter is whether ideological differences are evident in the public's beliefs about Social Security and Medicare—that is, whether the extent to which the level of liberal or conservative views that members of the public hold shape the way they feel about these programs.

Age: Younger versus Older Age Groups

An examination of recent literature on age differences in public opinion finds that older and younger respondents vary in their attitudes on a wide range of policies. These include punitive responses to crime (Payne, Gainey, Triplett, & Donner, 2004), education financing (Tedin, Matlin, & Weinher, 2001), affirmative action (Gimpel, Morris, & Armstrong, 2004), gay rights (Delli Carpini & Keeter, 1996; Gimpel, Morris, & Armstrong, 2004), abortion (Delli Carpini & Keeter, 1996), the role of women in society (Delli Carpini & Keeter, 1996), and social programs for the poor (Schlesinger & Lee, 1994).

However, two programs for which both younger and older Americans have consistently shown high levels of support in the past are Social Security and Medicare. Recent research has found that not only do younger Americans express considerable support for Social Security and Medicare (Huddy, Jones, & Chard, 2001), but they also do so at higher levels than seniors (Campbell, 2003). Studies using data from the General Social Survey in the 1980s, 1990s, and the year 2000 have found that younger Americans consistently exhibit more support for increasing or maintaining current levels of spending on Social Security than do seniors (Hamil-Luker, 2001; Street & Cossman, 2006).

Yet, the political debates of the last few years may have affected the solid support from the young that Social Security and Medicare experienced in the past. Despite the passage of the prescription drug package in the Medicare reforms of 2003 and the Bush administration's failure to win over voters to Social Security privatization schemes in 2004 and 2005, Social Security reform and Medicare reform have remained important issues on the political landscape. Recent debates overwhelmingly focus on whether or not current contributors will receive benefits once they become eligible to collect, and in so doing, often portray Social Security and Medicare as programs in crisis needing to be fixed (Baker & Weisbrot, 1999; Jerit, 2006). Many of the claims single out younger voters as having no confidence in the two programs. In particular, it is often claimed that young people are more likely to believe in UFOs than to think they will get Social Security when they retire (Cook, Barabas, & Page, 2002). In many of his public statements, President Bush made clear that the young were correct to doubt the viability of the current Social Security system (Bush, 2006).

According to research by Jerit (2006) and Page and Simmons (2000), the way in which these programs are framed in the media promotes a sense of crisis in the minds of individuals. Particularly targeted are younger Americans. In a telling example during the Democratic debate for the 2008 New Hampshire primary, the moderator prefaced a question to the candidates regarding Social Security by quoting alarming statistics linking what she described as the bleak future of Social Security and Medicare due to the swelling ranks of baby boomers and noted that "many young Americans simply assume there will be nothing left for them to guarantee the security of their old age" (Stark, 2008). With increasingly prevalent portrayals such as this, it may well be that younger adults have become less supportive over time.

RESEARCH METHODS

To address our research questions on the strength of the two pillars of public opinion for Social Security and Medicare—the belief in and commitment to their purposes and the belief that they are affordable public expenditures—we conducted a search of the archives of the Roper Center for Public Opinion Research using RoperExpress and iPoll (search functions provided by the Roper Center). All surveys had to meet our criteria that they were national random samples of adults aged 18 or older.

We found that the General Social Survey (GSS) conducted by the National Opinion Research Center (NORC) had conducted surveys at least every 2 years (and often more frequently) that consistently included a question asking respondents their preferences regarding Social Security spending. This consistency allows us to track trends in support for Social Security over time.

To examine support for Social Security by partisanship, ideology, and age, we conducted our own analyses of the 2006 GSS survey.

As for Medicare, we found no single series of surveys that consistently polled the American public on Medicare spending preferences over time as NORC has done for Social Security. Therefore, we had to rely on multiple surveys with similarly worded questions to gauge Medicare support over time. To find these surveys, we searched Roper archives for survey questions that contained the words "Medicare" along with "spending" or "funding" or "support" in order to be consistent with our examination of Social Security. We found similarly worded, though not identical, questions asking respondents whether spending on Medicare should be increased, decreased, or maintained at current levels.

In examining the effect of partisanship, ideology, and age on support for Medicare, we analyzed one of the most recent comprehensive surveys we found on Medicare policy preferences, the 2006 survey from the Kaiser Family Foundation and Harvard School of Public Health entitled, "The Public's Health Care Agenda for the New Congress and Presidential Campaign."

To find questions on what has been referred to as the second pillar of public support—the belief that Social Security and Medicare are affordable public expenditures—we searched the Roper archive for either Social Security or Medicare along with the words "trouble" or "problem" or "crisis" in addition to the words already included in the search.

ASSESSING THE STRENGTH OF THE TWO PILLARS OF PUBLIC SUPPORT

Support for the Purpose of Social Security and Medicare

Social Security

How much support exists for the first pillar of public opinion—a belief in the social purpose of Social Security and a commitment to the program?

Using data from the GSS from NORC, we operationalize commitment to the purpose of Social Security as believing that we are spending either the right amount or too little on Social Security. Specifically, the question in the GSS was:

> We are faced with many problems in this country, none of which can be solved easily or inexpensively. I'm going to name some of these problems, and for each one I'd like you to tell me whether you think we're spending too much money on it, too little money, or about the right amount. Are we spending too much money, too little money, or about the right amount on Social Security?

Operationalized this way, we find tremendous support over time for the purpose of Social Security (Fig. 14.1). Since 1984, more than 90% of respondents report that the United States spends too little or the right amount of money on Social Security. In 2006, the most recent year in which the question was asked, 95% of respondents favored maintaining or increasing program funding. When we disaggregate the support variable and raise the threshold by only considering whether Americans think that we spend too little on Social Security, we find that the majority of Americans think that we do not spend enough on this program. As shown in Figure 14.1, in 14 of the 16 years in which this question was asked since 1984, the majority of respondents said that too little was spent on Social Security.

The data in Figure 14.1 indicate that overall support for Social Security is extremely high. But is this indicative of a single public opinion, or do the politics of dissensus infiltrate the public view on Social Security spending such that there are marked differences between Republicans and Democrats, conservatives and liberals, and young and old? To learn the answer, in Table 14.1, we break down overall support along the three factors that often divide the public: partisanship, ideology, and age.

Looking first at partisanship, are the divisions as stark as some political scientists might predict? Commentators might interpret the findings differently. On the one hand, they might argue for few differences. Majorities of Republicans, Independents, and Democrats think that too little money is being spent on Social Security and less than 10% ever say that too much is spent. Further, when support is operationalized as thinking that the United States spends "too little" *or* "the right amount" on Social Security, 92% of self-identified Republicans support increasing or maintaining current levels of Social Security spending, compared to 95% of self-reported Independents and 98% of self-identified Democrats.

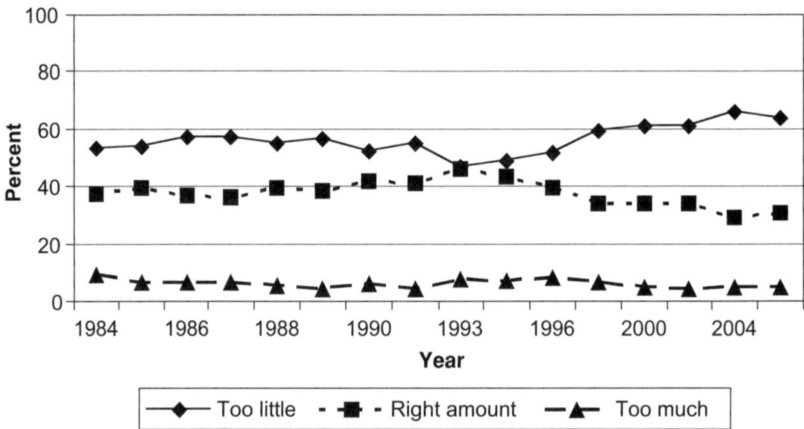

Figure 14.1 Support for Social Security, 1984–2006.
Source: The data are from NORC General Social Surveys. The question was: "We are faced with many problems in this country, none of which can be solved easily or inexpensively. I'm going to name some of these problems, and for each one I'd like you to tell me whether you think we're spending too much money on it, too little money, or about the right amount. Are we spending too much money, too little money, or about the right amount on Social Security?"
Note: This question was not asked in 1992, 1995, 1997, 1999, 2001, 2003, and 2005. These percentages do not include "Don't know" and other volunteered responses.

On the other hand, clear differences can be found when we compare Republicans and Democrats who think too little money is being spent. Democrats are 16% more likely than Republicans to think that too little money is being spent. A similar difference, though not as large, is found between Democrats and Independents. Here, then, are the divisions that the partisanship literature would lead us to expect. Do these marked differences mean that trouble is on the horizon regarding the first pillar of support for Social Security? We think not. Most of the Republicans and Independents who do not say that too little money is being spent are the very ones who report that "about the right amount" is being spent. We interpret this response as commitment to the program.

A second division seen to splinter consensus among the public is ideology. Liberals and conservatives are often at odds about a range of issues from capital punishment to welfare reform to universal health care, and so commentators might expect similar differences in regard to social insurance programs like Social Security and Medicare. As with the story on partisanship, commentators can see ideological divisions two ways. Majorities of conservatives, moderates, and liberals believe that too little is spent on Social Security. When we combine those who believe that either

Table 14.1

SUPPORT FOR SOCIAL SECURITY BY PARTY IDENTIFICATION, IDEOLOGY, AND AGE

	TOO LITTLE	ABOUT RIGHT	TOO MUCH
Party			
Republican	54%	38%	8%
Independent	65%	30%	5%
Democrat	70%	27%	2%
Ideology			
Conservative	57%	34%	8%
Moderate	70%	27%	3%
Liberal	64%	33%	2%
Age			
18–29	60%	32%	8%
30–49	69%	25%	6%
50–64	66%	32%	3%
65+	54%	43%	3%

Source: NORC General Social Survey. The question was, "We are faced with many problems in this country, none of which can be solved easily or inexpensively. I'm going to name some of these problems, and for each one I'd like you to tell me whether you think we're spending too much money on it, too little money, or about the right amount. Are we spending too much money, too little money, or about the right amount on Social Security?" N = 2,804, percentages do not include "Don't Knows."

"too little" or "about the right amount" is spent, 91% of conservatives, 97% of moderates, and 97% of liberals supported increasing or maintaining current levels of spending for Social Security. These majorities reflect strong commitment to the purpose of Social Security.

However, as with partisanship, differences emerge when we examine the majorities who think "too little" is being spent. As expected, liberals are more likely than conservatives to think too little is being spent, but somewhat surprisingly, moderates are more likely than both conservatives and liberals to report this view. So, those who argue that ideological beliefs predict social policy divisions have data to support their argument, but for our purposes, the vast majorities who favor current spending or worry about too little represent commitment to the program.

Finally, we examine differences by age. Conventional wisdom has become that the young are less likely to be supportive of Social Security than the old because they do not think it will be there for them when they retire. As Table 14.1 shows, the data dispute the conventional wisdom.

Not only do majorities of all age groups think that too little is spent on Social Security, but also young adults aged 18 to 29 are more likely than adults aged 65 and older to say too little is spent on Social Security.

Conventional wisdom can claim support from one finding shown in Table 14.1: Young adults are more likely than other age groups to say too much is being spent on Social Security. However, the differences are small (only 8% hold this view). The larger finding is that a resounding 92% of individuals between the ages of 18 and 29 support maintaining or increasing current levels of spending on Social Security. Similarly, 94% of individuals between the ages of 30 and 49, 98% between the ages of 50 and 64, and 97% of individuals aged 65 or older support maintaining current levels or increasing America's spending on Social Security.

Overall, it appears that public support for the first pillar of support on Social Security is overwhelmingly consensual. While there are disparities in the extent to which partisanship, ideology, and age affect views about whether or not there is too little money spent, the overall patterns of support are very similar by party identification, ideology, and age. Although we are only reporting data on these factors for the most recent year, 2006, these patterns are consistent in support over time since 1984.

Medicare

Similar to our operationalization of belief in and commitment to the purpose of Social Security, we measured level of commitment to the purpose of Medicare as support for increasing spending, maintaining spending, or decreasing spending. Unfortunately, we could only find exactly the same question asked by a survey organization in 3 years—1997, 2001, and 2002. (In each of these years, the Pew Research Group asked, "If you were making up the budget for the federal government this year, would you increase spending for Medicare, decrease spending, or keep spending the same?"). In other years between 1984 and 2006, we found 4 years in which similar but not identical questions were asked (Fig 14.2).

As was the case with Social Security, overall public support for Medicare spending was extremely high over the past 20 years. With the exception of 2 years, public support for increasing or maintaining current levels of spending on Medicare did not dip below 90%. And even in those 2 years, 1993 and 1997, public support was still high at 76% and 88% of the public supporting an increase or maintenance in current levels of spending on Medicare. The most current survey, 2006, indicates sustained support for Medicare spending with 91% of respondents favoring an increase or maintaining current levels in spending. Looking only at those who say they want to increase spending, 50% or more of the public in all but 1 year report that they would like to see the federal government spend more on Medicare. Only small percentages ever say they want to decrease spending (the average response in the years the question was asked was 7%). The exception was 1993, when 20% said they would like to decrease spending, but the question was a bit different that year and asked respondents if the federal government should spend more on Medicare "even if your own taxes should increase." Sixty-one percent wanted higher spending despite the consideration that their taxes might increase.

Clearly, these are high levels of support. But to what extent is this public support consensual? Using the 2006 survey from the Kaiser Family Foundation and Harvard School of Public Health, we examine the extent to which support for Medicare breaks down along partisan, ideological, and age divisions. Respondents were asked, "In order to help reduce the federal budget deficit, would you favor or oppose slowing the rate of growth in Medicare spending?" Note that slowing the rate of growth in Medicare is linked to reducing the federal budget deficit, raising the bar on support. We operationalize answers that *opposed* a slowing of the rate of growth in Medicare spending to be support for the purpose of the Medicare program.

In regard to partisanship, Medicare's enactment back in 1965 was seen as a victory for Democratic President Lyndon Johnson and a Democratically controlled Congress that resulted from massive electoral victories in 1964 (Marmor, 2000), and some still see the program in partisan terms despite a politics of consensus that existed for many years. With the increasing dissensus and disagreement about Medicare, have differences in support increased between Democrats and Republicans within the public? Table 14.2 shows differences in support by party identification. Democrats are 13% more likely to oppose cuts to Medicare than Republicans are. But the more important story is that the vast majority of Democrats, Independents, and Republicans all show high levels of support for Medicare, with 79% of Democrats, 78% of Independents, and 66% of Republicans reporting that they oppose cutting Medicare spending.

The story is much the same with ideology. Although a larger percentage of liberals and moderates oppose cuts to Medicare than do conservatives, the more important story is that large majorities of each group believe in and are committed to the program: 80% of self-identified liberals, 76% of self-identified moderates, and 68% of self-identified conservatives oppose cutting Medicare spending.

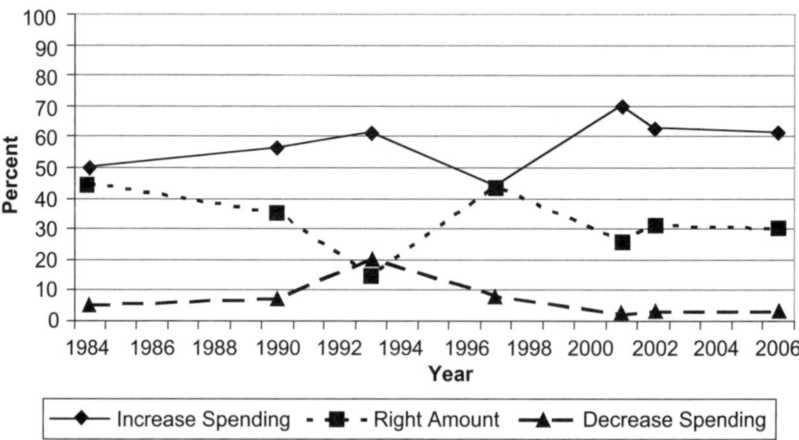

Figure 14.2 Support for Medicare, 1984–2006.
Source: Since we were unable to find a single series of surveys that consistently polled the American public on Medicare spending preferences, we had to rely on multiple surveys with similarly worded questions to gauge Medicare support over time. We report these questions, indicating the year and survey methodology associated with each.

For the 1984 survey, the question read, "Should federal spending on Medicare be increased, decreased, or kept the same?" Source: National Election Study, 9/5/84–1/5/84; N = 1,989.

For the 1990 survey, the question read, "Do you think that federal spending this year should be increased, decreased, or remain the same for each of the following?... Medicare" Source: Marist College Institute for Public Opinion, 1/29/90–1/31/90; N = 1,044.

For the 1993 survey, the question read, "Let's talk for a few minutes about government spending on various programs. I'm going to read you a list of programs. For each one just tell me, in your opinion, whether the federal government should spend more or should spend less on each program. (Even if your own taxes increase?)... Medicare" Source: Wirthlin Group, 12/5/93–129/93; N = 1,013.

For the 1997 survey, the question read, "If you were making up the federal budget this year, would you increase spending for... Medicare, decrease spending for Medicare, or keep spending the same for this?" Source: Pew Research Group, 5/15/97–5/18/97; N = 1,228.

For the 2001 survey, the question read, "If you were making up the budget for the federal government this year, would you increase spending for... Medicare... decrease spending for... Medicare... or keep spending the same for this?" Source: Pew Research Group, 4/18/01–4/22/01; N = 1,202.

For the 2002 survey, the question read, "If you were making up the budget for the federal government this year (2002), would you increase spending for... Medicare, decrease spending for... Medicare, or keep spending the same for this?" Source: Pew Research Center, 2/12/02–2/18/02; N = 1,199.

For the 2006 survey, the question read, "For each of the following budget items, please state whether you think the new budget should increase spending on this item from the previous budget, decrease spending on this item from the previous budget, or keep it the same... Medicare" Source: ICR, 1/4/06–1/9/06; N = 1,026.

Table 14.2

OPPOSITION AND SUPPORT FOR CUTTING MEDICARE SPENDING BY PARTY IDENTIFICATION, IDEOLOGY, AND AGE

	OPPOSE CUTS	SUPPORT CUTS
Party		
Republican	66%	34%
Independent	78%	22%
Democrat	79%	21%
Ideology		
Conservative	68%	32%
Moderate	76%	24%
Liberal	80%	20%
Age		
18–29	69%	31%
30–49	69%	31%
50–64	75%	25%
65+	78%	22%

Source: Kaiser Family Foundation and Harvard School of Public Health, "The Public's Health Care Agenda for the New Congress and Presidential Campaign, November 9–19, 2006. Question read, "In order to help reduce the federal budget deficit, would you favor or oppose slowing the rate of growth in Medicare spending?" N = 1,689, percentages based on those that answered and do not include "Don't Knows."

Finally, we consider the extent to which age groups differ in their support. Adults aged 65 and over are 9% more likely than young adults aged 18 to 29 to oppose cuts, with 78% of seniors opposing cuts as compared to 69% of those in the youngest age group. However, the differences across age are not great, and the big story is that clear majorities oppose cuts.

Although we do see differences by partisanship, ideology, and age, there is more support than opposition among all groups. The overall story gleaned from this examination is that regardless of partisanship, ideology, or age, the public seems relatively united in its support for Medicare.

Belief that Social Security and Medicare are Affordable Public Expenditures

Social Security

The second pillar of public support on which Social Security and Medicare rests, is the belief that the two programs are affordable public expenditures. In our extensive search of questions that have been asked about the two programs, we found no specific questions that asked respondents about how "affordable" they think the programs are. Specifically, respondents have been asked the following question about Social Security: "Which of the following do you think best describes the financial situation of Social Security today—it is in crisis, it is in serious trouble but not in crisis, it is in some trouble, or it is not really in trouble at all?"

Using four surveys with identical questions that were asked between January 2005 and October 2007, we measure perceived fiscal problems as answers of "crisis" or "serious trouble." The results suggest that Americans are alarmed about the future of Social Security. In January 2005, 14% of Americans said they thought Social Security was "in crisis." By October 2007, that figure had doubled. In 2007, 66% of Americans thought that the program was either in a "crisis" or in "serious trouble" (Table 14.3).

Medicare

Are the public's concerns equally strong for Medicare? To answer this question, we analyzed three surveys from August 2002, January 2003, and January 2005 to determine whether the public considers the Medicare program to be in danger (we were not able to find any surveys with a similar question after 2005). All surveys asked similarly worded questions gauging whether respondents thought that Medicare was in crisis, had major problems but not in crisis, had minor problems, or had no real problems. As was the case with Social Security, we measured perceived fiscal problems as answers of "crisis" or "major problems."

During the time period we examined, the results suggest that Americans are equally, if not more, concerned about the future of Medicare than they are Social Security. Compared to the 52% of Americans who thought Social Security was in a crisis or was in serious trouble in January of 2005, 64% of Americans felt that Medicare was in crisis or experiencing major problems. In fact, when *NBC News* and the *Wall Street Journal* surveyed the public in March 2005 and asked, "Which program do you believe is in more trouble and needs more attention from lawmakers—Social Security or Medicare? If you think that neither is in trouble, feel free to say so," 50% of respondents reported that Medicare was in more serious trouble, compared to 23% of Americans who thought Social Security needed more attention.[2] Tellingly, only 3% of Americans thought

---

[2] Survey by *NBC News*, *Wall Street Journal*. Methodology: Conducted by Hart and McInturff Research Companies, March 31–April 3, 2005 with a national adult sample of 1,002.

Table 14.3

PUBLIC FEARS ABOUT PROBLEMS IN SOCIAL SECURITY AND MEDICARE

	CRISIS	SERIOUS TROUBLE/MAJOR PROBLEMS	SOME TROUBLE/MINOR PROBLEMS	NOT IN TROUBLE/NO PROBLEMS
Social Security				
January 2005[a]	14%	38%	38%	7%
March 2005[b]	17%	37%	36%	7%
June 2005[c]	17%	38%	37%	5%
October 2007[d]	30%	36%	26%	5%
Medicare				
August 2002[e]	25%	49%	23%	1%
January 2003[f]	18%	52%	23%	2%
January 2005[g]	12%	52%	29%	2%

[a] NBC News, Wall Street Journal. Methodology: Conducted by Hart and McInturff Research Companies, January 13–17, 2005. N = 1,007.

Question wording for all Social Security questions: "Which of the following do you think best describes the financial situation of Social Security today—it is in crisis, it is in serious trouble but not in crisis, it is in some trouble, or it is not really in trouble at all?"

[b] NBC News, Wall Street Journal. Conducted by Hart and McInturff Research Companies, March 31–April 3, 2005. N = 1,002.

[c] CBS News/New York Times, June 10–15, 2005. N = 1,111.

[d] CBS News, October 12–16, 2007. N = 1,282.

[e] Survey by *Washington Post*, Henry J. Kaiser Family Foundation. Methodology: Conducted by Princeton Survey Research Associates, August 2–September 1, 2002. N = 2,886. Results are weighted to be representative of a national adult population.

Question wording for 1/2003 and 8/2002 Medicare question: "Now I have a few questions about Medicare, the government program that provides health insurance for seniors and some disabled people.... Please tell me which one of the following four statements comes closest to your view of the Medicare program. Would you say...the program is in crisis, the program has major problems, but is not in crisis, the program has minor problems, or the program has no problems?"

[f] *ABC News/Washington Post*, conducted by TNS Intersearch, January 30–February 1, 2003. N = 855.

[g] Quinnipiac University Polling Institute, January 25–31, 2005. N = 2,100, sample of nationally registered voters. Question worded, "Which of these statements do you think best describes the Medicare system?... It is in a state of crisis, it has major problems, it has minor problems, or it does not have any problems?"

neither program was in danger, whereas 19% of Americans thought both programs were equally troubled.

So far, we have seen that the first pillar of public opinion on which the two programs rest is strong: The vast majority of the public believes in and is committed to the programs as expressed by their willingness to spend money on them. However, the second pillar of public opinion is shaky. The majority of the public sees the financial situation as troubling for both Social Security and Medicare. So far, their concerns have not undermined their support. But as policy makers debate various changes that might be made to both programs, it is important to try to understand what it is exactly that the public is willing to sanction to strengthen the programs for the future.

Assessing What Changes the Public Favors

Various policy changes have been proposed for both Social Security and Medicare. Which changes does the public favor?

Social Security

During the late 1990s in the last years of the Clinton administration, several Republican Congress members proposed partially privatizing Social Security by allowing people to put part of their Social Security taxes into private accounts that would be invested in the stock market. In 2005, President Bush made privatizing Social Security the domestic policy centerpiece of his State of the Union address. Since the late 1990s, many claims have been made that the public supports private accounts (Cook, Barabas, & Page, 2002; Cook, 2005).

The facts are not so clear. There are two patterns. First, when not reminded of the risks associated with stock market investments or with the costs of transitioning to a privatized system, more members of the public support partial privatization (namely, being able to invest a portion of their Social Security taxes into personal retirement accounts) than oppose it. However, the level of support has diminished over time. The first third of Table 14.4 shows responses in seven surveys between June 1998 and May 2005. In June 1998, when the public was just hearing about the privatization proposal, 69% supported privatization while only 20% opposed it—a difference of 49 points. However, by 2005, support had declined considerably, and less than half the public supported it (although there were still more supporter than opponents by 47% to 40%). What caused support to plummet between 1998 and 2005? We think that support for privatization declined as the public learned more about it between 1998, when it was just being introduced, and 2005, when the concept had been around for awhile.

Second, when respondents are told more about privatization—either that it represents a change to the Social Security system or that risks are involved—their support for individual accounts declines markedly. In the middle segment of Table 14.4, the data show that the majority of respondents are opposed to partial privatization when the question to

Table 14.4

SUPPORT FOR PRIVATIZATION AS FRAMING OF POLICY OPTION CHANGES

	SUPPORT	OPPOSE	DIFFERENCE	N.O./D.K.*
Privatization[a]				
June 1998	69%	20%	49	11%
September 1999	70%	20%	48	8%
December 2004	54%	30%	24	16%
February 2005	46%	38%	8	16%
March 2005	44%	40%	4	16%
March 2005	46%	44%	2	10%
May 2005	47%	40%	7	13%
Privatization as a change to the system[b]				
December 2004	38%	50%	−12	12%
January 2005	40%	50%	−10	10%
March/April 2005	35%	55%	−20	10%
May 2005	36%	56%	−20	8%
July 2005	33%	57%	−24	10%
Privatization as a change to the system with risks[c]				
January 2005	40%	55%	−15	5%
February 2005	40%	55%	−15	5%
February 2005	36%	60%	−24	4%
March 2005	33%	59%	−26	8%
April 2005	33%	61%	−28	6%

* Represents "Do not know" and "No opinion" responses.

[a] Princeton Survey Research Associates International for Pew Research Center. Question read, "Generally, do you favor or oppose this proposal (which would allow younger workers to invest a portion of their Social Security taxes in private retirement accounts, which might include stocks or mutual funds)?" Surveys conducted June 4–8, 1998 (N = 1,012); July 4–September 9, 1999 (N = 3,973); February 16–21, 2005 (N = 1,502); March 17–21, 2005 (N = 1,090); March, 17–21, 2005 (N = 1,505); May 11–15, 2005 (N = 1,502).

[b] Hart and McInturff Research Companies for NBC News. Question read, "In general, do you think that it is a good or bad idea to change the Social Security system to allow workers to invest their Social Security contributions in the stock market?" Surveys conducted December 9–13, 2004 (N = 1,003); January 13–17, 2005 (N = 1,007); March 31–April 3, 2005 (N = 1,002); May 12–16, 2005 (N = 1,005); July 8–11, 2005 (N = 1,009).

[c] Gallup poll for CNN/USA Today. Question read, "As you may know, one idea to address concerns with the Social Security system would allow people who retire in future decades to invest some of their Social Security taxes in the stock market and bonds, but would reduce the guaranteed benefits they get when they retire. Do you think this is a good idea or a bad idea?" Surveys conducted January 7–9, 2005 (N = 1,008); February 4– 6, 2005 (N = 1,010); February 7–10, 2005 (N = 1,008); March 18–20, 2005 (N = 909); April 1, 2005-April 2, 2005 (N = 1,040).

them is framed this way: "In general, do you think that it is a good idea or bad idea *to change the Social Security system* to allow workers to invest their Social Security contributions in the stock market?" (italics added for emphasis). In other words, when they are told that investing their contributions in the stock market would mean changing the Social Security system, 57% said they were opposed, and only a third were in favor.

When respondents are told that investing some of their Social Security taxes in the stock market and bonds "would reduce the guaranteed benefits they get when they retire," 61% say they are opposed to individual accounts (see the responses in the bottom third of Table 14.4).

Clearly, then, in regard to support for partial privatization, question wording matters. Regardless of question wording, however, support for partial privatization has diminished since the 1990s, when few understood the implications of the proposal.

Some Social Security experts have recommended more incremental changes than the system-change of partial privatization—such as lowering cost-of-living adjustments or COLAs, reducing benefits for the wealthy elderly, increasing the payroll tax, raising the earnings ceiling or "cap" that exempts all income above a certain level from payroll taxation, raising the age of eligibility for full retirement benefits to 70, and raising the minimum age for receiving full benefits to 70, and raising the minimum age for receiving reduced benefits from 62 to 65 (see, for example, Baker & Weisbrot, 1999; Page & Simmons, 2000, chapter 3; Social Security Advisory Board, 1998, pp. 25–26). The results of four Princeton Survey Research Associates surveys about such options are given in Table 14.5. Only two of the six proposals—raising the earnings ceiling and reducing benefits for the wealthy elderly—received support from more than half the respondents (60% and 58%, respectively). Support and opposition are about equally divided on another proposal—increasing the early eligibility age from Social Security from 62 to 65.

Medicare

To address the financial problems facing Medicare, a variety of policy proposals have been suggested. In a survey conducted by International Communications Research (2006) for the Kaiser Family Foundation and Harvard School of Public Health, the public has been asked about nine of these: rolling back tax cuts to strengthen Medicare funding, requiring higher premiums from high income seniors, reducing doctor and

Table 14.5

PUBLIC SUPPORT FOR INCREMENTAL CHANGES IN SOCIAL SECURITY

POLICY OPTION	AUGUST 1998[a]	FEBRUARY 1999[b]	MAY 1999[c]	FEBRUARY 2005[d]
Raise Earnings Ceilings[e]				
Favor	60%	59%	61%	60%
Oppose	29%	28%	29%	33%
Reduce Benefits for the Wealthy[f]				
Favor	54%	54%	58%	58%
Oppose	40%	40%	37%	36%
Increase Early Eligibility Age from 62 to 65[g]				
Favor	47%	43%	46%	—
Oppose	47%	52%	48%	—
Increase Payroll Tax From 6.2% to 6.7%[h]				
Favor	40%	44%	44%	38%
Oppose	54%	50%	50%	56%
Lower COLA[i]				
Favor	34%	37%	40%	30%
Oppose	61%	56%	53%	64%
Raise Age of Social Security Eligibility to 70[j]				
Favor	23%	24%	22%	35%
Oppose	74%	74%	74%	64%

[a] Princeton Survey Research Associates (PSRA) data, 8/6/98-8/27/98, N = 2,008.
[b] Princeton Survey Research Associates (PSRA) data, 2/2/99-2/14/99, N = 1,000.
[c] Princeton Survey Research Associates (PSRA) data, 5/3/99-5/17/99, N = 1,001.
[d] Princeton Survey Research Associates (PSRA) data, 2/16/2005-2/21/2005, N = 1,502.

Question wording for 1998/1999 PSRA questions: "Now I'd like to get your opinion on some specific proposals for how Social Security might be changed in the future. If I ask you anything you feel you can't answer, just tell me. Do you favor or oppose the following proposals . . . (INSERT – READ AND ROTATE) . . . Do you strongly favor/oppose this proposal, or moderately favor or oppose it? Question wording for 2005 PSRA questions: "I am going to read you a list of some ways that have been suggested to address concerns about the Social Security program. Please tell me if you would favor or oppose each one . . . " See specific wording below.

[e] 1998/1999: " . . . Collecting payroll taxes on earnings up to $100,000 per year, instead of the current cut-off of about $72,000"; 2005: " . . . Collecting Social Security taxes on all of a worker's wages, rather than just the first $90,000 they earn per year."

[f] 1998/1999: " . . . Reducing Social Security benefits for people who have retirement incomes over about $60,000 per year"; 2005: " . . . Limiting benefits for wealthy retirees."

[g] 1998/1999: " . . . Gradually increasing the early retirement age for collecting reduced benefits from age 62 to 65."

[h] 1998/1999: " . . . Increasing the payroll tax that workers and employers each pay into the Social Security system from 6.2% to 6.7%""; 2005: " . . . Increasing Social Security payroll taxes for all workers."

[i] 1998/1999: " . . . Cutting the amount that Social Security benefits go up each year for changes in the cost of living"; 2005: " . . . Lowering the amount of Social Security benefits go up each year for changes in the cost of living."

[j] 1998/1999: " . . . Gradually raising the age when a person can collect Social Security benefits to age 70"; 2005: " . . . Raising the retirement age."

hospital payments for treating Medicare beneficiaries, reducing Medicare payments to HMOs and private insurers, increasing payroll taxes for workers and employers to fund Medicare, gradually raising the age of eligibility for Medicare from 65 to 67, limiting eligibility to low-income seniors rather than all seniors, cutting back Medicare drug benefits to save money, and requiring all seniors to pay larger shares of Medicare costs out of pocket.

A majority of the public support only one of these proposals—rolling back tax cuts to strengthen Medicare funding. As shown in Table 14.6, the public is fairly evenly split on another three of the proposals. On another five, the public is strongly opposed.

The public is concerned about the financial situation of both Social Security and Medicare, as the data in Table 14.3 clearly show. However, as the data in Tables 14.5 and 14.6 reveal, there are relatively few proposals to strengthen Social Security and Medicare that a majority of the public favors. We turn now to what these and our earlier findings can be taken to mean for the pillars of public opinion on which the two programs rest.

CONCLUSION

Social Security and Medicare have often been called two of America's most successful social programs. They have helped millions of Americans to be more financially secure in their old age and to receive necessary medical care (Page & Simmons, 2000). For many years, the politics of both programs were described as a "politics of consensus." However, beginning in the mid-1990s, the politics of consensus was replaced by a politics of dissensus. The debates have often been noisy and fractious with claims and counter claims made about the extent to which the programs were experiencing financial crises and near bankruptcy and about the actions that should be taken to deal with the problems. This chapter has asked whether the dissensus at the elite level has caused public support for Social Security and Medicare to weaken.

Two pillars of public opinion that have long undergirded support for Social Security and Medicare are, first, belief in and commitment to the purposes of the programs and, second, belief that the programs are affordable public expenditures (Marttila, 2005; Cook & Barrett, 1992). Using data from dozens of public opinion surveys over time, we have examined the extent to which these pillars remain strong in the face of

Table 14.6

PUBLIC SUPPORT FOR INCREMENTAL CHANGES IN MEDICARE

POLICY OPTION	FAVOR	OPPOSE
Roll back some tax cuts to strengthen Medicare funding	74%	23%
Require higher premiums from high income seniors	49%	47%
Reduce doctor and hospital payments for treating Medicare beneficiaries	47%	47%
Reduce Medicare payments to HMOs and private insurers	44%	45%
Increase payroll taxes for workers and employers to fund Medicare	38%	59%
Gradually raise age of eligibility from 65 to 67 for future retirees	28%	70%
Limit eligibility to low-income seniors rather than serving all seniors	24%	73%
Cut back Medicare drug benefits to save money	14%	84%
Require all seniors to pay larger share of Medicare costs out of pocket	9%	90%

Source: Kaiser Family Foundation/Harvard School of Public Health. Methodology: Conducted by International Communications Research, November 9 to November 16, 2006 and based on telephone interviews with a national adult sample of 1867. The question read, "I'm going to read you some proposals to keep the Medicare program financially sound in the future. Please tell me whether you would generally favor or oppose each one (First/Next) would you favor or oppose (Insert)? (To keep the Medicare program financially sound in the future?) Is that strongly or somewhat?" The policy options were divided and asked to approximately half of the respondents. The first group, N = 932, were asked the following policy options in the following order: "requiring higher income seniors to payer higher Medicare premiums", "Reducing payments to doctors and hospitals for treating people covered by Medicare", Increasing the payroll taxes workers and employers now pay to help fund the Medicare program", and "Gradually raising the age of eligibility for Medicare from 65 to 67 for future retirees". The second group, N = 935, were asked the following policy options in the following order: "Requiring all seniors to pay a larger share of Medicare costs out of their own pockets", "Reducing Medicare payments to HMOs and other private insurers", "Rolling back some tax cuts and using the money to help keep the Medicare program financially sound", "Cutting back the Medicare drug benefit to save money", and "Turning Medicare into a program that only serves low-income seniors instead of serving all seniors". "Strongly support" and "somewhat support" responses were combined to make a single "support" indicator; "strongly oppose" and "somewhat oppose" were combined to make a single "oppose" indicator. Responses do not include refusals and "do not know" responses.

sometimes fractious debate among policy makers, interest groups, and political commentators. The findings are revealing.

The public's belief in and commitment to the purposes of Social Security and Medicare are strong. The vast majority support the amount being spent on the programs with many actually wanting to increase spending. Only very small percentages—usually less than 10%—think too much is being spent and want to decrease spending. Moreover, this support is similar across many groups where we often find division. Regardless of party identification, ideology, and age, the pattern of support is very similar: Republicans and Democrats, conservatives and liberals, and young and old are united in their commitment to the two programs. Thus, the first pillar of public opinion on which Social Security and Medicare rest appears to be strong.

The second pillar of public opinion is weaker. The majority of Americans describe the financial situation of both Social Security and Medicare as either in crisis or serious trouble. So far, the weakening of the second pillar has not undermined support for the purposes of the program. Whether it will or not depends on a number of factors. One of these is surely whether Americans see their Congress members tackling the programs' financial difficulties in thoughtful, effective ways.

Do Americans see a clear pathway to strengthening the programs? Public support for partial privatization of Social Security was high when privatization proposals were first introduced in the late 1990s, but support plummeted as the public learned more about the tradeoffs that would be involved in implementing such reforms. Although some elites still call for reforms that would privatize Social Security benefits, our analysis finds that most members of the public are not in favor. Instead, they express support for incremental changes. For Social Security, the majority of Americans support raising the earnings ceiling and reducing benefits for wealthier older Americans. To keep Medicare financially sound in the future, a strong majority of Americans support rolling back tax cuts to strengthen financing. Both sets of these changes involve recalibrating existing policy instruments, rather than fundamentally changing the structure of the programs. Thus, although policy elites continue to debate the merits and detriments of privatization and marketization of Social Security and Medicare, the American public seems to be committed to the existing structures of these programs, preferring incremental changes to the system as it currently exists.

The findings of this chapter pose a real challenge to anyone who argues that support for Social Security and Medicare may be declining in the face of dissensus at the elite level. Clearly, support is high. However, the findings also point to the very real concern among the public about the financial future of the two programs. To address their financial concerns, members of the public have voiced support for a few incremental changes and opposition to a number of others. In order to overcome the current politics of dissensus, it behooves policy makers to take a careful look at where the public stands and build on that support.

DISCUSSION QUESTIONS

1. Cook and Czaplewski discuss two historical "pillars of support" for Social Security and Medicare. What are they, and how strong are they today?
2. Claims are often made that young people do not support Social Security because they do not believe it will be there for them when they retire. What do the polling data show about the opinions of young Americans?
3. What does the polling data say about the patterns in public opinion about the option of privatizing Social Security?
4. What are the kinds of changes Americans favor for addressing the fiscal situation of Social Security and Medicare?
5. What are some of the historical changes that contribute to what Cook calls a "politics of dissensus" around support for social insurance programs?
6. In 2005, when asked if he found the poll data on declining support for private accounts troubling, President Bush responded by saying:

   > Polls? You know, if a President tries to govern based upon polls, you're kind of like a dog chasing your tail. I don't think you can make good, sound decisions based upon polls. And I don't think the American people want a President who relies upon polls and focus groups to make decisions for the American people. (Bush April 28th, 2005)

   Please respond to this quote.

REFERENCES

Abramowitz, A. I., & Saunders, K. L. (2005). Why can't we all just get along? The reality of a polarized America. *The Forum*, 3(2), 1–22.

AssistGuide Information Services (2007). '08 Presidential candidates' on Social Security. Retrieved February 15, 2008, from http://carestation.agis.com/2007/11/27/08-presidential-candidates-on-social-security/

Baker, D., & Weisbrot, M. (1999). *Social Security: The phony crisis*. Chicago: University of Chicago Press.

Bartels, L. M. (2000). Partisanship and voting behavior, 1952–1996. *American Journal of Political Science*, *44*(1), 35–50.

Brewer, M. D. (2005). The rise of partisanship and the expansion of partisan conflict within the American electorate. *Political Research Quarterly*, *58*, 219–229.

Bush, President G. W. (2005, February 2). State of the union address. Washington, DC. Retrieved October 22, 2008, from http://www.presidentialrhetoric.com/speeches/02.02.05.html

Bush, President G. W. (2006, February 8). Address on the 2007 budget. Manchester, New Hampshire. Retrieved October 22, 2008, from http://www.presidentialrhetoric.com/speeches/02.08.06.html

Campbell, A. L. (2003). *How policies make citizens*. Princeton, NJ: Princeton University Press.

Campbell, A., Converse, P. E., Miller, W. E., & Stokes, D. E. (1960). *The American voter.* New York: John Wiley & Sons, Inc.

Converse, P. (1964). The nature of belief systems in mass publics. In D. Apter (Ed.), *Ideology and discontent* (pp. 206–261). New York: Free Press.

Cook, F. L. (2005). Navigating pension policy in the United States: From the politics of consensus to the politics dissensus about social security. *The Tocqueville Review*, *26*(22), 37–66.

Cook, F. L., Barabas, J., & Page, B. (2002). Invoking public opinion: Policy elites and Social Security. *Public Opinion Quarterly*, *66*, 235–264.

Cook, F. L., & Barrett, E. J. (1992). *Support for the American welfare state: The views of Congress and the public*. New York: Columbia University Press.

Delli Carpini, M. X., & Keeter, S. (1996). *What Americans know about politics and why it matters*. New Haven, CT: Yale University Press.

Fiorina, M. (2002). Parties and partisanship: A 40-year retrospective. *Political Behavior*, *24*, 93–115.

Gimpel, J. G., Morris, I. L., & Armstrong, D. R. (2004). Turnout and the local age distribution: Examining political participation across space and time. *Political Geography*, *23*, 71–95.

Glied, S. (1997). *Chronic conditions: Why health reforms fail*. Cambridge, MA: Harvard University Press.

Goren, P. (2004). Political sophistication and policy reasoning: A reconsideration. *American Journal of Political Science*, *48*, 462–478.

Hamil-Luker, J. (2001). The prospects of age war: Inequality between (and within) age groups. *Social Science Research*, *30*, 386–400.

Hetherington, M. J. (2001). Resurgent mass partisanship: The role of elite polarization. *American Political Science Review*, *95*, 619–631.

Huddy, L., Jones, J. M., & Chard, R. E. (2001). Compassionate politics: Support for old-age programs among the non-elderly. *Political Psychology*, *22*(3), 443–471.

International Communications Research. (2006). The Public's Health Care Agenda for the New Congress and Presidential Campaign. Survey conducted for The Kaiser Family Foundation/Harvard School of Public Health. November 9–19, 2006. Retrieved November 13, 2008, from http://www.kff.org/kaiserpolls/pomr120806pkg.cfm

Jacobson, G. (2000). Party polarization in national politics: The electoral connection. In J. R. Bond & R. Fleischer (Eds.), *Polarized politics: Congress and the president in a partisan era* (pp. 9–30). Washington, DC: CQ Press.

Jacobson, G. (2005). Polarized politics and the 2004 congressional and presidential elections. *Political Science Quarterly*, *120*, 199–218.

Jacoby, W. G. (1991). Ideological identification and issue attitudes. *American Journal of Political Science*, *35*, 178–205.

Jacoby, W. G. (1994). Public attitudes toward government spending. *American Journal of Political Science*, *38*, 336–361.

Jenkins-Smith, H., Mitchell, N. J., & Herron, K. G. (2004). Foreign and domestic policy belief structures in the U.S. and British publics. *The Journal of Conflict Resolution*, *48*, 287–309.

Jerit, J. (2006). Reform, rescue, or run out of money?: Problem definition in the Social Security reform debate. *The Harvard International Journal of Press/Politics*, *11*(6), 9–28.

Jost, J. T. (2006). The end of the end of ideology. *American Psychologist*, *61*, 651–670.

Kotlikoff, L., & Burns, S. (2004). *The coming generational storm: What you need to know about America's future*. Cambridge: MIT Press.

Lau, R. R., Brown, T. A., & Sears, D. O. (1978). Self-interest and civilians' attitudes toward the Vietnam War. *Public Opinion Quarterly*, *42*, 464–483.

Layman, G., Carsey, T. M., & Horowitz, J. M. (2006). Party polarization in American politics: Characteristics, causes, and consequences. *Annual Review of Political Science*, *9*, 83–110.

Marmor, T. R. (2000). *The politics of Medicare* (2nd ed.). Hawthorne, New York: Aldine De Gruyter, Inc.

Marmor, T. R., & Mashaw, J. L. (2006). Understanding social insurance: Fairness, affordability, and the 'modernization' of Social Security and Medicare. *Health Affairs*, *25*, 114–134.

Marttila, J. (2005). Are voters paying attention? *American Prospect*, *16*(2), 17–20.

Oberlander, J. (2003). *The political life of Medicare*. Chicago: University of Chicago Press.

Oliver, T. R., Lee, P. R., & Lipton, H. L. (2004). A political history of Medicare and prescription drug coverage. *The Milbank Quarterly*, *82*, 283–354.

Page, B. I., & Simmons, J. R. (2000). *What government can do*. Chicago: University of Chicago Press.

Payne, B. K., Gainey, R. R., Triplett, R. A., & Donner, M. J. (2004). What drives punitive beliefs?: Demographic characteristics and justifications for sentencing. *Journal of Criminal Justice*, *32*, 195–206.

Peterson, P. G. (2004). *Running on empty: How the democratic and republican parties are bankrupting our future and what Americans can do about it*. New York: Farrar, Straus, and Giroux.

Schlesinger M., & Lee, T. (1994). Is healthcare different? Popular support of federal health and social policies. In J. A. Monroe & G. S Belkin (Eds.), *The politics of health care reform* (pp. 297–374). Durham, NC: Duke University Press.

Sears, D. O. (1993). Symbolic politics: A socio-psychological theory. In S. Iyengar & W. J. McGuire (Eds.), *Explorations in political psychology* (pp. 113–149). Durham, NC: Duke University Press.

Sears, D. O., Huddy, L., & Schaffer, L. G. (1986). A schematic variant of symbolic politics theory, as applied to racial and gender equality. In R. R. Lau & D. O. Sears (Eds.), *Political Cognition* (pp 159–202). Hillsdale, NJ: Lawrence Erlbaum.

Social Security Advisory Board. (1998). *Why action should be taken soon*. Washington, DC: SSAB.

Stark, B. (2008, January 5). Democratic Presidential Debate. Manchester, New Hampshire. Retrieved October 22, 2008, from http://abcnews.go.com/Politics/DemocraticDebate/story?id=4092530=1

Street, D., & Cossman, J. S. (2006). Greatest generation or greedy geezers? Social spending preferences and the elderly. *Social Problems*, *53*, 75–96.

Tedin, K. L, Matlin, R. E., & Weinher, G. R. (2001). Age, race, self-interest, and financing public schools through referenda. *Journal of Politics*, *63*, 270–294.

Zaller, J. R. (1992). *The nature and origins of mass opinion*. New York: Cambridge University Press.

15 Restoring Confidence in Social Security: Our Obligation to Future Generations

HARRY R. MOODY

Gloom and doom about the future has been matched by a disturbing rise of pessimism about prospects for future generations (Rees, 2004). For example, by a two-to-one margin, people aged 65 and older expect today's children will be worse off when they grow up compared to people today (Pew, 2006). This attitude is a dramatic reversal of Americans' traditional belief in progress and an improved life for future generations. This broad pessimism has been accompanied by a trend identified by philosopher Jurgen Habermas (1988) as the "legitimation crisis," namely a pervasive decline of confidence in major institutions of our society such as Congress, the presidency, and the professions.

A similar pessimism has affected public attitudes toward social insurance programs. Here we see a paradox: There is widespread support for the programs (legitimation), yet declining confidence in the viability of these programs. Specifically, young people today support Social Security but lack confidence in its future, as any college professor can confirm by an informal poll of the students (Estes et al, 2008). Distressing numbers of students doubt that they will ever receive meaningful benefits themselves. Such global pessimism may be largely without foundation (as I believe), because funding in Social Security problems do not confront us immediately and can actually be resolved by taking fairly modest steps, as AARP outlined in its statement on "Reimagining America" (AARP,

2006). But to make those steps requires both recognizing a problem and being willing to make sacrifices to solve the problem.

The demand for political action and making sacrifices, poses a deeper question: How can we mobilize political will to insure the future of Social Security? On the one hand, privatization proposals amount to a cry of despair and a rejection of social insurance: "The public system is broken, so bypass it." This is the message that privatization advocates have been urging for years. But abstract endorsement of "solidarity" or the "interdependence of generations" (Kingson, Hirshorn, & Harootyan, 1987) is not sufficient to deal with pessimism. What is needed is acknowledgment that social insurance programs are part of an intergenerational compact and that justice requires sharing burdens and benefits across age groups and cohorts (Howse, 2004). A model for such intercohort distributive justice is found in the 1983 Social Security amendments, which not only redistributed burdens but also provided decades of stability. Once we acknowledge what Diamond and Orszag call a "legacy debt" in Social Security, we can take reasonable steps to modify both revenues and expenditures to make the system stable for future generations (Diamond & Orszag, 2005). Moves toward justice between generations are essential to fulfill an overriding goal—namely, to insure the survival and restore public confidence in the future of Social Security.

LOW CONFIDENCE IN SOCIAL SECURITY

An AARP national survey on Social Security was conducted in January 2005 among 1,000 persons aged 18 and older. According to that survey, a large majority of respondents held a favorable view of Social Security (62%), and two-thirds supported maintaining the program as close to the current system as possible (AARP, 2005). But there was a distinct gap between "support" for Social Security and "confidence" in the program. Only 37% of nonretired respondents were at least somewhat confident that "Social Security will be there for them when they retire." There were clear gaps depending on the age of respondents. Only 31% of Americans aged 18 to 39 years old believed Social Security would actually be there for them, compared with 82% of those aged 60 years and older.

Another review of public opinion on Social Security and Medicare concluded that by and large the public is not very attentive to specific funding arrangements for age-based entitlements. For example, most people have been unaware of the phased increase in Social Security's normal retirement age from 65 to 67, with many believing they will reach full eligibility before they can under current law (Paladino & Helman, 2003). Specifically, the idea of an "intergenerational compact" at the foundation of these programs seems to elude many American, and even among those who do appreciate this idea, there seems to be a combination of "denial and dread" about promises made for the retirement safety net in the future (Shaw & Mysiewicz, 2004).

This pervasive lack of confidence among younger people is an ominous sign for the future. The low level of confidence was present before George W. Bush's 2005 campaign on behalf of private accounts but was probably further weakened by messages telling the American people that the public system was broken and could only be "saved" by diverting payroll taxes to create new private accounts. There is no reason to think that since 2005 public confidence in the future of Social Security has improved. Today, we are dealing with residue of years of attack and doubt about the future of social insurance. Nancy Altman has put the matter succinctly:

> As long as the American people continue to support it, there's no reason why it can't provide benefits to our children, grandchildren and great-grandchildren. But public support is crucial. That's why I worry about the president's campaign, and especially about what it has done to undermine confidence among younger people. If we stop trusting Social Security, then of course we'll want to put our money somewhere else—and that starts the fatal snowball effect (Altman, 2005).

AARP, America's most prominent advocacy organization for older people, has long been aware of this problem, specifically the long-range impact of declining confidence among younger people and the fatal "snowball effect" that this could induce. For example, AARP's "Divided We Fail" (2007) Campaign that launched in 2007 urges public officials to act decisively to promote lifetime financial security. At the same time, the platform of "Divided We Fail" explicitly urges that, in coming up with solutions, policy makers should avoid "burdening future generations." In short, America's largest lobbying organization on behalf of older people has explicitly adopted concern about "justice between generations" into the most extensive lobbying campaign ever launched in its history.

The response by AARP appears to differ from the position taken by many other gerontologists and advocates for older people. Since the 1980s, there has been a commonly held belief that worries about "generational equity" are just a means of destroying public confidence in the legitimacy of age-based entitlements and social insurance. Two decades ago, at the time when groups like American for Generational Equity were beating the drum on these issues, such a purely defensive response was perhaps understandable. But today, issues about justice between generations are becoming unavoidable, especially as we consider the prospect of burdens posed on future generations by current environmental practices (Moody, 2008). Politically progressive defenders of Social Security need to recognize that issues of justice between generations are bound to arise when we transfer significant resources between age groups and birth cohorts.

Thus, for example, in contrast to some defenders of Social Security, Peter Diamond and Peter Orszag (2005) are not afraid to acknowledge the problem of justice between cohorts eligible for Social Security. They explicitly recognize an issue of justice between generations in the pay-as-you-go structure of the current system. Although rejecting proposals for privatization, they acknowledge what they term a "legacy debt." Legacy debt means simply that the first cohort receiving Social Security benefits received a "windfall" that was inevitable, to set the system in motion. That fact endures because of Social Security's operation as a pay-as-you-go system, which served to enrich earlier cohorts beyond what could be claimed on grounds of cohort equity alone. In short, some cohorts did better than others. But such "inequity" does not, in their view, imply that we should privatize the system, which would introduce further problems of equity and adequacy.

HISTORY OF RECENT SOCIAL INSURANCE REFORM EFFORTS

There are lessons to be learned from concern about justice between generations in social insurance programs. Anxiety about the future of population aging in the United States has long centered on the two big programs of age-based entitlement: Social Security and Medicare. President Bush's 2005 campaign to privatize Social Security only intensified that anxiety: Will these programs be sustainable for future generations? Can age-based entitlements be sustained to provide income and health security for future generations? When we look at the history of age-based entitlement reform from 1983 to 2005, we see a disturbing trend: Repeated failure, punctuated by a single success. The Social Security reform of 1983 was the great success. The Medicare Modernization Act of 2003 was a mixed result, dramatically expanding drug benefits, but introducing elements of privatization whose long-range outcome remains unclear. The lessons from this period of more than 2 decades of reform efforts are worth pondering, especially because the theme of justice between generations has been an integral element in the success or failure of entitlement reform.

The single greatest success in this period was first reform effort, the 1983 Social Security amendments re-establishing the solvency of Social Security. The 1983 amendments were the only policy initiative that explicitly aimed at long-term justice between generations—that is, applying a fair allocation of burdens and benefits across cohorts. This reform was the only initiative that clearly succeeded, in the sense that it became accepted public policy and, in retrospect at least, was properly judged to be "artful work" (Light, 1985; Light, 1994).

What about the other efforts at age-based entitlement reform during this period? These were the Medicare Catastrophic Coverage Act of 1988 (Himmelfarb, 1995), the Clinton Health Care Reform of 1994 (Skocpol, 1996), the Medicare Modernization Act of 2003 (Medicare Part D), and the Bush campaign to introduce private accounts into Social Security in 2005. All except Medicare in 2003 were clear failures, and the jury is still out on the long-range success of the Medicare reform that added prescription drug coverage for beneficiaries. A further point to be noted about the 2003 Act was the introduction of elements of privatization into the program. Both liberals and conservatives have expressed serious concerns about sustainability of Medicare Part D, because of the costs involved in the 2003 law, so reforms of different kinds, such as cost controls, seem possible in years to come.

Why did most of these initiatives fail? Partisan politics is an element, but it is not the whole answer. The 1983 amendments were passed by a Democratic-controlled Congress and signed into law by Republican President Ronald Reagan. The result was a bipartisan achievement. The Medicare Catastrophic law in 1988 was passed on a bipartisan basis, with overwhelming support, and the Medicare Modernization in 2003 was passed entirely by the Republican-controlled Congress, with no input or support from the Democrats. The Clinton Health Care Reform was also a partisan effort by Democrats, which failed to secure broader bipartisan support. Administration leaders of the initiative, at least initially, sought to bypass Congress but were ultimately unsuccessful. Finally, George W. Bush's campaign for private accounts never got any significant support from Democrats and eventually fell by the wayside.

These five efforts at age-based entitlement reform unfolded in a period when concern about "justice between generations" was gathering influence among policy elites, if not among the general public. During the 1980s, policy makers and elite voices gradually began to recognize that the elderly as a group could no longer be uniformly labeled simply as the "deserving poor," even if the public had yet to understand this fact. The truth was that, by the 1980s, the poverty rate for older Americans began to be substantially reduced. It would no longer be possible to base aging policy entirely on "compassionate ageism."

For aging advocates, reduction in poverty among the old had a downside. It was no longer possible to justify age-based entitlements on grounds of distributive justice if the criterion was one of need. If the old, as a group, could no longer be portrayed as needy, then why should we favor spending more money on them? Yet, social insurance programs such as Social Security and Medicare had never been constructed on the basis of targeting toward those in greatest need. Instead, social insurance was an age-based entitlement, without any means test or explicit targeting. Elements of progressivity, to be sure, were embedded in Social Security, but redistributive elements were obscured and balanced by a heavy dose of equity: Contributors who paid in more got out more from the system. This balance between adequacy and equity was a critical factor in the political success of Social Security. The balance assured that neither Social Security nor Medicare would fall victim to the politics of resentment that can fatally damage means-tested programs. This universalism was surely an important element in the long-term political success of age-based entitlements.

LESSONS FROM THE SUCCESS OF THE 1983 AMENDMENTS

As we look back at the history of the past 4 decades, it is important to draw lessons that can guide us in the future. Efforts at entitlement reform in the United States have not been notably successful, but one success does stand out: the 1983 Social Security amendments. This history shows, clearly, that it was only imminent disaster—the threat of insolvency and inability to send out checks—that finally mobilized key branches of the national government to work out a solution. That fact might be a gloomy or at least sobering lesson to draw from recent history: Namely, it is hard to make tough choices until the wolf is at the door. On the other hand, the character of the 1983 Social Security amendments give some hope that it is possible to address competing needs of different historical cohorts once we recognize that there are legitimate issues of distributive justice at stake. By striking a reasonable balance among competing demands, it was possible to reform the Social Security system in a way that led to surpluses and to solid foundation for a generation or more. That was no small achievement.

Throughout 1982, there was a financing crisis in Social Security, which worsened to the point where administrators warned that, within months, the system would no longer be able to send out checks. During the late 1970s, President Carter had signed legislation promising to make Social Security sustainable for a generation. But the promise proved hollow. The economic turbulence of the late 1970s and early 1980s eroded revenues needed to sustain the program, and by 1982, Social Security was again near bankruptcy. It was against this backdrop that legislators finally agreed to a compromise plan that restored solvency. Facing imminent catastrophe, a bipartisan commission came up with a solution to the financing of Social Security, a solution that involved benefit cuts, tax increases, and other reforms to insure that the program would be solvent for decades to come. The reform legislation was finally signed into law by President Reagan in 1983.

The Social Security crisis of the 1980s was a turning point in thinking about justice between generations. The 1983 Social Security reform was appropriately called "artful work," a triumph of bipartisan cooperation. Yet, just as in the late 1970s, public opinion persistently remained negative about the future of Social Security. In a national survey in 1985, only 35% felt confident in the future of Social Security, with 60% expressing lack of confidence: Virtually identical to the gloomy proportions in 1978. In 1987, partly in response to the lack of public understanding and growing lack of confidence, social insurance advocates established the nonpartisan National Academy of Social Insurance, aiming to deepen public understanding and appreciation of this distinctive achievement of America's social insurance programs.

The Social Security financing crisis brought attention to the issue of justice between generations in social insurance programs. Throughout the 1980s, critics would insist that Social Security was unfair to different birth cohorts. They warned that the program was unsustainable and would end up cheating future generations. It was argued that the system was unfair because young people would never get back what they paid in. This appeal to generational justice became a powerful element in arguments to end a public pension system altogether, as proponents of privatization maintained. These arguments never achieved acceptance by the public, but the critics did have a point: Social Security did provide unequal benefits and burdens to different historical cohorts. That fact could not be denied, but it did not necessarily follow that the system was unfair: Only that certain inequities needed somehow to be addressed.

ETHICAL ANALYSIS OF "DEDISTRIBUTIVE" REFORM OF 1983

Dedistributive policies are those that explicitly take away benefits from certain groups of people. One example here was the Social Security reform of 1983, which was made possible only by explicitly facing up to the demands of justice across different cohorts and making tough, "dedistributive" decisions for the sake of long-range sustainability. The reform measure finally approved required a sharing of burdens by present and future cohorts of beneficiaries, and it also required a balance between increased taxes and lower benefits. Current beneficiaries were required to accept a freeze or cut in cost-of-living support, whereas future cohorts were required to accept a gradual rise in the age of eligibility for the program, increasing to age 66 and then age 67 in the first decades of the 21st century. Table 15.1 provides a summary of the "dedistributive" structure in which burdens were allocated across different cohorts.

For purposes of simplicity, in this discussion we will refer to these three cohorts as "A" (1900–1920: roughly, the "G.I. generation"), "B" (1920–1940: roughly, the "silent generation"), and "C" (1940–1960: roughly, leading edge boomers). Our purpose here is not to vindicate, or criticize, the use of cohort analysis as an explanatory approach but to simply provide demarcations to illustrate the dedistributive effects of policy change on different generations.

As Table 15.1 shows, the 1983 Social Security amendments restored long-range fiscal stability to the system by the two strategies: cutting benefits and raising taxes. But the impact of different steps fell differently across the three cohorts. In 1983, Cohort A was already receiving Social Security benefits (average age 73). Their benefits were not directly cut, but the Cost-of-Living Adjustment (COLA) was delayed 6 months: Modestly painful but not devastating. However, delaying the COLA actually saved nearly $40 billion over the period required to bring Social Security into stability, so this seemingly small step had large consequences. Cohort A was also subject to taxation of Social Security benefits beyond a certain income threshold: But again, the impact here was modest because only

Table 15.1

DEDISTRIBUTIVE EFFECTS OF 1983 SOCIAL SECURITY REFORM[a]

CUTTING BENEFITS		RAISING TAXES	
DELAY IN COST-OF-LIVING ADJUSTMENT	RAISING AGE OF ELIGIBILITY	TAXATION OF BENEFITS	INCREASING THE PAYROLL TAX
1900–1920		1900–1920	
		1920–1940	1920–1940
	1940–1960	1940–1960	1940–1960

[a]Impact on three cohorts: Those born 1900–1920, 1920–1940, and 1940–1960.

a small percentage of beneficiaries were subject to the tax. In any case, it was not an example of a "means test" (e.g., Medicaid) but rather an "affluence test" (e.g., phase-out thresholds for IRA tax exemption). Other cohorts, B and C, would also bear the brunt of taxation of benefits. But because the income threshold was not indexed for inflation, gradually more and more beneficiaries would be subject to taxes on their benefits.

The other big cut was raising the age of eligibility for full Social Security benefits from age 65 to 67. This would be done gradually, after the 1990s, so that, by and large, the cut would not affect Cohort B but would affect Cohort C. Here, too, the rise in age of eligibility was done with decades in advance to plan for it and in such a way that there would be no abrupt changes.

Perhaps the most significant change in 1983 was raising the OASDI payroll tax from 10.4% (employee and employer combined) to its present level of 12.4%, which brought a huge infusion of revenues into the system. The purpose was not to create a truly "funded" social insurance system, but rather to build up a large reserve in the Trust Fund during the period when baby boomers were at their peak earning years. The increase in the payroll tax after 1983 affected Cohort B (average age 53), but only for a decade or so before they began to draw down benefits. Cohort C (older baby boomers at average age 33 in 1983) bore the lion's share of this tax burden.

What is striking about the 1983 amendments is the fact that all three cohorts—current beneficiaries (Cohort C) and current workers (Cohorts B and C)—bore different burdens. These were not necessarily "equal" burdens. But a standard of distributive justice will inevitably find it difficult to take account of all the shifting circumstances that affect different birth cohorts: For example, the G. I. generation bore the brunt of the Depression and W. W. II, while the older baby boomers were beneficiaries of a great post-War economic boom. One may argue that it should never be the purpose of public policy to remedy every type of "injustice" created by circumstances of history. Instead, the reasonable purpose of policy is to aim for "rough justice": In this case, some comparable sharing of burdens by different cohorts over time. In that respect, the 1983 Social Security amendments could well be a valuable model for future reform of Social Security: Shared burdens, rough justice, and incremental solutions that enhance the viability of the system.

OBLIGATIONS TO FUTURE GENERATIONS

In *Legitimation Crisis,* Habermas (1988) argues that under the regime of liberal capitalism, crises will inevitably appear in the form of unresolved "economic steering problems." Some assume catastrophic proportions such as economic depression and collapse. Others are less dramatic but engender pervasive loss of confidence in the political and economic systems, endangering social integration. The argument here is that the secular loss of confidence in social insurance programs is precisely such a danger to social integration across age groups and cohorts. Habermas' own solution is given in terms of his ideal of communicative ethics: "Only communication ethics guarantees the generality of admissible norms and the autonomy of acting subjects solely through the discursive redeemability of the validity claims with which norms appear. That is, generality is guaranteed in that the only norms that may claim generality are those on which everyone affected agrees (or would agree) without constraint if they enter into (or were to enter into) a process of discursive will-formation." If, following John Rawls (1971), we treat different age groups and birth cohorts as equally deserving of consideration, then the ideal of "justice between generations" compels our attention, whether in the environment (e.g., global warming) or in social welfare programs (e.g., the sustainability of Social Security).

It is reasonable, indeed, necessary, to aim for some kind of "rough justice" in the treatment of historical cohorts so that we avoid the spread of cynicism or disbelief in the fundamental equity and fairness of public programs like Social Security. Such a standard of "rough justice" is not a utopian ideal, but a very practical yardstick (Bedau, 1978; Vermeule,

2005). On the one hand, we avoid a strict criterion, such as that of treating every cohort with exact equality, as some economists have been tempted to do (Bommier, Lee, Miller, & Zuber, 2004). On the other hand, we avoid casual dismissal of justice between generations, as some aging advocates have tended to do, fearing, not unreasonably, that "generational equity" would simply become a stalking horse for those trying to undermine confidence in social insurance.

The problem, alas, is that confidence has already eroded at the same time that the "great risk shift" has transferred income security for retirement more and more to individuals (Hacker, 2006). The history of Social Security has always been a story of continual revision of the "generational compact" (Achenbaum, 1988), and the time will come for more revisions to take account of trends in population aging in the 21st century. John Myles, certainly no proponent of generational equity, is one of many voices who have recognized that justice requires reform of our public pension systems and a "new social contract" for an aging society (Myles, 2002; Myles, 2003). Now that AARP has joined in recognizing the challenge of justice between generations, there is no reason why we should delay in making changes in Social Security that will ensure its sustainability for future generations and restore public confidence in the system. The time to act is now.

DISCUSSION QUESTIONS

1. What is the legitimation crisis?
2. Explain why public support is so important for the future of social insurance programs.
3. Why, according to Moody, do most initiatives to change social insurance programs not succeed?
4. What does Moody mean by "justice between generations" or "generational equity," and how have various cohorts been affected by various social insurance reforms over the years? What does Moody suggest be done to provide for generational justice or equity?
5. Moody is the Director of Academic Affairs for AARP. How does the AARP approach to intergenerational concerns in social insurance programs differ from other recommendations in this volume?

REFERENCES

AARP. (2005). *Public attitudes toward Social Security and private accounts*. Washington, DC: AARP Knowledge Management.

AARP. (2006). *Reimagining America: How American can grow old and prosper*. Washington DC: AARP. Retrieved October 22, 2008, from http://assets.aarp.org/www.aarp.org_/articles/legpolicy/reimagining_200601.pdf

AARP. (2007). *Divided we fail platform*. Retrieved October 22, 2008, from http://www.aarp.org/issues/dividedwefail/about_issues/our_platform.html

Achenbaum, W. A. (1986). *Social Security: Visions and revisions*. New York: Cambridge University Press.

Altman, N. (2005, November). Nancy Altman: Drawing the line on Social Security *AARP Bulletin*. Retrieved November 10, 2008, from http://64.233.169.104/search?q=cache:ujRx76GFJ4MJ:www.thebattleforsocialsecurity.com/press/aarp_1105.php+%22fatal+snowball+effect%22+Social+Security+Altman=en=clnk=2=us

Altman, N. J. (2005). *The battle for Social Security: From FDR's vision to Bush's gamble*. Hoboken, NJ: John Wiley and Sons.

Bedau, H. A. (1978, December). Rough justice: The limits of novel defenses. *The Hastings Center Report*, *8*(6), 8–11.

Bommier, A., Lee, R., Miller, T., & Zuber, S. (2004). *Who wins and who loses? Public transfer accounts for US generations born 1850 to 2090*. Cambridge, MA: National Bureau of Economic Research.

Diamond, P. A., & Orszag, P. R. (2005). *Saving Social Security: A balanced approach*. Washington, DC: Brookings Institution Press.

Estes, C. L., Grossman, B. R., Rogne, L., Hollister, B., & Solway, E. (2008). *Teaching social insurance in higher education*, Washington, DC: AARP Office of Academic Affairs.

Habermas, J. (1975). *Legitimation crisis* (T. McCarthy, Trans.). Boston: Beacon Press

Hacker, J. (2006). *The great risk shift*. Oxford: Oxford University Press.

Himmelfarb, R. (1995). *Catastrophic politics: The rise and fall of the Medicare Catastrophic Coverage Act of 1988*. University Park, PA: Pennsylvania State University Press.

Howse, K. (2004). What has fairness got to do with it? Social justice and pension reform. *Ageing Horizons*, *1*, 1–16.

Kingson, E. R., Hirshorn, B., & Harootyan, L. K. (1987). *The Common Stake: The Interdependence of Generations*. Washington, DC: Gerontological Society of America.

Light, P. (1985). *Artful Work*. New York: Random House.

Light, P. (1994). *Still artful work: The continuing politics of Social Security reform*. New York: McGraw-Hill.

Moody, H. R. (2008, Spring). Environmentalism as an aging issue. *Public Policy and Aging Report*, 1–7.

Myles, J. F. (2002). A new contract for the elderly. In G. Esping–Anderson, D. Gallie, A. Hemerijk, & J. Myers (Eds.), *Why we need a new welfare state*. Oxford: Oxford University Press.

Myles, J. F. (2003). What justice requires: Pension reform in ageing societies. *Journal of European Social Policy*, *13*, 264–270.

Paladino, V., & Helman, R. (2003). Findings from the 2003 retirement confidence survey (RCS) and minority RCS. *EBRI Notes, 24*(7), pp. 1–6.

Pew Foundation. (2006). Once again, The future ain't what it used to be. Pew Research Center Publications. Retrieved October 22, 2008, from http://www.mcgraw-hill.com/footer/contacts.shtml

Rawls, J. (1971). *A theory of justice*. Oxford: Oxford University Press.

Rees, M. J. (2004). *Our final hour: A scientist's warning: How terror, error, and environmental disaster threaten humankind's future in this century*. New York: Basic Books.

Shaw, G. M., & Mysiewicz, S. E. (2004). Polls-trends: Social Security and Medicare. *Public Opinion Quarterly, 68*(3), 394–423.

Skocpol, T. (1996). *Boomerang: Clinton's health security effort and the turn against government in U.S. politics.* New York: W.W. Norton.

Vermeule, A. (2005, September). Reparations as rough justice (Public Law and Legal Working Paper No. 5). Chicago: University of Chicago.

PART IV

Critical Perspectives on Social Insurance Reform

Part IV: Critical Perspectives on Social Insurance Reform

Introduction

CARROLL L. ESTES

This section is comprised of four chapters, each of which presents a critical perspective on one or more aspects of social insurance, social justice, and social inequalities related to the allocation of program benefits and costs. Historical and contemporary issues and comparisons in Western industrialized states are described, with attention to the earliest forms of social insurance programs and changes in them over time and directions of current reform efforts. Concepts of interdependence, risk sharing, fairness, equality, and justice are threaded through the chapters.

In chapter 16, Alan Walker focuses on the birthplace of social insurance, contrasting the two archetypal forms found in Western Europe (Germany and the United Kingdom). Although there were basic differences in the originating principles of the two programs, similar pressures for reforms in their social insurance programs confront not only these nations, but also other European countries as well. The chapter concludes with a discussion of the future of social insurance in Western Europe, sounding its wider implications.

In chapter 17, Chris Phillipson covers historical and contemporary developments from the post–World War II period to the present, focusing on the pension crisis arising from the neoliberal social policies from the late 1970s on (Phillipson, 1988). With Britain as an example and with comparisons to the United States and other countries, Phillipson examines the role of pensions in constructing the experience of dependency and exclusion in old age (Estes, 1979; Walker, 1986; 2006) and the negative effects in recent pension reforms that have produced deeper inequalities through the individualization of risk and the shift of pension plans in the United Kingdom from defined benefits to defined contributions. Phillipson locates these changes within the new economic globalization and urges a new global discourse with older people themselves as key participants.

In chapter 18, Phoebe S. Liebig and Bernard A. Steinman examine the taxation of Social Security benefits and the policy implications for the true costs of an aging society. After 1984, when the policy was implemented that Social Security benefits could be taxed (for those whose income exceeded a certain amount), revenue generated from taxation of Social Security benefits was deposited in the Social Security Trust Fund. Thus, general revenues (from income taxes) are now in the Trust Fund along with payroll taxes. Liebig and Steinman show that the consequences of the ways in which the U.S. government and the individual states tax (or do not tax) Social Security benefits generally favors higher income elders. The authors describe how and why Social Security income is treated differently in various states, including the fact that some states have no personal income taxes. The authors explore the implications of the ways in which Social Security benefits and pensions are taxed (or not taxed) in terms of equity among those who are more and less economically advantaged.

In chapter 19, Debra Street examines tax expenditures as a form of social welfare because they involve government revenues, whether foregone or extracted, direct and indirect. Tax expenditures are a mechanism for the distribution of public resources. Two types of such tax expenditures are identified—occupational welfare (employment-based "private" benefits) and fiscal welfare (redistribution through the tax code). In the case of the United States, the public costs to taxpayers lie in the redistribution of resources from the less economically advantaged to the more advantaged. This outcome fosters both a "pension elite" and the "pretence" that retirement income is a private individual accomplishment when, in fact, it is tax-subsidized through fiscal welfare.

REFERENCES

Estes, C. (1979). *The aging enterprise.* San Francisco: Jossey Bass.

Phillipson, C. (1998). *Reconstructing old age.* London: Sage.

Walker, A. (1986). Pensions and the production of poverty in old age. In A. Walker, & C. Phillipson (Eds.), *Ageing and social policy* (pp. 184–216). Aldershot, England: Gower.

Walker, A. (2006). Reexamining the political economy of aging: Understanding the structure/agency tension. In J. Baars, D. Dannefer, C. Phillipson, & A. Walker (Eds.), *Aging, globalization and inequality: The new critical gerontology* (pp. 59–80). Amityville, New York: Baywood Publishing Co.

16

Social Insurance in Europe

ALAN WALKER

This chapter focuses on the birthplace of social insurance and, after a brief introduction to its background and different manifestations, contrasts the two archetypal forms found in Germany and the United Kingdom. Although their basic architecture diverges, the direction of recent reforms to both of these social insurance schemes (and those of other European countries) has been similar, mainly because similar forces are driving them. The final part of this chapter reflects on the future of social insurance in Europe. In this context, "Europe" refers to Western Europe.

FORMS OF SOCIAL INCLUSION IN EUROPE

The general European term *social protection* covers not only income maintenance but also health and other services in which the state plays a major role as a provider and/or funder. Social insurance comprises one of three approaches to social protection, the others being: (1) social assistance and (2) universal benefits and services. Due to the central role of the state, all three are distinct from models of social protection based on private insurance. The term *social assistance* refers to means-tested schemes, aimed at poverty relief, but universal benefits and services are provided to everyone, such as all citizens, residents, or members of a particular group (usually a demogrant), regardless of an individual's circumstances or needs. In contrast, entitlements under social insurance are not needs-based or a social right (as under universalism) but depend on compulsory contributions paid to a fund or funds when in employment. Social insurance differs from its private counterpart in that contributions are compulsory and benefits/payments are not determined by reference to risks.

The first social insurance schemes were introduced in Europe in the late 19th and early 20th centuries following the landmark German legislation in 1889. They were, however, very limited in their coverage of the industrial risks such as sickness, invalidity, and old age. Moreover, initially they were opposed by many trade union activists because it was feared that they would undermine existing workers' support schemes and, with them, working class solidarity (Clasen, 1997). However, from the perspective of the conservative and liberal elites and social democratic reformers, they came to be regarded as a key mechanism for the integration of the growing working class into the existing economic social and political order. Early trade union opposition was reversed when the potential of social insurance to enhance socioeconomic security was realized and, crucially, the schemes themselves proved to be popular with workers. Thus, in the first 2 decades of the 20th century there was a remarkable common trend among European countries in the introduction of social insurance schemes:

> From the frozen shores of Norway down to the sunny clime of Italy, from the furthest East and up to Spain, all Europe, whether Germanic, Saxon, Latin or Slav, follows the same path. Some countries have made greater advance than others, but none have remained outside of the procession, unless it be a few of the more insignificant principalities of the Balkan peninsular. The movement for social insurance is one of the most important world movements of our times. (Rubinow, 1913, p. 26)

Although not stated explicitly in this American commentator's rather colorful observation, the proximity of the countries in question suggests that an important role for foreign evidence in the making of national social policy – the pensions, health care and so on – was born in this period. Thus, social insurance was regarded as an expression of national solidarity: The application of what had been hitherto community-based mutualism on a national scale. This expansion of social insurance was one of the main engines behind the growth and institutionalization of the major European welfare states. It was hoped, at the time, that this would embed a broad class coalition in support of social progress that would facilitate a decline in social problems, especially poverty, and also in the application of selective means-tested approaches. Although this optimism was well founded in most European countries between the 1950s and the 1980s, by the latter and, more so, in the 1990s, it had good reasons to diminish severely. As we will see, one of the main reasons given for the demise of social insurance is its essential link with paid employment. First, let us examine the two contrasting approaches to social insurance in Europe.

BEVERIDGE AND BISMARCK: TWO MODELS OF SOCIAL INSURANCE

This fault line in approaches to social inclusion in Europe originates in the different historical and institutional legacies of Britain and Germany and the sociopolitical coalitions dominant at the time their systems were introduced. On the one hand, there was the British liberal tradition, emphasizing a minimal role for the state in providing a floor on which individuals could build their own personal savings. On the other hand, there was the conservative German approach, shaped by the church with a strong emphasis on traditions including the class and status structure, focused on the maintenance of status differentials by ensuring that the benefits provided by the state preserved an individual's previous standard of living (*Lebensstandardsicherung* or status maintenance). As well as differing in the forms of payments, the organization of the systems differs between the two countries. In Britain, there is a single National Insurance fund, operated by the state, which collects employers' and employees' contributions (the National Health Service is a universal service that is funded directly from taxation). German social insurance consists of five different branches—pensions, accident, unemployment, health, and long-term care—and these funds are controlled by nonstate agencies.

As with all simplifications, there is a danger of making too much of this classic contrast between Beveridge and Bismarck. First, German Chancellor Bismarck had intended the state to have a major role in the finance and administration of the system (Hennock, 1987). Then, after the World War II, the Allied Forces were planning the introduction of a Beveridge style "universal system" (Baldwin, 1990). The election of the conservative Christian Democratic Union in West Germany's first election in 1949, however, resulted in the reinstatement of the previous administration and framework. Second, the original Beveridge system was modified in the 1960s and 1970s to add earnings-related benefits. Third, both countries finance their social insurance systems primarily on a pay-as-you-go (PAYGO) basis and, in both, wage labor is the prime determinant of social rights.

Despite these caveats, however, the Beveridge/Bismarck distinction is helpful in indicating the fundamental difference between a flat rate and an earnings-related principle as applied in Britain and Germany, particularly with regard to retirement pensions. Moreover, these contrasting core institutional principles are characteristic of the overall welfare regimes of the two countries. On the one hand, there is the liberal welfare regime, of which Britain is an example, wherein the market and the family are emphasized. As a result, social rights are rather limited and Social Security benefits are modest at best. On the other hand, the corporatist-conservative regime, led by Germany, puts social insurance at the heart of the Social Security system and ensures that occupational status is paramount in determining the benefit amount (Esping-Andersen, 1990).

The British and German old-age income security systems are shown in Table 16.1. Both of them are three-pillar systems with the mandatory social insurance pension scheme occupying the first pillar. In Britain, it is the national Insurance Basic Pension (BP) and, in Germany, the Gesetzliche Rentenversicherung (GRV). In addition to these statutory schemes, there is social assistance provision in both countries that covers pensioners (see Table 16.1).

THE REFORM OF SOCIAL INSURANCE: CONTRASTING IMPACT OF NEOLIBERALISM

The creation of Europe's social insurance systems represented the heyday of the continent's welfare states, but in the 1990s, they became prime targets for reform as a general wave of neoliberalism engulfed policy makers in all countries. Although specific national reforms have followed their own paths and there is considerable variation between them, the common trend among European countries is unmistakable: A scaling

Table 16.1

PENSION SYSTEMS IN BRITAIN AND GERMANY

	BRITAIN	GERMANY
First Pillar	**Mandatory** ■ Basic State Pension	**Mandatory** ■ Statutory pension insurance scheme (GRV) ■ Old-age security system for self-employed ■ Means-tested basic pension (since 2002)
Second Pillar	**Mandatory** ■ State second pension (DB) ■ *or* final salary occupational pension (DB) ■ *or* money purchase occupational pension (DC) ■ *or* personal pension	**Voluntary** ■ Occupational (private companies and public sector)
Third Pillar	**Voluntary** ■ Personal pension ■ *or* additional voluntary contributions to second pillar (DC)	**Voluntary** ■ Private Insurance, ■ Officially certified private provision (since 2002) Riester-Rente

Source: Ginn, Fachinger and Schmäll (2009).

back of social insurance coupled with an increasing role for both social assistance and private provision. Britain and Germany will provide the case studies after an initial overview of the key factors behind the reforms to social insurance.

Accounts of the decline in popularity of social insurance among policy makers, if not by any means the general public, usually emphasize changes in the nature of the economy and society that have undermined their effectiveness (Baldwin & Falkingham, 1994). Although these changes are important and they are considered shortly, it is impossible to understand this policy shift without reference to the ideological transformation that took place in Europe on policy making during the 1990s. In fact, the first wave of neoliberalism to hit the continent came in the early 1980s and, as it swept across the Atlantic, it was the Anglo-Saxons that were the most receptive. The election of a right wing (New Right) government, led by Margaret Thatcher, which shared the neoliberal ideology of the Reagan administration in the United States, provided the major impetus to reform. The welfare state is always a target for attacks by neoliberals, because it offends their beliefs in the sovereignty of the free market and corrosive influence of government intervention. As a result, Britain's welfare state reforms predated those of most other European countries by a decade, and in global terms, were more in tune with Japan and the United States on this score. With the National Health Service a political livewire, the brunt of the neoliberal social policy reform agenda was borne by social insurance and, as is outlined below, the Thatcher Governments radically restructured it. In doing so, they undermined its effectiveness and added to the existing doubts about whether it is an appropriate form of social protection for the late-modern or postmodern society.

Some of the factors called in rhetorical aid to legitimize this unprecedented attack on the welfare state heartland are the same ones that are usually employed to demonstrate the outmoded nature of social insurance. Not all of them, however, can be taken at face value. For example, it is commonly asserted that changes in the so-called dependency ratio (particularly between those of working and pension ages) have rendered PAYGO an unsustainable basis on which to fund social protection. This assertion was used extensively by the Thatcher Governments in crisis of ageing rhetoric that effectively stifled public debate (Walker, 1990). Pensions and, by implication, older people were portrayed as a "burden" and a threat to Britain's future economic performance (Walker, 1991). Echoing the similar proposition advanced by the Americans for Generational Equity interest group in the United States, the idea of generational equity was used for the first time to try to legitimize the government's opposition to social insurance:

> Our belief in One Nation (sic) means recognising our responsibilities to *all* the generations represented within it. . . . it would be an abdication of responsibility to hand down obligations to our children which we believe they cannot fulfil. (DHSS, 1985a, p. 18)

In practice, there was no public debate about what the advantages and disadvantages of PAYGO as a financing method, nor about the disadvantages of private schemes even in the wake of a major misselling scandal involving agents who were paid commissions for every sale. The assertion, as common today as it was then, that PAYGO is unsustainable and, therefore, that private funding is better than social insurance, is an ideological one without supporting evidence.

Without indulging in an extensive excursion, it is critical in such discussions to acknowledge that the transfer from PAYGO to private prefunding does nothing to reduce the cost to society of compensating for lost income and, arguably, it increases the cost to individuals and families because of the higher administrative burden associated with private provision. This argument usually focuses on pensions because they are the largest item of social protection expenditure and the failure of the private sector to provide unemployment insurance. With regard to pensions, in any society, these must be paid for from the economic product of the working population, regardless of whether the method of pension financing is PAYGO or prefunding (Barr, 2000). Nor should it be assumed, as it frequently is, that saving to prepare for demographic ageing is the prerogative of the private sector, as the recent examples of Belgium, Canada, and France demonstrate. In practice, however, such rational points are not allowed to obstruct the path of a policy backed by an ideological steamroller. Thus, in the 1980s, the Thatcher Government was explicit about its intentions:

> The purpose of these proposals is to achieve a steady transition from the present dependence on state pension to a position where we as individuals are contributing directly to our own additional pensions and in which we can exercise greater choice in the sort of pension provision we make. (DHSS, 1985b, p. 6)

This essentially neoliberal ideological perspective was echoed 3 years later in an OECD report that paved the way for the global critique of public pensions and that created the second wave of neoliberal policy prescriptions to affect Europe:

> Under existing regulations the evolution of public pension schemes is likely to put a heavy and increasing burden on the working population in coming decades. Such a financial strain may put inter-generational solidarity—a concept on which all public retirement provisions are based—at risk. (OECD, 1988, p. 102)

In exactly the same mould, the World Bank (1994) report that followed 6 years later became the leading reference point for the pension reforms that took place globally in the 1990s (Walker & Deacon, 2003).

Apart from the demographic changes, two other socioeconomic developments have cast doubt in the key role of social insurance, both currently and in the future. First, there are changes in the labor market and the nature of employment that have called into question the core nexus between social insurance and wage labor. All of Europe's social insurance systems were embedded within their national welfare states and labor markets in the period of full employment following World War II. Thus, the idea that eligibility for social protection should be determined by full-time, continuous, and long-term participation in paid employment was not given a second thought. Barely 2 decades later, the doubts began to mount as a result, on the one hand, of persistently high unemployment in the 1970s and 1980s, and on the other hand, a bifurcation in the labor market between a core of secure jobs and a growing group of insecure discontinuous and other "nonstandard" or "atypical" forms of employment, especially part-time work. This latter group is increasingly excluded from social insurance because either the earnings of the workers are too low or they work too few hours per week. This excluded group is predominantly women. For example, in Britain, although 92% of men qualify for an NI Basic Pension, less than 50% of women do so. In Germany, barely 50% of the total workforce is covered by GRV insurance.

Second, since the 1970s, the concept of the "male breadwinner" has been subject to fierce criticisms led, not surprisingly, by feminists (Land, 1978; Lewis, 1992). The idea that men alone were the wage earners and women and children their dependents, although it reflected the contemporary conditions when many social insurance systems were originated, became anachronistic, at least as far as women are concerned, with the rapid increase in their labor force participation from the 1960s and the wide acceptance of their equal status. Whether or not these major socioeconomic changes should necessarily undermine the principle of social insurance is a matter that is discussed in the final section of this chapter.

With these socioeconomic and demographic factors in the background, the foreground impact of neoliberal ideology on social insurance in Europe (and many other branches of social policy) came in two waves, in the 1980s and the 1990s, but it was not spread evenly across the continent. As indicated previously Britain, under the New Right Thatcher Government, led the way and the rest of Europe followed a decade later. Moreover, the formers' reforms were far more radical than in the vast majority of other European countries (excluding those of the former communist block in Central and Eastern Europe). Although the role of social insurance undoubtedly came under question in most countries in the 1990s and was both restructured and, to a greater or lesser extent, cut back in favor of greater selectivity or means testing and/or private provision, the British reforms were far more thoroughgoing and seriously threatened the future of the country's social insurance system. This difference can be illustrated with reference, again, to Britain and Germany particularly with regard to pension reforms: The former representing a radical neoliberal strategy, an outlier in Europe, and the latter the more restrained European mainstream response to neoliberalism.

PENSION REFORM IN BRITAIN

As noted previously, the basic flat-rate benefit principle of the Beveridge system was transgressed in the 1960s when earnings related contributions and benefits were introduced. This was extended substantially in the 1970s by the introduction of a new state second pillar earnings related pension: The State Earnings Related Pensions Scheme (SERPS). The 1980s, however, witnessed a sharp reversal in the fortunes of the pension system and, indeed, the whole of the social insurance system.

The Thatcher Government's first white paper on public expenditure established the following rationale for subsequent attacks on social insurance and other parts of the welfare state: "public expenditure is at the heart of Britain's present economic difficulties" (Treasury, 1979, p. 1). Needless to say, because the BP is the largest single item of social expenditure, it was one of the earliest targets. Thus, immediately on taking office, the government broke the annual uprating link between pensions and average earnings and substituted a retail price index one. This meant that, year by year, as the average wage escalator outpaced the prices one, the relative value of the BP shrank. In effect, the basic social insurance pension was being residualized by the continuous rise in average earnings and inequalities between the employed and retired increased rapidly (Walker, 1991). This policy also advanced the second main strand of the government's social security strategy in this period. In addition to cutting overall expenditure, it sought to increase the use of means tests at the expense of social insurance (Piachaud, 1997). In the government's own euphemistic terms, this meant restraining social security spending to "what the economy can afford" and "targeting" benefits on those in greatest need (DHSS, 1985a). The main aim of this strategy was successful in its own terms: The numbers receiving social insurance pensions (based on contributions when in employment) rose by 12% between 1978/1979 and 1986/1987 and expenditure increased by a modest 16%. In contrast, the numbers receiving means-tested social assistance rose by 62% and spending by 161%. Taking a longer time frame, in 1979, 4.4 million people were receiving social assistance, and in 1995, the figure was 9.8 million or one sixth of the population (Hills, 1997). Although beyond the scope of this chapter the "targeting" euphemism was little more than that as an estimated 900,000 pensioners failed to claim their social assistance entitlements.

The second flank of this opposition to social insurance pensions in the 1980s was the dismantling of SERPS. Introduced with cross-party backing in Parliament in 1978, this state earnings related scheme was not due to mature fully until 1998. In the mid 1980s, the OECD advised the British government that there was no need to take any action to limit the cost of pensions until 2010 at the earliest, mainly because of the relatively low level, and therefore low cost, of its pensions compared to other European countries. The government took a different view: "The certain and emerging cost of the state earnings-related pension should give everyone—of whatever persuasion—pause for thought" (DHSS, 1985a, p. 21). So, the 1986 Social Security Act made substantial cuts to the value of SERP benefits by altering the basis of the calculation of entitlement from the best 20 years to lifetime earnings and, at the same time, encouraged (through tax reliefs and National Insurance contribution rebates) contracting out of the state scheme in favor of contributing to a private personal pension or an occupational one (Table 16.1). The best 20 years entitlement criteria for SERPS was introduced to try and improve the pension rights of women and, therefore, its removal had the biggest impact on them. The Act also cut out other attributes of the scheme that favored women—the right of spouses to inherit the full SERPS entitlement and home responsibility credits for those looking after children.

During the 1980s in Britain, social insurance for retirement was a major target for a government intent on reducing the size of the public sector and promoting the private one. As a result, the "continental" tendency toward earnings-related social insurance was cut back substantially, and the system was regressed back to its Beveridgean origins as a minimum pension worth less than one fifth of average earnings (currently 17%). This ensures that means-tested supplementation is essential if dire poverty is to be avoided. This must count as one of the most extraordinary chapters in the annals of social insurance and general pension reform.

Perhaps the most extraordinary aspect stemmed from the government's pursuit of the classic twin neoliberal goals—reduction in the role of the state and promotion of the private sector. When advanced with evangelical fervor the results can be shocking. In this case, the opportunity and open encouragement for workers to opt out of SERPS (a defined benefit scheme) and into personal (defined contribution) pensions, in return for tax reliefs and social insurance contribution rebates, led to a major mis-selling scandal. In effect, the government passed its social responsibility for pensions to a poorly regulated private sector in which overzealous agents and insurance companies, with direct personal pecuniary interests, were able to promote the sale of largely inferior and more costly personal pension schemes in place of SERPS. Estimates vary but at least 3 million people were missold private pensions when they would have been *better off* remaining in the state social insurance scheme.

The attack on social insurance ranged more widely than pensions and spread over 2 decades. For example, with regard to unemployment benefit. First, in 1984, at a time of high unemployment, the eligibility criteria were made more stringent and child additions were abolished. Then, in 1996, both the National Insurance unemployment benefit and social assistance for the unemployed were replaced by the Job Seekers Allowance (JSA), the first structural change to Britain's unemployment benefit system since the 1930s. Accompanying this change was a reduction in the payment period of the social insurance contribution based component of JSA from 1 year to a maximum of 6 months. At the time of its introduction, more than half of the unemployed benefit recipients had been out of work for more than 6 months. This radical restructuring of social security for the unemployed not only cut spending on this group but also blurred the boundaries between the purposes of social insurance and social assistance with the result that few of the unemployed qualified for the insurance based benefit. As with the residualization of social insurance pensions, although pensioner's benefits are higher than those of the unemployed, for both claimants and analytical purposes, it makes little sense to assess independently social insurance and social assistance.

The 1990s and early 2000s saw further changes to the state pension infrastructure, but nothing to compare with the damage done in the 1980s. Perhaps most surprisingly, the New Labor Governments have done nothing to reverse the previous policies and their impact on pension rights and pensioners, such as restoring the earnings link to the BP, as called for repeatedly by the pensioner's movement. In fact, the trend toward an increasing role for means tests, at the expense of social insurance, has been reinforced by linking the uprating of the social assistance benefit for pensioners (currently called Pension Credit) to earnings rather than prices. From 1980, the earnings escalator has been widening the income gap between wage earners and pensioners, whereas it is now is creating a gulf between the value of social insurance and social assistance benefits for pensioners. Despite a series of high-profile take-up campaigns by the government, there are approximately 600,000 pensioners who do not claim their social assistance entitlement. SERPS has been replaced by the State Second Pension (S2P), which is now aimed only at those with relatively modest earnings and, therefore, represents a downgrading of the aims and aspirations of social insurance, as embodied in SERPS, to match and in some respects exceed private sector provision. In another echo of the more-rampantly neoliberal policies of the 1980s, the New Labor Government attempted to encourage the private sector to introduce low-cost personal pensions, called stakeholder pensions, for those with low earnings. But regulation proved a barrier because providers baulked at the 1% ceiling on administrative charges.

PENSION REFORM IN GERMANY

The social insurance pension reform process in Germany contrasts directly with Britain's with regard to its timing and degree. As noted previously, Germany and most other continental European countries, implemented reforms a decade later than Britain. Also, there was not the same overt neoliberal fervor as in Britain, and, therefore, although the overall direction of travel is similar and reflects the World Bank's (1994) blueprint, the reforms are nowhere near as radical nor do they undermine the basic principles of social insurance. In this context, the background demographics and socioeconomic factors can be seen more in the foreground than in the British reforms.

Germany commenced its public pension reforms in the early 1990s and this has been a, more or less, continuous process ever since. The federal government has been explicit repeatedly about its aims with regard to the country's social insurance pension (GRV), which are to reduce the rise in contribution rates paid by employees and to reduce the level of the pension. The overarching goal is to adapt the GRV to the demographic and labor market transitions to ensure its future sustainability (BMFSFJ, 2006). Thus, in this case, neoliberal policy prescriptions are adjusted to national circumstances: The GRV is a socially embedded and popular scheme but the government seeks to limit its scale primarily to moderate the increase in labor costs, in the interests of international competitiveness, and to promote employment.

Over the past 15 years, the reform measures introduced have been parametric ones aimed at adjusting the scheme to achieve the above goals. Of course, all of these "adjustments" consist of cuts in pension levels or greater restrictions on eligibility. The most important ones are as follows:

- Extending the qualification period for pensions by the introduction of a new formula that attempts to balance the contributors against the pension recipients.
- Introducing taxes on high pensions and other sources of income of pensioners, such as interest or rent.
- Removing contribution credits for pension entitlements for periods of education and training.
- Reducing the uprating of pensions.
- Raising statutory pension ages.
- Introducing actuarial cuts in pensions for those who retire early.
- Providing tax incentives to encourage the enlargement of private and occupational pension schemes and to entice workers to join them (Naegele & Walker, 2007, p. 155).

As well as these measures that have cut back the social insurance pension, there have been some parallel enhancements. For example, in 2002, Germany's first basic means-tested pension system was introduced for those excluded from the GVR, such as full-time mothers, disabled people, and older workers with small pensions. This is separate from the country's social assistance system and was designed to prevent older people with pension entitlements below the poverty line from being dependant on it. The second pillar has also been enhanced since 2005 by the introduction of a right for employees to build up entitlements to occupational pensions schemes by transferring part of their earned income into such schemes. This has led to a rapid spread of occupational pensions to around 80% of German companies, covering some 60% of the private sector workforce. They are more common, however, in the old rather than the new *länder* and women are underrepresented as members (Naegele & Walker, 2007).

In common with other European countries, Germany has increased its pension age as a way of improving the sustainability prospects of its social insurance system. (In Britain, this policy option is complicated by the fact that the pension ages for men [65] and women [60] are currently being equalized over a 20-year period as a result of an Equal Treatment ruling by the European Court of Justice in 1995). In Germany, this change was originally announced in 1992, and in 2002, the pension age was raised to 65; in 2012, it will be 67. Early exit is still possible at the former early retirement ages of 60 and 63 but with stiffer actuarial penalties designed as a deterrent. Thus, if people choose, or are forced, to retire prematurely, they have to accept a significant cut in the value of their pension amounting to 0.3% for every month of early exit. So, for example, a person retiring at the age of 60 will experience an 18% reduction in their GRV pension.

In a similar vein to the earlier British approach, although in a more careful and regulated form, Germany has introduced a private defined contribution supplementary pension scheme, on January 1, 2002 (the *Atersvermögensergänzungsgesetz*). Although the aim is undoubtedly to encourage the development of an additional pillar of private insurance, in line with World Bank (1994) prescriptions, it is not, openly at least, regarded as a potential replacement for the main social insurance scheme, as was the case in the Thatcher policies of the 1980s. Instead, like the British second pension introduced at roughly the same time, this supplementary pension is aimed at those with a low income or families with young children to encourage them to make voluntary contributions to an occupational or personal pension, in addition to their GVR entitlement, so that by 2030 their overall pension replacement ratio will reach a 67%/68% target. Thus, the new supplementary pension provides some potential compensation to future pensioners for the loss in the value of their social insurance pension as a result of the cost containment measures outlined above. In other words, the German policy is affecting a small transfer, with public subsidies, from social insurance to the private sector, or from the state to the individual. Individuals are being provided with public subsidies as incentives, either in the form of tax relief or direct payments for those who would not benefit form such relief. Some EUR 10 billion has been allocated in 2008, the final phase of the scheme, to encourage these private pension investments. At the moment, this supplementary pension scheme covers all those who pay compulsory contributions to the GVR and it is planned to extend it to civil servants and other public sector employees.

Although this policy is clearly one of state-sponsored privatization, the step-by-step build up of private pension products alongside the social insurance system is in direct contrast to the free-for-all seen in Britain in the mid-1980s, the costs of which are still being born by millions of people. In Germany, private pension products must fulfill specific requirements to qualify for the financial incentives; for example, they have to be arranged before the age of 60, they cannot be used to secure a loan, and there must be a fixed or graduated monthly allowance guaranteed for the rest of the investor's life. In the cases of private funded pensions and bank savings plans, there must be approved payment plans. The supplementary pension consists of a person's own contributions together with public tax reliefs or direct payments. A minimum contribution is required to qualify for the public subsidies that consist of a basic allowance, for an adult, and one for children. Expenditure on this new scheme, both personal contributions and tax allowances, started in 2002 at a ceiling of 1% of the social security contribution ceiling for the GVR and climbed to 4% in 2008. It is permitted to save less, but the state allowances are reduced.

These two case studies of recent social insurance pension system reforms illustrate the big difference in style and approach adopted by the originators of the two archetypal systems in Europe. The German case is more representative of the overall European reform trend than the British one, apart that is, from the former communist bloc countries. In general, the reform of social insurance has been an incremental process with the EU itself, playing an increasingly important role in facilitating the exchange of policy information and experience between Member States as well as in setting standards. Yet, another direction of social insurance pension system reform is provided by Sweden, which decided to follow not the original World Bank (1994) multipillar model, but its revised one, favoring notional defined contributions (Holzmann & Stiglitz, 2001). In this model rather than privatizing parts of the social insurance pension system, as in the extreme and mild forms found in Britain and Germany, the individual notional account is created alongside the social insurance system. In Sweden, for example, a 2.5% slice of the total 18.5% pension contribution is paid into a separate individual premium reserve. This approach preserves the fundamental features of the social insurance pension system, but makes part of the benefit dependant on prevailing economic conditions and adds a disincentive to early exit.

THE FUTURE OF SOCIAL INSURANCE

Having reviewed the recent reform trends in Europe's major social insurance system, what can be said about the future of social insurance?

Without indulging in any ungrounded speculation, the most likely future is a continuation of existing trends, which broadly follow the well-trodden paths of the welfare regime types in Europe and the specific historical and institutional features of each country. It is likely, moreover, that the changes in the labor market and family mentioned earlier will be presented as good reasons to limit the role of social insurance in the overall social protection system. Arguably, however, this strategy is largely driven by an ideology that seeks to replace solidarity with individual responsibility because it would be a relatively straightforward matter to adjust, or modernize, social insurance to contemporary circumstances. To illustrate this, a quick reminder of the advantages and disadvantages of social insurance may be helpful.

On the plus side, social insurance systems thrived because they provide a relatively cost-effective and straightforward method of ensuring social protection for periods of absence from the labor market. The contingency basis of social insurance is administratively simple for both claimants and administrators, hence the universally high take-up rates; and the close association between poverty risks and the labor market makes sense as long as paid employment is the primary source of socioeconomic security. Because social insurance is a method of wage substitution, it supports the operation of the labor market by providing workers with security via national risk pooling, and with benefits set below wages, there are no disincentive effects. There is little or no stigma attached to social insurance in contrast to assistance benefits based on a means test. In addition, although the link between contributions and benefits is tenuous in PAYGO schemes, the ideas of "horizontal equity" and social rights to benefits paid for by contributions are enduringly popular. This, in turn, reinforces social cohesion especially when the national system is highly regarded, as in Germany. The contributions also made by employers add to a general sense that there is an obligation on both sides of the labor market to provide not only for themselves but also for the wider workforce. In addition, the idea of a social contract for solidarity underpinning pensions is impossible to generate in the absence of social insurance (Walker, 1997). Finally, social insurance is far cheaper to administer than either social assistance or private insurance (in the United Kingdom, the cost ratio of insurance to assistance is at least one to 10).

On the down side, as noted previously, the wage labor nexus was appropriate at a time of full- or near full-time employment but, increasingly, less so as the labor market has been restructured. This means that any social insurance system that retains its original form is bound to exclude increasing numbers of "nonstandard" workers. Similarly, with changes in family structure, the strict contribution conditions that govern access to social insurance are a guarantee of the social right they have earned but also a barrier to those unable to reach the required standard. This particularly applies to women who are more likely than men to both spend periods outside of the labor force and in part-time work. Some contingencies remain outside of social insurance schemes, such as lone parenthood and long-term care (but later discussion).

Although the insurance contributions secure the right to benefits in practice, under PAYGO systems, there is only a very tenuous link between an individual's contributions and their benefits. In fact, it is up to governments to ensure that there are sufficient resources in the fund to pay the benefits of current recipients. Finally, although the administrative costs for the state are comparatively low, they may be significant for employers, especially small ones.

Some may argue also that another disadvantage of social insurance is that the rich receive benefits as well as the poor, but this entirely misses the fundamental point of social insurance as a collective endeavor. Leaving aside such ideologically driven arguments that, in line with pure neoliberal principles, would sweep away state interventions such as social insurance, do the disadvantages outweigh the advantages and, therefore, establish a bleak future for social insurance in Europe? I do not think so, but if social insurance is to have a future commensurate with its illustrious past, it must be adapted to current socioeconomic and demographic conditions. In fact, this is precisely what has been happening in a number of European countries. For example, with regard to the demise of the male breadwinner model, the approach of most systems is to offer individual protection for both men and women. In the case of new family obligations, Germany has led the way in Europe by adding a long-term care fund to its social insurance system. The exclusion of women from social insurance was recognized in the British SERPS, but this was demolished first by a Conservative and then by a Labor Government.

The major requirement for the modernization of social insurance—modification of the contribution conditions to allow the inclusion of those groups not entitled to (full) social insurance benefits—has not been addressed. This would mean, on the one hand, providing insurance credits for a wide range of contingencies (such as education, training, and caring) and, on the other hand, universalizing provision to include those with only partial contribution records, again mainly women. These steps would transgress the core principle of social insurance but, in PAYGO systems, this is largely fictitious anyway. Moreover, without such a fundamental reform, social insurance would gradually become the right, ironically, only of those with full-time, secure employment. Apart from the recent major addition to social insurance in Germany, however, the governmental preference in most reforms—although acknowledging gaps in coverage—has been to fill them by means of selective social assistance or private insurance. This suggests that the future of social insurance is primarily a matter of political will and, at the moment in Europe, the political tide is running against major enhancements of social insurance.

CONCLUSION

This review of the past, present, and future of social insurance leads to five main conclusions. First, the differences in the original systems are due to particular traditions, sociopolitical coalitions, and institutional structures prevailing before, and at the time of, their creation. Second, partly for this reason, these systems have proved remarkably resilient (their popularity with contributors is also a key factor in their survival). Third, however, although they have been subjected to continuous reforms, the two waves of neoliberalism in the 1980s and 1990s had the greatest structural impact. Fourth, the extent of this impact is a function of the depth of belief in its basic principles held by governments and the strength of popular support for the insurance system. Finally, the future of social insurance in Europe does not look like an expanding one but, rather, a continuing story of limited reforms to reduce its scale and scope.

DISCUSSION QUESTIONS

1. What is the history of the development of social insurance in the United Kingdom and Germany? How do the two plans differ?
2. What suggestions does Walker give to make the systems more equitable for women or for part-time workers?
3. According to Walker, what is the relative role of changes in the labor market and family structure and ideologically driven arguments in driving changes in pension programs in the United Kingdom and Germany?

REFERENCES

Baldwin, P. (1990). *The politics of social solidarity*. Cambridge, England: Cambridge University Press.

Baldwin, P., & Falkingham, J. (Eds). (1994). *Social security and social change*. Hemel Hempstead: Harvester-Wheatsheaf.

Barr, N. (2000). *Reforming pensions: Myths, truths and policy choices*. Washington, DC: World Bank.

BMFSFJ. (Ed.). (2006). *Fifth report on the situation of the elderly in Germany*. Berlin, Germany: Bundesministerium für Familie, Senioren, Franen und Jugen.

Clasen, J. (Ed.). (1997). *Social insurance in Europe*. Bristol, England: Policy Press.

DHSS. (1985a). Reform of social security (Cmnd 9517). London: HMSO.

DHSS. (1985b). Reform of social security: Programme for change (Cmnd 9581). London: HMSO.

Esping-Andersen, G. (1990). *Three worlds of welfare capitalism*. Oxford: Polity Press.

Ginn, J., Fachinger, U., & Schmäll, W. (2009). Pension reform and socio-economic status of older people. In G. Naegele & A. Walker (Eds.), *Social policy in ageing societies*. Hampshire, England: Palgrave.

Hennock, E. (1987). *British social reforms and German precedents: The case of social insurance 1880-1914*. Oxford: Clarendon Press.

Hills, J. (1987). Whatever happened to spending on the welfare state? In A. Walker, & C. Walker (Eds.), *The growing divide* (pp. 88–100). London: Child Poverty Action Group.

Holzmann, R., & Stiglitz, J. (Eds.). (2001). *New ideas about old age security*. Washington, DC: The World Bank.

Land, H. (1978). Who cares for the family? *Journal of Social Policy*, *7*(3), 257–284.

Lewis, J. (1992). Gender and the development of European welfare regimes. *European Journal of Social Policy*, *2*(3), 159–173.

Naegele, G., & Walker, A. (2007). Social protection: Incomes, poverty and the reform of pension systems. In J. Bond, S. Peace, F. Duttmann-Kohli, & G. Westerhoff (Eds.), *Ageing and Society* (pp. 142–166). London: Sage.

OECD. (1998). *Reforming public pensions*. Paris: OECD.

Piachaud, D. (1997). The growth of means testing. In A. Walker, & C. Walker (Eds.), *Britain divided* (pp. 75–83). London: Child Poverty Action Group.

Rubinow, I. (1913). *Social insurance*. New York: Williams and Norgate.

Treasury. (1979). *The Government's Expenditure Plans 1980-81*. London: HMSO.

Walker, A. (1990). The economic 'burden' of ageing and the prospect of intergenerational conflict. *Ageing and Society*, *10*(2), 377–396.

Walker, A. (1991). Thatcherism and the new politics of old age. In J. Myles, & J. Quadango (Eds.), *Labor markets and the future of old age policy* (pp. 19–36). Philadelphia: Temple University Press.

Walker, A. (Ed.). (1997). *The new generational contract*. London: UCL Press.

Walker, A., & Deacon, B. (2003). Economic globalisation and policies on ageing. *Journal of Societal and Social Policy*, *2*(2), 1–18.

World Bank. (1994). *Averting the old age crisis*. Washington, DC: World Bank.

17

Pensions in Crisis: Aging and Inequality in a Global Age

CHRIS PHILLIPSON

INTRODUCTION

A major goal for social policy, across all industrialized countries, has been the achievement of income security for older people. Initially, the focus was on relieving poverty and destitution—especially among those in late old age. Gradually, aspirations shifted toward achieving replacement of preworking incomes at a level that would allow continuity of lifestyles from work to retirement. Countries varied in terms of the development of pension support: Europe introduced embryonic national insurance and pension schemes from the late 19th century onward (e.g., Bismarck's system of worker insurance in Germany in 1889, noncontributory old-age pensions in the United Kingdom in 1908). The United States created its own national retirement program in 1935 with the passing of the Social Security Act (Title 2 of the Act creating old-age insurance). In the United Kingdom, the 1942 Beveridge report laid the basis for legislation on social insurance in 1948. In general, though, at least until the early 1950s, support for older people in most Western countries remained extremely limited, resting on legislation, which essentially spoke the language of "poor relief" as opposed to that of "social insurance" (Blackburn, 2002).

In a European context, Tony Judt (2005, p. 73) emphasizes the extent to which the Second World War transformed both the role of the modern state and the "expectations placed upon it." He goes on to note that "the change was most marked in Britain, where Maynard Keynes correctly anticipated a 'post-war craving for personal and social security.'" Memories of the injustice and insecurity experienced during the economic depression of the 1930s were crucial in this regard, with the development of the welfare state, an attempt to institutionalize "a deeper sense of community and mutual care" (Lowe, 1993, p. 21) or "social citizenship" in the influential reading of T. H. Marshall (1950). Older people were integral to this theme of a more inclusive society, one seeking to erase the historical link between old age and images of poverty and decrepitude.

The purpose of this chapter is to examine developments in the field of pensions, taking Britain as an example, but with reference to the United States and other countries for comparison. The theoretical framework adopted draws on that of critical gerontology, exploring the role of pensions in constructing experiences of dependency and exclusion in old age (Estes, 1979; Walker, 1986, 2006). To develop a critical analysis of contemporary issues around pensions, this chapter will, first, sketch the evolution of pensions in industrial countries over the postwar period; second, summarize the impact of neoliberal social policies from the late 1970s onward and the new context of economic globalization; third, review the pensions crisis arising from the individualization of risk and welfare (Phillipson, 1998); finally, indicate new areas for policy discussion and debate in the field of pensions.

POSTWAR DEVELOPMENTS IN PENSIONS

Public provision for pensions[1] has been a contested area within social policy. Until the 1950s, pensions provided through social insurance tended to be modest in scope, both in the amount of money provided and in respect of the groups covered within the working population. In the majority of cases, replacement rates barely reached 20% of the average wage (13% in the United Kingdom in 1939; 17% in Canada; 21% in the United

---

[1] In the context of the United Kingdom, *Private pension income* refers to income from all nonstate pensions, including (unless otherwise stated) public sector occupational pension schemes. *State benefit income* refers to retirement pension (the Basic State Pension and additional state pensions provided through social insurance) plus income from related benefits such as pension credit, disability living allowance, attendance allowance, incapacity allowance, and winter fuel allowance.

States). The level of support itself reflected the underlying goal of public sector schemes, namely, that of providing bare subsistence and reducing the overall level of poverty (World Bank, 1994).

The period from the early 1950s through the mid-1970s was, if not exactly a "golden age" for retirees (Hannah, 1986), certainly one of progress in respect of the development of pensions. The rapid expansion of occupational (employer-based) schemes was a major element in this regard.[2] In the United Kingdom, employers used pensions (especially in the 1950s and 1960s) to cultivate a loyal workforce in a context of widespread shortages of skilled labor (Phillipson, 1982). Whiteside (2006) notes how some European countries, faced with the social and economic devastation arising from World War II, introduced citizenship pensions (illustrated by Sweden and the Netherlands) to prevent the spread of destitution. In the United States, economic prosperity fostered the expansion of employer-based pensions but with labor unions, such as the United Mine Workers, also influencing the adoption of pensions as a key item in collective bargaining (Sass, 1989).

In the case of the United Kingdom, postwar government policy increasingly emphasized the need for public provision to be supplemented by other forms of support. Pemberton, Thane, and Whiteside (2006) see this as integral to a view of state pensions as playing a residual role in comparison with commercial providers, personal savings, or employment. In reality, this was always going to penalize substantial groups in the population, notably those in poorly paid employment, those engaged in full-time personal care, the self-employed, and those in unstable employment (or as Pemberton, Thane, and Whiteside [2006, p. 7] remark "the majority of the population"). Little wonder that, after the burst of optimism about the impact of reform was over, it was the poverty of older people that was thrust into the limelight, with studies in the United Kingdom such as the *Poor and the Poorest* (Abel-Smith & Townsend, 1965) and in the United States, *The Other America* (Harrington, 1963) highlighting the scale of financial problems facing elderly people.

Pensions also became associated, from the 1950s onward, with the emergence of retirement and the development of what Walker (1980) identified as the "social creation of dependency" through the process

---

[2] *Scheme status*: an occupational pension scheme may be open, closed, frozen, or winding up. An open scheme admits new members. A closed scheme does not admit new members but may continue to accrue pension rights. In a frozen scheme, benefits continue to be payable to existing members, but no new members are admitted, and no further benefits accrue to existing members.

of economic exclusion. Income from employment gradually reduced in importance for older people over the postwar period; indeed, with the spread of earlier retirement from the 1970s onward, the period spent outside the labor market was substantially increased. At the same time, pensions provided through social insurance continued to be set below average earnings. In the United Kingdom, occupational pension provision in the private (as opposed to public) sector actually peaked in terms of membership in 1967, declining substantially thereafter (with in any event most schemes providing relatively small amounts and with significant groups, such as blue collar workers and women excluded from membership).

Any gains in pension provision were subsequently challenged by the neoliberal agenda affecting social policy from the late 1970s. In the 1950s, as Johnson and Falkingham (1992) observe, the move from a fully funded to a pay-as-you-go (PAYGO) public pension system slipped through without controversy. Economic growth provided a sense that state support for pensions could be guaranteed, so long as income and expenditure were kept roughly in balance each year. The 1970s were, however, to bring the initial questioning of the PAYGO system, as social security now came to be viewed as an obstacle rather than aid to economic efficiency. Given the level of expenditure on pensions, they inevitably came into the front line of the debate about the future of the welfare state (Myles, 1984). In the United Kingdom, plans for pension reform and for strengthening the public sector were abandoned in the 1980s to be replaced by a substantially weakened state pension system, an extension of means testing, and accelerated pension privatization (Walker, 1991).

In a climate stressing the economic threat associated with demographic aging, together with possible conflict between workers and pensioners over resources (Johnson, Conrad, & Thompson, 1989), the desirability of limiting reliance on PAYGO quickly assumed a degree of orthodoxy (Vincent, 2003). This was reinforced with the publication by the World Bank (1994, p. 21) of *Averting the Old Age Crisis*, which set out the case for moving away from what was viewed as an "ever more costly public pillar," underpinned by "high tax rates that inhibit growth and bring low rates of return to workers." Apart from recommendations to increase the retirement age, limit rewards for early retirement and downsize benefit levels (reforms that were already underway in many countries), the World Bank advocated launching of a "second (private) pillar with appropriate contribution and regulatory structures" (World Bank, 1994, p. 22). The benefits of this were presented by the World

Bank as threefold: First, an increase in long-term saving, capital market deepening, and growth through the use of full funding and decentralized control in the second pillar; second, diversification of risk through a mix of public and private management; third, insulation of the pensions system from pressures for design features that would be both inefficient and inequitable.

The World Bank (1994) built on an existing appetite for reform given a context of neoliberal social and economic policies. Through the 1990s and into the 2000s, benefits linked to social insurance declined in value—a process set to continue through the coming decades. PAYGO remained in place in maturing pension systems, but the ages at which benefits could be drawn were usually increased, as well as modifications to the contribution periods required. At the same time, almost everywhere traditional defined benefit schemes (DB) were abandoned in favor of the "portability" associated with defined contribution (DC) schemes, with the burden of risk and decision making transferred onto the shoulders of the individual worker.[3]

GLOBALISATION AND PENSIONS

The drive toward pension reform was given additional impetus by the trends associated with globalization, notably the increasing influence of global actors and institutions on nation-state-based economic and social policy. A key dimension, in this regard, has been the way in which intergovernmental organizations (IGOs) such as the World Trade Organization (WTO) and World Bank (WB) contributed to what has been termed the "crisis construction and crisis management" of policies for older people (Estes & Associates, 2001). This process created a worldview of aging as a worldwide economic and social "problem," with the accompanying ideology of globalization challenging existing programs of social insurance.

Deacon (2000) suggests that globalization generates a global discourse within and among global actors on the future of social policy, with

[3] *Defined benefit* (DB) *scheme* refers to a pension scheme in which the rules specify the rate of benefits to be paid. The most common defined benefit scheme is a salary-related scheme in which the benefits are based on the number of years of pensionable service. *Defined contribution* (DC) *scheme* refers to a pension scheme in which the benefits are determined by the contributions paid into the scheme, the investment returned on those contributions, and the type of annuity purchased upon retirement. DC pensions are sometimes referred to as "money purchase schemes."

pension provision a major area of attention. Yeates (2001, p. 122) observes that "both the World Bank and International Monetary Fund have been at the forefront of attempts to foster a political climate conducive to [limiting the scope of] state welfare . . . promoting [instead] . . . private and voluntary initiatives." This position has influenced both national governments and transnational bodies such as the Organisation of Economic Cooperation and Development (OECD), with an emerging consensus supporting minimal public pension provision, an extended role for individualized and capitalized private pensions, and the raising of the age of retirement.

In Deacon's (2000) terms, this debate amounts to a significant global discourse about pension provision and retirement ages, but one that has largely excluded perspectives, which might suggest an enlarged role for the state and those which might question the stability and cost effectiveness of private schemes. The International Labour Organisation (2002) has concluded that "investing in financial markets is an uncertain and volatile business: under present pension plans people may save up to 30 per cent more than they need—which would reduce their spending during their working life; or they may save 30 per cent too little—which would severely cut their spending in retirement" (p. 1). Add in, as well, the crippling administrative charges associated with the running of private schemes and the advocacy of market-based provision hardly seems as persuasive as most IGOs have been keen to present (Blackburn, 2006). John Vincent (2003) suggests that the focus on aging as a "demographic time bomb" reflects a particular ideological standpoint. He goes on to conclude that:

> "The function of such arguments is to create a sense of inevitability and scientific certainty that public pension provision will fail. In so far as this strategy succeeds it creates a self-fulfilling prophecy. If people believe the 'experts' who say publicly sponsored PAYG systems cannot be sustained, they are more likely to act in ways that mean they are unsustainable in practice. Certainly in Britain and elsewhere in Europe the state pension is an extremely popular institution. To have it removed or curtailed creates massive opposition. Only by demoralising the population with the belief that it is demographically unsustainable has room for the private financiers been created and a mass pensions market formed." (Vincent, 2003, p. 86)

Globalization gave impetus to a new conception of managing growing old, one based around what Ferge (1997) referred to as the "individualization of the social." On the one side, growing old was viewed as a global problem and concern; on the other side, the pressures were around individualizing the risks linked to movement through the life course. These were no longer seen as requiring the collective solutions of a mature welfare state. Indeed, as Blackburn (2006, p. 4) notes, individuals and institutions had now to be "weaned from the teat of public finance and learn how to be 'responsible risk takers' . . . rejecting the old forms of dependence of which the old age pension was a prime example" (see, also, Walker, 2006). Globalization has, in fact, introduced a new paradox to the experience of aging. Growing older seems to have become *more* secure, with longer life expectancy and enhanced lifestyles in old age. Set against this, the pressures associated with the achievement of security are themselves generating fresh anxieties among older people as well as younger cohorts. The language of social insurance has been displaced by the personalization of risk. Dannefer (2000) summarizes this process in the following way:

> Corporate and state uncertainties are transferred to citizens—protecting large institutions while exposing individuals to possible catastrophe in the domains of health and personal care finances, justified to the public by the claim that the pensioner can do better on his or her own. (p. 270)

What evidence is there, however, that the individual pensioner is doing "better"? What has been the record since the process of pension reform started back in the 1980s? Has the aspiration of the World Bank for more efficient and equitable pensions been achieved? The next section of this chapter examines the record to date, with a focus on evidence from the United Kingdom, but with reference to other countries as well.

PRIVATIZING PENSIONS: MANAGING RISK

Securing a supplementary pension to one provided through social insurance has become essential given that the latter—across many industrial countries—is set to reduce in value as a proportion of average income. But developing a robust private alternative is proving fraught with dangers for large groups of workers. In the United Kingdom, confidence in the pension system was damaged early in the privatizing process. The number of people with a personal pension increased rapidly from 3.4 million in 1988 to 5.6 million in 1994/1995 (Department of Social Security,

1997). Unfortunately, this expansion brought major problems, with the misselling of pensions on a huge scale. In the measured tones of *The Times* (July 16, 1997, p. 29):

> The life insurance companies saw the handing over of pensions provisions in the private sector as a golden opportunity to deprive the public of £4 billion. Life insurance salesmen, earning hundreds of thousands in commission, encouraged miners, nurses and other public sector workers to leave schemes with guaranteed benefits to take out plans where the charges in some cases meant that none of the policyholders' contributions were invested for up to four years.

It is estimated that between 1988 and 1993, approximately 1.5 million pension policies were wrongly sold in the United Kingdom, with the worst affected those who were duped into leaving attractive index-linked pensions for private plans. Years later, thousands were still unaware of the mistake they had made and that they could be missing out on thousands of pounds for their old age. A report by the U.K. Office of Fair Trading (OFT) (1997) concluded that many personal pensions were of poor value, with benefits eroded by the high costs of marketing and fund management. The OFT found that up to 30% of a fund could be eaten up by charges over 25 years, with salesmen making inflated claims for the returns from active management of personal pensions to distract attention from high charges.

Little wonder that a survey conducted in 2006 found that among those with a current personal pension or who had had one in the past, 60% took the view that they were "too much of a risk" (Clery, McKay, Phillips, & Robinson, 2007). The same survey (drawn from a nationally representative sample of adults) found nearly one in two (47%) of respondents (not yet retired) reporting that they "had no idea" what their retirement income would be (just 10% had a "good idea"). This was not unconnected to the fact that in 2005/2006 as many as 44% of working age employees did not contribute to a private pension (Department for Work & Pensions [DWP], 2007)—even though one survey found that nearly three quarters of respondents did not expect the state pension system to provide them with an adequate level of income in retirement (DWP, 2008a). Membership of a personal pension (including occupational pension scheme) varies substantially among different groups. For example, 86% of men working in public administration contribute to a pension (81% of women);

among those working in hotel and catering, just 16% of men and 15% of women do so. Among those on low to average wages (defined here as £5,000 [$8,000] to £25,000 [$38,000]), 51% are not saving for a pension.

Despite the ambitious claims for the virtues of market as opposed to collective provision, the proportion of working-age people in the United Kingdom saving for their retirement actually *declined* over the period from 1999/2000 to 2005/2006 (DWP, 2007). This reflects the long-term fall in occupational pension provision, yet to be offset by the growth of personal (DC) pensions (DWP, 2008a). There has been a substantial (and—in terms of rapidity—largely unforeseen) decline in membership of DB schemes: In 2000, active members (i.e., current employees accruing new benefits) in nongovernment (private sector) DB schemes totaled *4.1 million*; this figure had dropped to *1.3 million* by 2007 (Office of National Statistics (ONS), 2008a). This figure was actually below the modeling assumptions used in the U.K. Pensions Commission (2004) *First Report*, which suggested a long-term floor of approximately 1.6 to 1.8 million members. Seventy percent of final salary DB schemes in the United Kingdom are now (2008) closed to new employees, compared with just 17% in 2001.

On the other side, personal pensions provide income to a relatively small group of pensioners—20% of pensioner couples and just 7% of single pensioners. The income provided is also small—median amounts of £42 (approximately $63) per week for pensioner couples and £32 ($48) per week for single pensioners (2006–2007) (DWP, 2008b). Indeed, total pension income (defined as private—including occupational—pensions plus state benefit income) continues to provide “only modest levels of income for many pensioner households” (ONS, 2008b). Some 20 years of market-led reforms have left nearly two thirds (61%) of single pensioners in the United Kingdom with a total annual income of less than £10,000 ($15,000) and nearly one in two (45%) of pensioner couples with less than £15,000 ($23,000) (ONS, 2008b). Governmental sources of income remain crucial to sustaining the lives of older people: In 2006 through 2007 state benefits accounted for 44% of pensioners’ income, occupational pensions comprised 25%, earnings 17%, investment income 10%, and personal pensions 3%.

Widening inequalities are, however, the other significant dimension to pension privatization. The distribution of pensioners’ incomes in the United Kingdom has become broader since 1979, with the increasing value of occupational pensions and investments leading to a faster growth in incomes toward the top end of the income distribution (DWP, 2008b). Twelve percent of pensioner couples had an annual pension income of £30,000 ($45,000) or more in 2006/2007, whereas 5% of single pensioners had annual pension incomes of £20,000 ($30,000) or more. At the bottom end of the distribution, there are substantial groups with very low levels of annual pension income of less than £5,000 ($8,000) (approximately 10% of single women pensioners falling into this category).

Building a pension system around assumptions of increased private provision poses acute problems for women. Price and Ginn (2006) make the point that "in depending so heavily on private pension accumulation over a full-time working lifetime, the pension structure does not take into account lifetime working patterns interrupted and/or affected by caring and domestic responsibilities, nor the low earnings of women, nor the low wage economy and large inequalities of earnings" (p. 78). As a consequence, women continue to shoulder a disproportionate share of poverty—both across the life course, but especially in old age.

Single women pensioners are especially disadvantaged, with more than two-thirds (64%) receiving private pension income of less than £5,000 ($8,000) (2006/07 figures). Taking the period from the mid-1990s through to 2006/2007, women's dependence on benefit income (i.e., the state pension plus income-related means-tested benefits) has hardly changed: From 67% of gross income to 61%. This situation looks set to continue, given continued gender inequalities in private pensions, with a particular problem facing women working part-time where (in 2006) only 36% were currently enrolled in an employer's pension scheme. Again, among women employed part-time, only a small proportion is paying into a personal pension (less than one in 10 in 2006). These differences persist even among the self-employed (a fast-growing sector of the working population), where men are much more likely to be contributing to a personal pension in comparison both with full-time and part-time women. Ginn (2006) argues that new patterns of pension disadvantage are emerging among women, influenced by factors such as the rise in divorce (with lone motherhood among younger women much more common now than in the past); greater vulnerability of women from particular ethnic groups (e.g., first-generation women from Pakistan and Bangladesh); and the persistence of low pay and poor working conditions affecting women combining care work with paid work (see also, Meyer & Herd, 2007).

PENSION PRIVATIZATION IN CRISIS

The trends identified above clearly reflect continuing problems in the provision of pensions for key groups among the working and retired populations. Blackburn (2006) concludes from his analysis that "pension provision is a field where commercial provision has been tested and found wanting. After nearly fifty years during which more than half the working population has paid into such schemes—and during which they enjoyed . . . vast subsidies—the modest (US) or miserly (UK) public old-age pension is still the most importance source of income for 60 per cent of those in retirement in those countries" (p. 118). In addition, developments over the past 10 years suggest a more fundamental shift in approach toward financial support for retirement. This point is spelled out by Robert Peston (2008) as follows:

> What has happened to corporate pensions funds reflects a change in the culture of the U.K., the abandonment of the notion that companies have a moral obligation to promote the welfare of their employees after a lifetime of service. It is part and parcel of the death of paternalism and the rise of individualism. Company directors are no longer asking what it costs them to provide a comfortable retirement for staff. Instead, the majority of big companies are investigating the price of ridding themselves of any responsibility for their retired workforce. This is a less conspicuous but hugely important example of how the wealth of the many is being eroded, while that of the super-rich has soared. (p. 255)

Similarly, in the United States, Munnell observes that "we [are] seeing a brand-new phenomenon: healthy companies are closing their pension plans to existing employees and new employees . . . Employers want out of the benefits game. They just do not want the responsibility of providing pensions" (cited in Greenhouse, 2008). This process looks set to be accelerated with the economic crisis that began in 2007 with the collapse in the value of mortgage-backed securities—the so-called subprime crisis (Blackburn, 2008; Polivka, 2008). Brummer (2008, p. 50) notes how bondholders, including pension funds that had bought subprime mortgage bonds, suffered huge financial losses. This came at a time when pension funds had begun to return to surplus after a period of experiencing substantial deficits in many cases. The impact of stock market volatility was reflected in £15 billion being wiped off the value of U.K. pension schemes in the first 3 weeks of 2008. In the *Financial Times*,

Cohen (2008, p. 14) reported an aggregate shortfall in the plans of the FTSE 350 largest companies, compared with a £10 billion surplus at the end of 2007.

For individual employees, faced with pressures associated with higher mortgage repayments and rising interest rates on credit cards, cutting back on pension contributions has become a serious option. One U.K. survey found one in 10 (almost 2.4 million) pension savers expecting to take a break in pension payments during 2008, with those aged 25 to 34 most likely to do so (Brewin Dolphin, 2008). Women were more likely to pause or reduce their pension payment than men—a worrying aspect given the low number saving for a personal pension in the first place.

The developments identified above, illustrate the move toward the individualization of risk associated with the neoliberal current within social policy. The three aspects that can be highlighted in terms of continued problems of pension provision for those working and those in retirement include (1) difficulties associated with DC schemes, (2) problems of long-term and persistent poverty in old age, and (3) continued pressures associated with globalization.

On the first aspect, the growth of DCs will almost certainly extend inequalities among already disadvantaged groups with women, low-paid workers, and minority groups being especially penalized. In the United States, Hacker (2008) views the replacement of DB with DC schemes (401[k]s) as part of what he terms the "Personal Responsibility Crusade," with the move (as noted earlier) to transfer economic risk from government to workers themselves. Blackburn (2006) summarizes the besetting problems of DC schemes in terms of "uneven coverage, high charges and weak employer commitment" (p. 117). Wolff (2007) highlights research linking the rise in DC with greater wealth inequality and limited coverage among low-wage, part-time, and minority workers. Women have particular problems with DCs, with the longevity risk transferred to individual contributors rather than pooled among different groups. Zaidi (2006, p. 9) observes here that although "countries have tended to legislate that gender-neutral mortality tables are utilised, there have been practical problems of implementing these annuity regulations with insurance companies reluctant to offer them and the market proving difficult to kick-start. Thus, the net outcome of these reforms increases the risk that women will continue to have lower pension incomes" (see, Blackburn, 2006).

Timmins (2008) highlights the views of one U.K. investment provider that hundreds of thousands of employees who have been switched out of final-salary pension schemes and into money-purchase products could be on their way to being "private pension paupers" in old age—with these schemes only replacing approximately 38% of current salary. This reflects the extent to which employers often contribute fewer resources to their DC plans than were characteristic of traditional DB schemes. Indeed, the switch to DCs is invariably accompanied by a review of contribution levels—usually to the detriment of employees (see Timmins, 2008).

DC schemes are a particular problem given findings on people's limited understanding of pensions—with research in the United Kingdom reporting two thirds of respondents claiming their knowledge as "very patchy" or that they "know little or nothing" about pensions (cited in DWP, 2008a). In the United States, Munnell (cited in Greenhouse, 2008) observes that "workers have to decide whether to join the (DC) plan, how much to contribute, how much to allocate to what plan, when to change contribution formulas, how to handle things when they move from one job to another. The data show very clearly that many people make mistakes every step of the way" (p. 286). Zaidi (2006), summarizing evidence from Hungary and Poland on the switch from DB to DC schemes, cites surveys that showed how most people felt they were well informed and that information on pension reform was readily available, but that surveys also showed that "knowledge of the pension system was limited to slogans rather than a deep understanding" (p. 10). Research conducted by the World Bank also concluded that "a significant proportion of people simply joined the pension of the first agent they came across" (Zaidi, 2006, p. 10).

Second, the evidence reviewed in this chapter suggests that problems of cumulative deprivation will be a major feature of aging in the 21st century. The interlocking features here include (1) the growth of low-paid employment, especially associated with the collapse of manufacturing industry and the decline of labor unions, (2) the large proportion of workers either excluded from the private pension system or accumulating very small amounts for old age (especially in a context of increasing longevity and—in the United States—rising health care costs), and (3) insecurity associated with the marketization of pensions, with DC schemes leading to uncertainty about the level and adequacy of postretirement income. In the United Kingdom, a substantial minority of older people—1.2. million (11% of older people)—experience severe poverty (below the 50% line of contemporary earnings); 2.2 million (21%) of older people live below the 60% line before housing costs. Modeling of the future income position of pensioners suggests that unless policies change, the United Kingdom will face the same level of pensioner poverty in 2017 as it does in 2008 (Brewer, Brown, Emmerson, Goodman, Muriel, & Tetlow, 2007).

Finally, globalization will almost certainly influence ideologies and policies relating to aging (Phillipson, 2006). This will reflect four main factors: First, the growth of neoliberalism is one obvious dimension, this propagating hostility toward collective provision by the state or at the very least, a view that private provision is inherently superior to that provided by the public sector (Yeates, 2001; Walker & Deacon, 2003). Second, politicization has also arisen from the way in which globalization fosters awareness about the relative economic position of one nation state compared with another. George and Wilding (2002) make the point here that "globalization has created an economic and political climate in which national states become more conscious of the taxes they levy and their potential economic implications. Neo-liberal ideology feeds and justifies these concerns" (p. 58). Third, the ideological debate has been promoted through key supranational bodies such as the OECD, WTO, World Bank, IMF, and transnational corporations (notably pharmaceutical companies), all of which contributed to a distinctive worldview about the framing of policies for old age. Fourth, globalization will almost certainly create new forms of inequality for older people. Walker (2007) identifies a new politics of old age, driven by global-level institutions, which is now assuming increasing importance in determining the nature of financial provision for old age. Significant variations can be found across different countries, notably among the Member States of the European Union (EU). But Walker (2007) notes the impact of global institutions such as the World Bank on the countries of central and eastern Europe, with pressure on these countries to privatize existing pension systems or to follow the private, prefunding route in building pensions, often as the condition for the award of a loan (see, Zaidi, 2006).

CONCLUSION: REBUILDING PUBLIC PENSIONS

This chapter has illustrated a number of instabilities affecting pensions in the United Kingdom, but with many of the examples relevant to the United States as well as countries across Europe. Unsurprisingly, indeed, as this volume bears testimony, a lively debate is underway about the provision of support for old age (see, Blackburn, 2006; Munnell & Sass, 2008; Ghilarducci, 2008). In the U.K. context, substantial legislation has been passed—the Pensions Act, 2007—or is under discussion—the Pensions

Bill, 2008—with the aim of ensuring security for older people. In the case of the Pensions Act, 2007, the State Pension Age (SPA) for men and women will rise to 68 by 2046, and the Basic State Pension (BSP) will be indexed to National Average Earnings "some time after 2012." And the number of years needed to contribute to a full (BSP) is to be reduced. In the case of the Pensions Bill, 2008, proposals include introducing a new pension saving scheme of portable individualized saving accounts from 2012, automatic enrolment into a qualifying workplace pension, and a national minimum contribution from employers.

Viewed from a critical gerontological perspective, these reforms raise a number of concerns. First, they take as axiomatic the desirability of working additional years, this viewed as acceptable given increased life expectancy and necessary as a means of reducing the cost of pensions. But this measure (now largely accepted across a range of industrial countries) is especially unfair on working class groups whose lower life expectancy means they will draw their pension for a significantly shorter period in comparison to those from managerial and professional groups. Blackburn (2006) summarizes the issues as follows:

> The unfairness of class differentials is compounded by the fact that most manual workers, having missed out on further education, started work three or four years earlier than the more long-lived graduate employees, so that those with the longest contribution records receive fewer benefits. Any increase in retirement ages will simply increase these injustices. (p. 53)

Second, the United Kingdom proposals continue to rest on assumption about the stability and equity of defined contribution schemes to supplement public pension provision. But the record here—over the past 2 decades—does little to inspire confidence that those who most need additional income—women, those on low incomes, minority groups—will benefit from such provision. Indeed, one U.K. analyst describes the kind of personal accounts to be introduced in 2012 as a "scandal in the making," with lower-paid workers receiving "negative returns" on their contributions once means-tested benefits are taken into account (*Financial Times*, June 9, 2008, p. 2).

Third, despite recognition of time spent in unpaid care, it will almost remain the case that many groups of women will continue to fare less well in comparison with men under the changes proposed. Low pay and limited private pensions for part-time workers will continue to reflect the predominance of what Meyer and Herd (2007) refer to as "market-friendly" rather than "family-friendly" social and economic polices (see also, Estes, 2006).

What are some of the responses that might be made to the issues identified in this chapter? We will conclude with four points: First, it is essential to rebuild confidence that governments can provide protection and support in old age—fundamental elements to any system of social insurance. In the United Kingdom, just 14% of respondents in a national survey were "confident" that the government would provide them with sufficient income in retirement (Clery, McKay, Phillips, & Robinson, 2007). This reflects the deep-rooted crisis in the pensions system as described in this chapter, with many working age people (and older people themselves) caught between doubts about government provision on the one side, and market-generated support on the other. Restoring belief that adequate protection for old age is achievable is a fundamental task for any society, but one that many prosperous industrial societies are failing to achieve at the present time.

Second, public provision such as the Basic State Pension in the United Kingdom and Social Security in the United States remain fundamental building blocks in financing a secure old age. However, it is essential here that the pension provided not only eliminates poverty, but also provides an adequate replacement rate in relation to previous wages and salaries. This raises a fundamental challenge given the direction of policy at the present time. In the United States, benefits from Social Security are likely to replace only 30% of preretirement income for a retiree in the middle of the income distribution by 2030, compared with 40% in 2008. Similarly, in the United Kingdom, the reforms introduced in 2007 will mean that an individual on median earnings retiring in 2055 can expect to achieve a replacement rate of just 32% from the BSP. For both countries, large groups of workers will struggle to achieve a decent standard of living if reliant on public pension alone. Achieving a higher level of income replacement through public provision, one that compensates for periods of caring and low wages, remains a fundamental goal for an equitable social policy.

Third, a new global discourse on pensions is required, one that challenges the view that government provision should be reduced, and reliance on the market should be increased. The experience thus far indicates that market provision has led to a deepening of inequalities among different groups of workers and pensioners, that significant groups are likely to remain without the support of a viable additional pension, and that the volatility of the market is in direction contradiction to the need for security and certainty in old age. This discourse will need to challenge the neoliberal consensus around pensions, adopted in IGOs such as the World Bank, the International Monetary Fund, and the Organisation of Economic Co-operation and Development (Estes & Phillipson, 2002). These bodies have been able to exert considerable influence on the pension debate, but one that has marginalized views regarding the necessity of substantial public sector provision.

Finally, generating a new debate on pensions will require the construction (or reconstruction) of a politics of aging that draws on the energies of older people themselves, a group largely excluded from discussions around the future of social insurance. One of the most serious consequences of the privatization of pensions has been the undermining of confidence in the possibility of security in old age. Doubts about the point of planning or saving for retirement are now widespread—certainly in the United Kingdom, but in many other countries as well. This is, however, hugely corrosive in the context of rebuilding a new type of aging. The outcome will almost certainly be a "free enterprise old age" with large groups excluded from any kind of dignity and security, albeit with a minority able to carry forward much of their lifestyles in their middle years into retirement. Challenging the new social divisions in later life is set to be a key issue for social policy, and critical gerontology in particular, in the years ahead. Providing retirement security under the conditions posed by economic globalization will demand critical theoretical and empirical research if this challenge is to be met.

DISCUSSION QUESTIONS

1. What does Phillipson say about the evolution of pensions in the post-World War II period in Europe and the United Kingdom?
2. What are the basic tenets of a "neoliberal ideology" and how have globalization and intergovernmental organizations such as the International Monetary Fund and the World Bank influenced policy and undermined confidence in public pension systems?
3. How has the shift to defined contribution pension plans affected equality in the United Kingdom, especially in relation to women, minorities, and low-waged workers? What other consequences

of the shift from collective to individual risk related to retirement security does Phillipson describe?

4. What response does Phillipson recommend to the threats to social insurance he outlines in the chapter? From a critical gerontology perspective, how should older people be involved in these issues?
5. The Concord Coalition (www.concordcoalition.org) is one of a number of U.S. organizations advocating social insurance reform, including a shift to individual responsibility and private accounts. In contrast, the National Committee to Preserve Social Security and Medicare (www.ncpssm.org) advocates collective responsibility for economic and health security and recommends the preservation of Social Security and Medicare as social insurance programs. In light of Phillipson's account of the recent experience with pension reform in the United Kingdom, how would you evaluate the respective arguments about social insurance of these two U.S. advocacy organizations?

REFERENCES

Abel-Smith, B., & Townsend, P. (1965). *The poor and the poorest.* London: Bell.

Blackburn, R. (2002). *Banking on death.* London: Verso Books.

Blackburn, R. (2006). *Age shock: How finance is failing us.* London: Verso Books.

Blackburn, R. (2008, March/April). The subprime crisis. *New Left Review, 50*, 63–108.

Brewer, M., Browne, J., Emmerson, C., Goodman, A., Muriel, A., & Telow, G. (2007). *Pensioner poverty and the next decade: What role for tax and benefit reform.* London: The Institute for Fiscal Studies.

Brewin Dolphin. (2008). *Pensions at risk from debt repayments.* Retrieved October 23, 2008, from http://www.brewindolphin.co.uk/PensionCalculator/PensionBreak.aspx

Brummer, A. (2008). *The crunch: The scandal of Northern Rock and the escalating credit crisis.* London: Business Books.

Clery, E., McKay, S., Phillips, M. & Robinson, C. (2007). *Attitudes to pensions: The 2006 survey* (Research Report 434). London: Department for Work and Pensions.

Cohen, N. (2008, January 26). Financial turmoil puts pensions deficits back in the in-tray. *Financial Times*, p. 14.

Dannefer, D. (2000). Bringing risk back in: The regulation of the self. In K. W. Schaie & J. Hendricks. (Eds.), *The evolution of the aging self* (269–280). New York: Springer Publishing.

Deacon, A. (2000). *Globalization and social policy: The threat to equitable welfare.* Globalization and Social Policy Programme, UNRISD. (Occasional Paper No 5). Retrieved June 1, 2008, from http://www.org.unrisd/http://www.org.unrisd

Department for Work & Pensions. (2007). *Family resources survey 2005-06.* London: Department for Work and Pensions.

Department for Work & Pensions. (2008a). *Pensions bill – impact assessment.* London: Department for Work and Pensions.
Department for Work & Pensions. (2008b). *The pensioners' income series 2006-07.* London: Department for Work and Pensions.
Department of Social Security. (1997). *Welfare reform focus file.* London: Central Office of Information.
Estes, C. (1979). *The aging enterprise.* San Francisco: Josey Bass.
Estes, C. (2006). Critical feminist perspectives, ageing and social policy. In J. Baars, D. Dannefer, C. Phillipson, & A. Walker. (Eds.), *Aging, globalization and inequality: The new critical gerontology* (59–80). Amityville, New York: Baywood Publishing Co.
Estes, C. (Ed.). (2001). *Social policy: A critical perspective.* New York: Sage.
Estes, C., & Phillipson, C. (2002). The globalization of capital, the welfare state and old age policy. *International Journal of Health Services*, *32*(2), 279–297.
Felsted, A. (2008, June 9) A pension scheme 'scandal in the making'. *Financial Times*, p. 2
Ferge, Z. (1997). A Central European perspective on the social quality of Europe. In W. Beck, L. van der Maesen, & A. Walker. (Eds.), *The social quality of Europe* (89–108). The Hague: Kluwyer International.
George, V., & Wilding, P. (2002). *Globalization and human welfare.* London: Palgrave.
Ghilarducci, T. (2008). *When I'm sixty-four: The plot against pensions and the plan to save them.* Princeton: Princeton University Press.
Ginn, J. (2006). Gender inequalities: Sidelined in British pension policy. In H. Pemberton, P. Thane, & N. Whiteside. (Eds.), *Britain's pensions crisis* (91–111). Oxford: Oxford University Press.
Greenhouse, S. (2008). *The big squeeze: Tough times for the American worker.* New York: Knopf.
Hacker, J. (2008). *The great risk shift.* New York: Oxford University Press.
Hannah, L. (1986). *Inventing retirement.* Cambridge: Cambridge University Press.
Harrington, M. (1963). *The other America.* Baltimore: Penguin
International Labour Organisation. (2000). Press Release, April 28. Geneva: ILO.
Johnson, P., & Falkingham, J. (1992). *Ageing and economic welfare.* London: Sage.
Johnson, P., Conrad, C. & Thomson, D. (Eds.). (1989). *Workers versus pensioners: Intergenerational justice in an ageing world* (92–112). Manchester: Manchester University Press.
Judt, T. (2005). *Postwar: A history of Europe since 1945.* London: Heinemann.
Lowe, R. (1993). *The welfare state in Britain since 1945.* London: MacMillan.
Marshall, T. H. (1950). Citizenship and social class, and other essays. Cambridge: Cambridge University Press.
Merrell, C. (1997, July 16). Simple, low cost plans came to late for victims of industry's abuses. *The Times*, p. 29.
Meyer, M. H., & Herd, P. (2007). *Market friendly or family friendly? The State and gender inequality in old age.* New York: Russell Sage Foundation.
Munnell. A., & Sass, S. (2008). *Working longer: The solution to the retirement income challenge.* New York: Brookings Institute Press.
Myles, J. (1984). *Old age in the welfare state: The political economy of public pensions.* Lawrence, KS: University Press of Kansas.

Office for National Statistics. (2008a). *Occupational pensions schemes survey* 2007. London: ONS.
Office for National Statistics (2008b). *Pension trends.* London: ONS.
Office of Fair Trading (1997). *Inquiry into pensions.* London: OFT.
Pemberton, H., Thane, P., & Whiteside, N. (2006). Introduction. In H. Pemberton, P. Thane, & N. Whiteside. (Eds.), *Britain's pensions crisis* (1–27). Oxford: Oxford University Press.
Pensions Commission (2004). *Pensions: Challenges and choices. The first report of the Pensions Commission.* London: The Stationery Office (TSO).
Peston, R. (2008). *Who runs Britain?* London: Hodder.
Phillipson, C. (1982). *Capitalism and the construction of old age.* London: Macmillan.
Phillipson, C. (1998). *Reconstructing old age.* London: Sage
Phillipson, C. (2006). Aging and globalisation: Issues for critical gerontology and political economy. In J. Baars, D. Dannefer, C. Phillipson, & A. Walker. (Eds.), *Aging, globalization and inequality: The new critical gerontology* (43–59). Amityville, New York: Baywood Publishing Co.
Polivka, L. (2008). Back to the future: Restoring economic security for workers and retirees. *The Gerontologist, 48*(3), 404–412.
Price, D., & Ginn, J. (2006). The future of inequalities in retirement income. In J. Vincent, C. Phillipson, & M. Downs. (Eds.), *The futures of old age.* (76–84) London: Sage.
Sass, S. (1989). Pension bargaining: The heyday of US collectively bargained pension arrangements. In P. Johnson, C. Conrad, & D. Thomson. (Eds.), *Workers versus pensioners: Intergenerational Justice in an ageing world* (92–112). Manchester: Manchester University Press.
Timmins, N. (2008, May, 30). 'Paupers' warning over private pensions. *Financial Times,* p. 4.
Vincent, J. (2003). *Old age.* London: Routledge.
Walker, A. (1980). The social creation of dependency in old age. *Journal of Social Policy,* 9(1), 45–75.
Walker, A. (1986). Pensions and the production of poverty in old age. In A. Walker & C. Phillipson. (Eds.), *Ageing and Social Policy* (pp. 184–216). Aldershot: Gower.
Walker, A. (1991). Thatcherism and the new politics of old age. In J. Myles & J. Quadagno. (Eds.), *States, labor markets and the future of old age policy* (pp. 19–35). Philadelphia: Temple University Press.
Walker, A. (2006). Rexamining the political economy of aging: understanding he structure/agency tension. In J. Baars, D. Dannefer, C. Phillipson, & A. Walker. (Eds.), *Aging, globalization and inequality: The new critical gerontology* (pp. 59–80). Amityville, New York: Baywood Publishing Co.
Walker, A. (2007). The new politics of old age. In H. Wahl, W. Tesch-Römer, & A. Hoff. (Eds.), *New dynamics of old age* (pp. 307–324). Amityville, New York: Baywood Publishing Co.
Walker, A., & Deacon, A. (2003). Economic globalization and policies on aging. *Journal of Societal and social Policy,* 2(2), 1–18.
Whiteside, N. (2006). Occupational pensions and the search for security. In H. Pemberton, P. Thane, & N. Whiteside. (Eds.), *Britain's pensions crisis* (pp. 125–140). Oxford: Oxford University Press.

Wolff, E. (2007). The adequacy of retirement resources among the soon-to retired, 1983–2001. In D. Papadimitriou. (Ed.), *Government spending on the elderly* (pp. 315–342). London: Palgrave.

World Bank. (1994). *Averting the old age crisis.* Oxford: Oxford University Press.

Yeates, N. (2001). *Globalization and social policy.* London: Sage.

Zaidi, A. (2006). *Pension policy in EU25 and its possible impact on elderly poverty.* Vienna: European Centre of Social Welfare Policy and Research.

18

Federalism, State Taxation of OASDI Benefits, and the Economic Well-Being of Older Americans

PHOEBE S. LIEBIG AND BERNARD A. STEINMAN

When assessing the well-being of older Americans, the extent of budget outlays and their impact on elders' levels of income attract the greatest attention; effects of federal and state tax policies are often overlooked. However, government policies can and do influence the levels of income not only via transfer programs, such as Social Security, through which current younger workers pay in to provide income support to current retirees, but also by taxation policies that may be less obvious in their influence on the net incomes of retired workers.

Understanding the economic well-being of older Americans thus requires scrutiny of tax credits, deductions, and exemptions. These *tax expenditures*, also known as tax preferences, are not subject to the same level of review as other government programs that compete for funding; they also reduce revenues by departing from the standard tax base (Kenyon, 2006; Liebig, 2001a; Mackey & Carter, 1994). For example, more than $81 billion in revenue is forgone by exempting contributions to pensions and self-employed retirement plans from present tax obligations (Liebig, 2001b). Similarly, pension compensation is not subject to payroll taxes to finance Social Security and Medicare (Clark, 2001). However, tax expenditures increase the amount of money available for household spending (Clark, 2001), a major component of the U.S. economy today.

The purpose of this chapter is to outline the federalist relationship between state and federal levels of government, with respect to changes in taxing Social Security benefits and other tax expenditures provided to older Americans. We begin the discussion by describing the basic structure and history of old-age retirement security in the United States, with a focus on Old Age Security and Disability Insurance (OASDI) as a social insurance program that has positively impacted the economic status of older retirees. We describe changes in federal rules regarding the taxation of OASDI benefits and the impacts these changes have had on the basic funding structure/mechanism of the program, including a shift toward an increased tax-burden on higher-income beneficiaries.

Next, we introduce basic concepts of federalism as they relate to state income taxation of Social Security benefits and other tax breaks provided to older retirees. We emphasize the great degree of variability that exists between state and federal rules that is characteristic of a federalist system. We conclude the chapter with a discussion about why older Americans are provided with special tax breaks, as well as some implications of state tax policies for social insurance, the economic well-being of older individuals themselves, and revenues in states that enact them.

SOCIAL SECURITY

Old Age and Survivors Insurance and Economic Well-Being of Elders

The Old Age and Survivors Insurance (OASI) program, commonly called Social Security, contributes significantly to the economic well-being of older Americans. Prior to its enactment, traditional sources of retirement income were labor, assets, family, and charity (DeWitt, 2003). In the early 20th century, public (federal, state, and local) and private employer pensions were a source of income for a small minority of retirees. For example, only about 3% of the elderly were actually receiving benefits from state old-age programs (DeWitt, 2003). After the enactment of Social Security, the "three-legged stool" with Social Security supplemented by pensions and asset income has become the norm (Myers, 2001). For 20% of elders—primarily the young-old—earnings constitute a fourth leg.

Older Americans may differ in their sources and levels of retirement income and their ability to continue working, but Social Security is unquestionably a primary source of their income—90% of all elderly households receive some Social Security benefits. Although asset income, pensions, and earnings are more important for higher-income elders, Social Security is the major source of income for 40% of older Americans (Clark, 2001; Clark, Burkhauser, Moon, Quinn, Smeeding, 2004). As the level of income decreases, dependence on Social Security increases.

Social Security Disability Insurance (SSDI)

Older Americans also have benefited from the Social Security disability program (SSDI). First established in 1956 to protect the incomes of older people unable to work due to physical and mental impairments, SSDI now covers younger workers as well, some of whom are aging with a long-term disability (Sheets & Liebig, 2005). Nevertheless, the average age of SSDI beneficiaries remains over age 50 (Social Security Administration [SSA], 2007a), emphasizing SSDI's role as a potential substitute for OASI benefit options. In most cases, older adults begin collecting Social Security after becoming eligible for early or normal retirement (Rust & Phelan, 1997); timing decisions are influenced by age-related individual factors, such as health status and income. After age 62, the likelihood of applying for SSDI benefits drops dramatically (Benitez-Silva, Buchinsky, Chan, Rust, & Sheidvasser, 1999).

Although SSDI may be more advantageous than OASI early retirement, due to eligibility for Medicare, uncertainty of acceptance seems to deter many aged 62 and older from applying. In addition, prospective applicants must weigh "hassle costs" relative to their circumstances. Currently, a 5-month waiting period from determination of eligibility is required before benefits are paid. When eligibility is not clear-cut, SSDI can be delayed much longer, due to a complicated hearing/appeals process (Hu, Lahiri, Vaughan & Wixon, 2001; SSA, 2005). As a result, many older workers may forego applying, despite the possibility of entitlement. By contrast, younger workers must weigh "delay costs" associated with lost benefits from postponing their applications against their expectations for greater returns over longer periods of time (Benitez-Silva et al., 1999).

State and federal policies also influence individual decisions to apply for SSDI. For instance, *acceptance rates* have been shown to influence the rate of SSDI applications. Despite nationally standardized eligibility criteria, stringency of screening, and determination processes by state-based Social Security Disability Determination Services departments may vary greatly due to divergent administrative standards (Hu et al., 2001), different demands on resources, and interstate/regional differences in economic circumstances that can affect the length of backlogs and hinder the flow of cases. More applications are likely to be denied as the number of applicants increases (Benitez-Silva et al., 1999), resulting in lower overall acceptance rates. More lenient acceptance rates by states could increase the likelihood of older workers near retirement applying for SSDI, with more stringent rates reducing applications. *Benefit rates* also are a key factor in SSDI application decisions (Burkhauser, Butler, & Gumus, 2003). *Benefit rates* are likely to be higher for older disabled workers, because they are indexed to earnings and years worked. Older workers with disabilities are likely to have reached peak earnings earlier in their careers, leading to higher monthly replacement rates compared to younger workers.

Social Security and Income Levels of Older Americans

In 1933, approximately 50% of elders were poor. The OASI program has reduced poverty among the elderly significantly, from 35% in 1959 (Crown, 2001) to 9% today (Federal Interagency Forum on Age-Related Statistics [FIFARS], 2008). Major improvements in benefits during the 1960s and 1970s (e.g., automatic cost-of-living adjustments [COLAs] in response to inflation, expanding coverage to more workers) were largely responsible for this change. The SSDI program, also subject to COLAs, has had similar impacts on older adults with disabilities who are, however, likely to have reduced annual incomes compared to workers without disabilities, in part, due to their reduced earnings prior to entering Social Security rolls (Charles, 2003). Still, workers with disabilities, such as spinal cord injury, who may have more consistent work histories (partly due to the Americans with Disabilities Act), can be members of higher-income groups in retirement.

The significant income gains for elders during the last third of the 20th century in absolute terms, when adjusted for inflation and compared to the rest of the population, demonstrate the effectiveness of Social Security (Liebig, 2006). The annual median, pretax income of household incomes for elders (stated in 2006 dollars) grew to $27,798 in 2006, compared to $19,086 in 1974 (FIFARS, 2008). Furthermore, the proportion of elders with high incomes (greater than 400% of poverty) has increased from 18% in 1974 to 29% in 2006 (FIFARS, 2008), partly due to receipt of pension income. Knowledge about the wide range of income among the elderly was certainly a factor in the decision to tax OASDI benefits.

FEDERAL TAXATION OF SOCIAL SECURITY

Until 1983, Social Security benefits were not taxed. This and other reforms (e.g., gradual increase in the age of eligibility, coverage of federal employees, postponement of COLAs, more stringent SSDI eligibility requirements) were designed to ensure the long-range viability of the OASDI system. These changes also appeared to respond to caricatures about the elderly as "greedy geezers," many of whom were seen as not really needing Social Security benefits.

Rules for Taxing Social Security

As of 1984, the federal government began taxing a portion of OASDI and Railroad Retirement benefits of higher-income beneficiaries, if their "provisional income" exceeded thresholds of $25,000 for individuals and $32,000 for married couples filing jointly.

Provisional income was defined as the sum of federal adjusted gross income (excluding Social Security and deductions for student loan interest), tax-free interest income (often a steady source of income for risk-aversive elders and of some interest to the states that exempt their own state and local bond payments from income taxes), and one half of Social Security benefits. The amount of Social Security subject to taxes was the lesser of one half of the excess of provisional income over the threshold or one-half of Social Security and Railroad Retirement Social Security equivalent benefits (Baer, 2001). A portion of SSDI benefits are also taxable, based on the same criteria that determines the taxable portion of OASI benefits (Morton, 2006).

Under the Omnibus Budget Reconciliation Act (OBRA) of 1993, the thresholds were changed—between $25,000 and $34,000 for single filers and between $32,000 and $44,000 for married persons filing jointly. At those levels, up to 50% of Social Security was taxable. However, the proportion of taxable benefits rose to 85% for elders whose provisional income exceeded the higher thresholds. The amount subject to tax is the lesser of 85% of Social Security and Railroad Retirement Social Security equivalent benefits, or 85% of income over the higher threshold, plus the smaller of $4,500 for single filers, $6,000 for married joint filers, or 50%

of the Social Security benefit amount (Baer, 2001). Seniors with incomes below the thresholds pay no tax on Social Security and SSDI benefits.

Outcomes of Federal Taxation of Social Security

Taxing Social Security has resulted in several outcomes that directly influence the financial well-being of older Americans. Although the OASI Trust Fund was originally financed exclusively by payroll taxes imposed via the Federal Insurance Contributions Act (FICA), since 1984, general revenues from personal income taxes levied on Social Security benefits of higher-income individuals and households are also credited to the trust fund (Clark et al., 2004). Thus, payroll taxes are no longer the sole financing mechanism for Social Security, with the personal income tax acting as a form of "back door" financing.

Another less visible aspect of taxing Social Security has been the impact of inflation. Levels and types of inflation, such as increases for medical care or housing, have differential impacts on the economic well-being of different groups of elders (Liebig, 2001a). For example, medical inflation continues to drive increases in Medicare Part B monthly premiums ($96.40 in 2008) and income-related monthly adjustments that include tax-exempt interest income and IRA withdrawals, based on the prior year's income tax for higher-income households. However, in setting the income thresholds for taxing Social Security/SSDI, Congress made *no provision for indexing for inflation* (Baer, 2001; Myers, 2001), similar to the Alternative Minimum Tax (AMT). Each year, more beneficiaries are likely to pay taxes as their total incomes increase. In 1984, about 8% of beneficiaries paid taxes on their Social Security benefits; 16 years later, that proportion had quadrupled (Baer, 2001). Nearly three quarters of 12.1 million tax returns listing Social Security as income reported paying taxes on those benefits (Baer, 2001). This taxation of OASI and SSDI benefits for higher-income elders since 1984 has tended to smooth out income inequality among elders and result in a slight shift in the tax burden from younger to older households (Crown, 2001; Liebig, 2001b). All in all, federal tax treatment of older persons has become somewhat less favorable since the 1980s (Crown, 2001).

In addition, because of the formula used to phase in taxing Social Security benefits, one result is that over certain ranges of income, the marginal tax rate on an extra dollar of non-Social Security income is higher than on an extra dollar of benefits (Penner, 2002). Recipients are also subjected to very high marginal tax rates on extra earnings or extra income from investments, with every dollar of such income having a double impact on a person's tax bill. By taxing Social Security and SSDI benefits, their net value is reduced, essentially operating as an indirect approach to means testing, with the largest tax burden falling on the most affluent beneficiaries (Penner, 2002, pp. 1410).

In summary, federal taxation of OASDI benefits largely reflects growing concern over the last 3 decades for the solvency of programs that have provided significant income security to older Americans. In light of demographic circumstances that portend an increasingly narrowed dependency ratio, recent changes to OASDI taxation policies have resulted in what amounts to benefit reductions for higher-income retirees while leaving the lowest-income beneficiaries relatively unaffected. In addition, increased incomes driven primarily by inflation have increased the proportion of beneficiaries who surpass thresholds at which benefits become taxable. But federal taxation of OASDI benefits has also affected tax policy more broadly, a topic to which we now turn.

FEDERALISM AND TAX POLICY

Principles of Federalism

Federal taxation of OASDI has also impacted state income tax policy (Liebig, 2001b). Although not all states tax income, the majority of those that do base their tax codes on federal rules—the amount reported on federal tax forms, federal adjusted gross income, or federal taxes paid (Baer, 2001; Institute on Taxation and Economic Policy [ITEP], 2006). States that follow Washington's lead automatically generate increased state income tax revenues, unless their legislatures explicitly decouple personal income tax from the federal standard (Kenyon, 2006).

The relationship between state and federal tax systems exemplifies the concept of *federalism*, as practiced in the United States. Federalism is a type of political organization that unites separate polities into an overarching political system that allows each entity to maintain its fundamental political integrity and distributes power among general and constituent governments (Elazar, 2006). Federalism is characterized by a written constitution; decentralization of power; contractual sharing of public responsibilities; and common involvement in policy making, financing, and administration at multiple levels of government (Elazar, 2006). The U.S. Constitution provides numerous guarantees to the states and also places restrictions on their activities; resulting tensions are sometimes resolved by the courts. For example, state and local government employees were not required to join Social Security when it was enacted. Court decisions determined that those subnational governments *may* opt for participation. Subsequent laws passed in the 1950s allowed state and local governments to enter into *voluntary agreements* with the federal government under Section 218 of the Social Security Act to cover their employees (SSA, 2007b). Only 70% of state and local workers are covered by Social Security (Munnell & Soto, 2008), but under Section 218, employees who are qualified members of a public retirement system are provided Medicare-only coverage, if hired prior to April 1, 1986. The OBRA of 1990 mandated full Social Security coverage, including Medicare, for the approximately 3.8 million public sector employees—usually part-time, seasonal, and temporary workers—who are not members of a retirement plan system (National Conference of State Legislatures [NCSL], 2008).

Over the years, the states have played many roles in our federal system, including acting as a testing ground for policies subsequently adopted at the national level. For example, 30 states had income-maintenance policies for elders before the Economic Security Act was enacted in 1935. Similarly, several developed their own employee pension systems before the federal government enacted pensions for its civilian employees. This "bubble up" (as opposed to "top down") policy making became more widely recognized during the late 1980s and 1990s (Liebig, 2006). In addition, states implement federal policies (e.g., age discrimination, SSDI as noted above), but often in conformance with their own policy goals and relationships with their local governments. States also "borrow" policies from each other but allow for differences in their traditions and historical preferences (Elazar, 2006). For example, California's Ham and Eggs and Townsend Movements had impacts on other states' old-age pensions, as well as influencing the enactment of Social Security. This diffusion of policies across states has shaped their fiscal policies, enabling them to compete for business and foreign investment, *as well as for retirees*, by providing a wide array of tax breaks (Mackey, 1995; Penner, 2002; ITEP, 2006).

Fiscal federalism centers on the allocation of spending and taxing powers among the federal, state, and local levels of government, characterized by the division of responsibilities and of revenue-raising powers (also known as "tax assignment") and by grants-in-aid (Kenyon, 2006). In particular, states' abilities and willingness to raise revenues by taxing some areas (e.g., property, sales) and not others (e.g., personal income), help them determine what kinds of programs and services they will offer to their residents, such as state additions to federal Supplemental Security Income (SSI) benefits or federally mandated Medicaid services. However, for states choosing to use federal taxable income as the guide for their own income tax policies, the result is a double-edged sword. Although this action simplifies filing and administering state income taxes for taxpayers and state administrators, it also results in states automatically allowing some federal tax breaks to reduce state revenues (ITEP, 2006).

STATE TAX POLICIES FOR RETIREMENT INCOME

Variation in State Income Tax Policies

Under the principles of federalism, states can choose to follow federal templates, counterbalance what happens at the federal level, and/or break their own ground in policy making. The tax policies of the 50 states and the District of Columbia exemplify these patterns. Although personal income taxes are the second most important source of state revenue (after the sales tax), not all states have this revenue source (Mackey & Carter, 1994)—they are not bound by Amendment XVI to the U.S. Constitution, which empowers Congress to impose a tax on any source of income. In all, seven states do not levy such a tax; two others collect income tax only on interest and dividend income (see Table 18.1). By excluding/limiting the personal income tax, these nine states must look to other sources such as sales, inheritance/estate, and property taxes to finance state policies and activities.

The other 41 states and the District of Columbia have enacted a broad-based personal income tax. They do not, however, all follow the federal lead in tax exemptions, deductions, and credits. Considerable variation in tax preferences occurs among this group of states. These differences are evident in how they tax OASDI and other sources of retirement income.

State Taxation of OASDI

State tax treatment of Social Security is a critical issue for elders because it is a vital leg of the three-legged stool in maintaining a preretirement standard of living and peace of mind in the retirement years. Individual and regional differences are evident among the states. As noted above, a group

Table 18.1

STATE TAXATION OF OASDI

STATE	STATE PERSONAL INCOME TAX	STATE SOCIAL SECURITY TAX
Alabama	Yes	Exempt
Alaska	No	No
Arizona	Yes	Exempt
Arkansas	Yes	Exempt
California	Yes	Exempt
Colorado	Yes	Yes**
Connecticut	Yes	Yes‡
Delaware	Yes	Exempt
Dist. of Columbia	Yes	Exempt
Florida	No	No
Georgia	Yes	Exempt
Hawaii	Yes	Exempt
Idaho	Yes	Exempt
Illinois	Yes	Exempt
Indiana	Yes	Exempt
Iowa	Yes	Yes†
Kansas	Yes	Yes*
Kentucky	Yes	Exempt
Louisiana	Yes	Exempt
Maine	Yes	Exempt
Maryland	Yes	Exempt
Massachusetts	Yes	Exempt
Michigan	Yes	Exempt
Minnesota	Yes	Yes*
Mississippi	Yes	Exempt
Missouri	Yes	Yes*
Montana	Yes	Yes***
Nebraska	Yes	Yes*
Nevada	No	No
New Hampshire	Limited	No
New Jersey	Yes	Exempt
New Mexico	Yes	Yes*
New York	Yes	Exempt
North Carolina	Yes	Exempt
North Dakota	Yes	Yes*
Ohio	Yes	Exempt
Oklahoma	Yes	Exempt
Oregon	Yes	Exempt
Pennsylvania	Yes	Exempt
Rhode Island	Yes	Yes*
South Carolina	Yes	Exempt
South Dakota	No	No
Tennessee	Limited	No
Texas	No	No
Utah	Yes	Yes ±

STATE	STATE PERSONAL INCOME TAX	STATE SOCIAL SECURITY TAX
Vermont	Yes	Yes*
Virginia	Yes	Exempt
Washington	No	No
West Virginia	Yes	Yes*
Wisconsin	Yes	Yes†
Wyoming	No	No

Note. From *Individual Income Tax Provisions in the States (Informational Paper 4)*, by F. Russell & L. Hanson, 2007, Madison, WI: Wisconsin Legislative Fiscal Bureau.
* Same as federal
** Age 55 to 64, up to $20,000/person federally taxable Social Security excluded; $24,000 for ages 65 and older.
*** Separate state calculation of taxable amount
‡ Exempt if income is below $50,000 ($60,000 for married or head of household)
† Up to 50% of benefits are taxable
± Under age 65, deduct $4,800; age 65 and older, deduct $7,500

of nine states (Alaska, Florida, Nevada, New Hampshire, South Dakota, Tennessee, Texas, Washington, Wyoming) do not tax Social Security because they have no/limited personal income tax (PIT). In addition, the 27 states and the District of Columbia with a personal income tax (PIT), do not tax Social Security. Thus, Social Security benefits of residents in 36 states and the federal district (or 71%) are exempt from state taxes. When it comes to following federal income tax policy, these two groups of states clearly go their own way in creating their own tax structure, as well as counterbalancing the effects of federal taxation of Social Security. One result is their older residents, especially better-off elders, have more income for household consumption of goods and services, thereby promoting state economies.

Even among the 15 states with a PIT that have chosen to tax Social Security, variation exists. Eleven use the federal Social Security taxation formula—four have opted for their own policy. Both Iowa and Wisconsin have not adopted the higher tax rate (85%) enacted in OBRA 1993. Instead, they have retained the 50% tax rate enacted in 1983. Several states, including Colorado, Connecticut, and Utah, have developed a more complicated formula. In Colorado, up to $20,000 of federally taxable Social Security benefits are excluded for ages 55 to 64—for those aged 65 and older, up to $24,000 is excluded (Baer, 2001; Russell & Hanson, 2007). These maximum amounts are combined limits for pension income and federally taxed Social Security. Connecticut exempts Social Security benefits from state taxation if income is below $50,000 ($60,000 for married individuals/head of household); if those income limits are exceeded, only up to 25% of their benefits can be taxed (Baer, 2001; Russell & Hanson, 2007). Utah allows state taxpayers to deduct up to $4,800 of the federally taxable portion per person if younger than age 65, and $7,500 if age 65 or older. This phases out for higher-income taxpayers (Russell & Hanson, 2007).

Regional patterns of state taxation of Social Security can be identified. Of the six New England states, only two exempt Social Security. By contrast, all six Middle Atlantic states (including the District of Columbia) have this exclusion. Among the five Great Lakes states, only Wisconsin taxes Social Security. Of the seven Plains states, all tax Social Security (except South Dakota, which has no PIT), and three of the Far West states fully exclude Social Security from state taxation (Alaska and Washington have no PIT). Finally, of the nine Southwestern and Rocky Mountain states, only two (Arizona and Idaho) fully exclude Social Security benefits (Nevada, Texas, and Wyoming have no PIT); and of the 12 southeastern states, nine fully exempt Social Security (Florida and Tennesse have no PIT). These patterns have implications for whether retirees may choose to relocate to other nearby states or regions that have more favorable tax preferences.

Other Tax Breaks for Seniors

State governments provide various tax benefits for seniors besides lack of OASDI taxation. Many provide higher *personal exemptions* than the federal government. Slightly more than one fifth of the states (21) give seniors an extra exemption/exemption credit, sheltering twice as much income as nonelderly taxpayers can claim (ITEP, 2006). Some allow exemptions only for low-income individuals, with a phase-out for higher-income persons. For example, homestead exemptions and "circuit breaker" programs are targeted to low-income households and are often both age- and disability-related. However, most states have elder tax breaks for all income levels (Mackey, 1995; ITEP, 2006).

Even more important is state provision of *exemptions for certain types of income,* which include pension income (private, public, federal civilian, and military) that is critical for the 43% of older Americans—usually higher-paid individuals—receiving that source of retirement income. In all, 73% of the states allow exemptions for private/public pensions (ITEP, 2006), usually tax deductions that are more beneficial to higher-income persons. Unlike the federal income tax policy that regards all pension income as the same, most states provide less-favorable tax treatment for private pension income than public pensions (NCSL, 2003).

In keeping with principles of federalism, the states are generally free from federal control in how they tax pensions. The Supreme Court, however, has held that states cannot discriminate against federal civil service or military pensions by providing more favorable tax treatment for state pensions. In addition, they cannot tax pensions earned in their own state employee plans if recipients have become permanent residents of another state (NCSL, 2003). Federal law also prohibits the states from taxing Railroad Retirement benefits.

Why Do Seniors Get So Many State Tax Breaks?

Several reasons have been advanced to explain why seniors get greater tax breaks at the state level. One might be called the *magnet argument*. States seek to become retirement havens and entice elders "to vote with their feet" by not taxing OASDI and pension income and by offering lower estate and inheritance rates and property taxes (Mackey, 1995; Penner, 2002). The lack of an income tax or exempting significant portions of retirement income is also attractive to "snowbirds" who live in Sun Belt states during the winter months and return to their homes in the north the rest of the year. Due to this split-year residence pattern, they are less likely to be large consumers of publicly supported senior services.

Political clout of the elderly also has been suggested as a reason for senior tax concessions (see Myers, 2001; Penner, 2002). However, the influence of organized seniors at subnational levels has been questioned (e.g., see Andel & Liebig, 2002; Nownes, Thomas & Hrebnar, 2008). One way to test this argument is to compare the influence ratings of state-level interest groups (Thomas & Hrebnar, 2004) with state taxation of Social Security. In 2002, Iowa and New Mexico were the only states with senior interest groups in the highest rank—both states tax Social Security. In the same year, nine states with senior groups ranked as second in influence included California, Delaware, Georgia, Indiana, New York, Oklahoma, South Carolina (none tax Social Security), Missouri, and Rhode Island (tax Social Security), indicating a somewhat weak relationship between senior influence and Social Security taxation. Five years later, Nownes, Thomas, and Hrebnar (2008) found that no senior interest groups were listed in the top rank in any state. Among the 12 states where seniors were ranked second in influence, a similar relationship is evident: Arkansas (no PIT), Colorado, Connecticut, Iowa (Social Security tax, own formula), Kansas,

Missouri, Rhode Island (Social Security tax), Michigan, New York, Oklahoma, South Carolina (no Social Security tax), and Tennessee (limited PIT). Paralleling this pattern, over the past 6 years, Nownes, Thomas, and Hrebnar found that overall the influence of senior groups in the states dropped, from 31st to 39th out of a total of 40 groups ranked.

Lack of visibility of senior tax breaks may be another reason. As noted earlier, tax expenditures are far less obvious than budget outlays, even in states undergoing huge budget crunches. For example, in California with its $16 billion to $20 billion deficit, the estimated $1.8 billion revenue loss by not taxing Social Security receives little attention. In addition, many states have part-time legislatures, with limited time for legislative policy making. Coupled with stringent term limits, state legislators—despite some intermittent analysis of tax policy affecting seniors (see ITEP, 2006; Mackey & Carter, 1994)—may focus less on the extent of tax breaks for seniors. It may also be an instance of "let sleeping dogs lie"; deciding to tax Social Security could prove to be a rallying call for senior advocates. In addition, in states that tax Social Security by following federal tax policies, publicizing the effects of nonindexing might also become a flashpoint, as has occurred with the AMT.

IMPLICATIONS OF STATE TAX POLICIES FOR SENIORS

There are several implications of state preferential tax policies for seniors. *Geography can matter.* Although AARP and others, in their advice on relocation in retirement, focus some on tax matters as a decision criterion, the nontaxation of Social Security benefits and of pensions—the second leg of the retirement income stool—clearly should be an important factor in retiree decision making. However, it has been pointed out that with the resulting loss of revenue, states and localities may have fewer dollars to meet the needs of their citizens (Mackey, 1995). This is especially true of states and the District of Columbia with higher than average rates of poverty among persons aged 65 and older, such as Kentucky, New York, and Texas (Kaiser Family Foundation, 2006), all of which do not tax OASDI.

Loss/lower levels of publicly funded services may be one result of tax breaks for seniors that *usually benefit better-off older taxpayers*. Although these higher-income individuals may be able to purchase services, the overall well-being of other older and younger citizens may suffer. Still, the closing of emergency rooms and inadequate first responder infrastructure in many localities are but one example that money may not guarantee one's access to services. In addition, poorly targeted tax breaks for elders shift the cost of funding public services for seniors and other age groups toward nonelderly taxpayers (ITEP, 2006).

Equity is one of the key principles of a good tax system (Mackey & Carter, 1994). Tax treatment of income from both intergenerational and intragenerational perspectives deserves attention. In those states that exempt Social Security as well as pension income, tax equity issues arise between younger and older households (Mackey, 1995; NCSL, 2003). Greater benefits accrue to seniors than to the general population because state income tax exemptions for nonelderly taxpayers generally do not discriminate between wages and other income sources (ITEP, 2006). Special tax breaks for Social Security and pensions, but not for salaries and wages also shift the costs of public services away from retirees and onto working taxpayers. This latter group includes seniors who still work, often because they cannot afford to retire completely. In those states that do tax Social Security, these equity issues may be less severe.

Congruence of state tax policies with principles of *social insurance* is another consideration. The policy in 27 states of not taxing Social Security benefits adheres more closely to the multitiered retirement system envisioned in the Economic Security Act. This includes supporting a variable standard of living by paying benefits without regard to other resources, and not having one's benefits cut back as a result of having arranged for additional retirement income (Bethell, 2000). By contrast, the practice of income taxation of Social Security benefits adopted by 15 states (especially the 11 that have explicitly copied the federal rules) can be viewed as a backdoor approach to means testing (see Penner, 2002).

Finally, *tax expenditures for seniors obscure the true costs of an aging society* (Liebig, 2001b). During the 1980s and 1990s when the proportion of elders was 13%, state legislatures focused on fixed-income elders, often via tax breaks that did not carry the stigma of handouts funded under direct expenditure programs. The effects of the coming demographic boom on the states, however, will go well beyond the cost of Medicaid services and adding to SSI. By 2030, nearly 20% of the U.S. population will be aged 65 and older, but some states are "aging" faster than others (e.g., Iowa). States may wish to assess the distribution of tax benefits among low-, medium-, and upper-income elders to see if the distribution of tax relief is in accordance with policy makers' original intent of helping lower income persons. This evaluation may lead current policy makers to make changes that will better target the neediest seniors, so as to achieve a more equitable and sustainable tax system.

DISCUSSION QUESTIONS

1 What are "tax expenditures," and how are they related to Social Security?
2 What is the history of taxation of Social Security benefits, and what beneficiaries are taxed?
3 Discuss the variation among states in how Social Security benefits are taxed.
4 To what extent is the taxation of Social Security benefits consistent with the general guiding principles of social insurance? What compromises are made when we begin taxing benefits?

REFERENCES

Andel, R., & Liebig, P. S. (2002). The city of Laguna Woods: A case of senior power in local politics. *Research on Aging, 24*, 87–105.

Baer, D. (2001). *State taxation of social security and pensions in 2000* (Issue brief #55). Washington, DC: AARP Public Policy Institute.

Benitez-Silva, H., Buchinsky, M., Chan, H. M., Rust, J., & Sheidvasser, S. (1999). An empirical analysis of the social security disability application, appeal, and award process. *Labour Economics, 6*, 147–178.

Bethell, T. N. (Ed.). (2000). *Insuring the essentials: Bob Ball on Social Security.* New York: Century Foundation Press.

Burkhauser, R. V., Butler, J. S., & Gomus, G. (2003). *Dynamic modeling of the SSDI application timing decision: The importance of policy variables.* Bonn, Germany: Institute for the Study of Labor.

Charles, K. K. (2003). The longitudinal structure of earnings losses among work-limited disabled workers. *Journal of Human Resources, 38*, 618–646.

Clark, R. L. (2001). Economics. In G. L. Maddox (Ed.), *The encyclopedia of aging, I,* (pp. 319–321). New York: Springer.

Clark, R. L., Burkhauser, R. V., Moon, M., Quinn, J. F., & Smeeding, T. M. (2004). *The economics of an aging society.* Malden, MA: Blackwell.

Crown, W. H. (2001). Effects of government policy on the incomes of younger and older households. In G. L. Maddox (Ed.), *The encyclopedia of aging, I,* (pp. 321–324). New York: Springer.

DeWitt, L. (2003, March). *Historical background and development of social security.* Retrieved October 26, 2008, from http://www.ssa.gov/history/briefhistory3.html.

Elazar, D. J. (2006). Federalism. In J. R. Marbach, E. Katz, & T. E. Smith (Eds.), *Federalism in America: An encyclopedia, I,* (pp. 223–242). Westport, CT: Greenwood Press.

Federal Interagency Forum for Age-Related Statistics (FIFARS). (2008). *Older Americans 2008: Key indicators of well-being. Federal Interagency Forum on Aging-Related Statistics.* Washington, DC: U.S. Government Printing Office.

Hu, J., Lahiri, K., Vaughan, D. R., & Wixon, B. (2001). A structural model of Social Security's disability determination process. *The Review of Economics and Statistics*, 83, 348–361.

Institute on Taxation and Economic Policy (ITEP). (2006). *State income taxes and senior citizens* (Policy brief #30). Washington, DC: Author.

Kaiser Family Foundation. (2006). *Poverty rate by age, states (2005–2006), U.S.*, Retrieved October 26, 2008, from http://www.statehealthfacts.org/comparebar.jsp?ind=10&cat=1

Kenyon, D. (2006). Fiscal federalism. In J. R. Marbach, E. Katz, & T. E. Smith (Eds.), *Federalism in American: An encyclopedia, I,* (pp. 252–258). Westport, CT: Blackwell.

Liebig, P. S. (2001a). Inflation impact and measurement. In G. L. Maddox (Ed.), *The encyclopedia of aging, I,* (pp. 538–541). New York: Springer.

Liebig, P. S. (2001b). Tax policy. In G. L. Maddox (Ed.), *The encyclopedia of aging, II,* (pp. 1001–1004). New York: Springer.

Liebig, P. S. (2006). The purview and sweep of aging policy. In D. J. Sheets, D. B. Bradley, & J. Hendricks (Eds.), *Enduring questions in gerontology* (pp. 225–269). New York: Springer.

Mackey, S. (1995, May). Time to talk about senior tax breaks? *State Legislatures*, 12–13.

Mackey, S., & Carter, K. (1994). *State tax policy and senior citizens.* Denver: National Conference of State Legislatures.

Morton, D. A. (2006). *Nolo's guide to Social Security disability: Getting and keeping your benefits.* Berkeley, CA: Nolo Press.

Munnell, A. M., & Soto, M. (2008). *State and local pensions are different from private plans.* Boston: Center for Retirement Research. Retrieved January 8, 2008, from http://crr.bc.edu/images/stories/Briefs/slp_1.pdf?phpMyAdmin=43ac483c4de9t51d9eb41

Myers, R. J. (2001). Social Security. In G. L. Maddox (Ed.), *The encyclopedia of aging, II,* (pp. 947–955). New York: Springer.

National Conference of State Legislatures (NCSL). (2003). *State personal income taxes of pension and retirement income: Tax year 2003.* Denver: Author. Retrieved October 26, 2008, from http://parca.samford.edu/State%20Personal%20Income%20Taxes%20on%20Pensions%20and%20Retirement%20Income%20Tax%20Year%202003.htm.

National Conference of State Legislatures (NCSL). (2008). *Mandatory Social Security coverage of state and local government employees.* Retrieved October 26, 2008, from http://www.ncsl.org/standcomm/sclaborecon/sclaborecon_Policies.htm#MandatorySocialSecurity

Nownes, A. J., Thomas, C. S., & Hrebnar, R. J. (2008). Interest groups in the states. In V. Gray & R. L. Hanson (Eds.), *Politics in the American states: A comparative analysis* (9th ed., pp. 98–126). Washington, DC: CQ Press.

Penner, R. (2002). Taxation. In D. J. Eckert (Ed.), *Encyclopedia of aging* (pp. 1409–1415). New York: Macmillan Reference.

Russell, F., & Hanson, L. (2007). *Individual income tax provisions in the states* (Informational paper 4). Madison, WI: Wisconsin Legislative Fiscal Bureau.

Rust, J., & Phelan, C. (1997). How Social Security and Medicare affect retirement behavior in a world of incomplete markets. *Econometrica, 65*, 781–831.

Sheets, D. J., & Liebig, P. S. (2005). The intersection of aging, disability, and supportive environments: Issues and policy implications. *Hallym International Journal of Aging, 7*, 142–165.

Social Security Administration. (2005). *Flow of cases through the disability process*. Retrieved October 26, 2008, from http://www.ssa.gov/disability/od_process.pdf

Social Security Administration. (2007a). *Fast facts and figures about Social Security, 2007.* Retrieved February 18, 2008, from http://www.ssa.gov/policy/docs/chartbooks/fast_facts/2007/fast_facts7.pdf

Social Security Administration. (2007b). *State and local government employers information.* Retrieved October 26, 2008, from http://www.ssa.gov/slge/

Thomas, C. L., & Hrebnar, R. L. (2004). Interest groups in the states. In V. Gray & R. L. Hanson (Eds.), *Politics in the American states: A comparative analysis* (8th ed., pp. 100–128). Washington, DC: CQ Press.

19 Social Justice and Tax Expenditures

DEBRA STREET

For all but the wealthiest Americans, Social Security benefits are the critical foundation for dependable retirement income. Social Security embodies the concept of "middle class incorporation," (Esping-Andersen, 1990) characteristic of programs that provide high quality benefits to citizens across the income spectrum, creating cross-class interests and intergenerational solidarity, and sustaining political legitimacy (Street & Cossman, 2006). Because of its scope, the importance of its income guarantee, and the size of the soon-to-retire baby boom generation, the future of Social Security appropriately takes center stage in public policy debates. But Social Security provides modest levels of income replacement and, for beneficiaries who rely on it exclusively, many have retirement income levels near or not much greater than poverty. Access to occupational pension benefits or individual savings and wealth usually spells the difference between having enough income to meet all needs and some wants, and experiencing financial insecurity in old age (Harrington Meyer & Herd, 2007; Street & Wilmoth, 2001).

Just as Social Security legislation authorizes public pensions, law and regulation authorizes indirect expenditures for selective "private" benefits—tax expenditures that subsidize occupational pensions and eligible retirement savings plans. Tax expenditures were defined in the Congressional Budget Act of 1974 as "revenue losses attributable to provisions of the Federal tax laws which allow a special exclusion, exemption, or deduction from gross income or which provide a special credit, a preferential rate of tax, or a deferral of tax liability" (Congressional Budget and Impoundment Control Act of 1974). Stanley Surrey introduced the concept of tax expenditures as an important, and often overlooked component of the federal budgetary process, and regarded them as spending programs embedded in the Internal Revenue Code (Surrey, 1973; Surrey & McDaniel, 1985). By taking advantage of tax expenditures, workers can shelter some of their earnings from taxes they would otherwise have to pay. They qualify for special tax treatment, for example, by saving in specialized accounts for retirement, or by acquiring health insurance through an employer. Individuals who do not or who cannot participate in those activities that qualify for tax expenditures pay taxes on all of their taxable income.

In contrast to overwrought debates about the future affordability of Social Security, the increasingly extensive and expensive role of tax expenditures attracts little media attention. Tax expenditures mystify and complicate understanding of the full magnitude of public investment in retirement income security, and they obscure the social welfare outcomes of different welfare state programs. Yet reaching important policy goals of income security and adequacy in retirement requires evaluating all public investment in retirement income, whether direct or indirect. At stake is informed decision making about how to optimize retirement income and garner political support for various programs that impact it—how to sustain affordable systems of benefits, rooted in equitable and socially just outcomes, providing adequate resources for all retirees.

THE STRUCTURE OF PUBLIC EXPENDITURES FOR RETIREMENT INCOME

Hybrid public/private systems characterize social provision in all wealthy modern welfare states (see Béland & Gran, 2008). Each welfare state has a distinctive framework of tax rules and public expenditure policies that shape the redistribution of resources and the degree of income inequality in that country. How tax systems treat different sources of income (the balance of income and consumption taxes, the complexity and progressivity of tax codes), the degree of reliance on direct and indirect expenditure, rules for eligibility, and the universal or selective nature of programs determine whether income stratification is merely reproduced or is altered by social welfare policies. Distinctions in these patterns of national social welfare practices coincide with different types of welfare states (Esping-Andersen, 1990).

Welfare state policy making recognizes a collective need to maximize social welfare through mechanisms that smooth out the peaks (during earning years) and valleys (during unemployment, illness, or retirement) of income over the life course. Welfare state policies that accomplish this important social welfare goal include unemployment benefits, disability insurance, and public pensions; progressivity in tax rates (higher rates for high earners) and benefits (proportionately higher benefits for those with greater need); and public administration to promote oversight, efficiency, and equity in public programs operations. Policies are expected to avoid employment disincentives[1] and to promote individual self-sufficiency in all welfare states, but especially in liberal ones like the United States (Esping-Andersen, 1990).

Social insurance values emphasize shared experience and public accountability in broad-based programs like Social Security (Estes, 2004). Value principles and ideological perspectives are also implicit components of social welfare regimes used to frame arguments for and against public or private solutions for income security (Estes, 2004; Street & Ginn, 2001; Quadagno & Street, 2005). Neoliberal ideology, recently in ascendance on the political scene, has emphasized market principles over social insurance principles, favoring minimal redistribution and private solutions for social welfare (Estes, 2004; Street & Ginn, 2001). Moral economy assumptions arise from norms of reciprocity that inform welfare state policies, either shaping expectations for public programs delivering high levels of social welfare anchored in citizenship rights (as in social democratic systems such as Sweden), or for dominantly market-driven, private and individualistic approaches (as in liberal welfare states like the United States) (Hendricks, 2005; Minkler & Cole, 1999)

The Role of Public Investment in "Private" Retirement Income

Operating alongside direct expenditures for social insurance and social assistance, there are two systems of selective, indirect public expenditures

[1] For example, the Personal Responsibility and Work Opportunity Act (PRWORA) (1996) departed from social welfare policies that, since the 1930s, had provided public assistance to poor mothers and their children. It replaced Aid to Families with Dependent Children (AFDC) with Temporary Assistance for Needy Families (TANF), which limited public benefits an individual could receive to 5 years over a lifetime. The intent was to remove "work disincentives" that critics claimed entitlement to public benefits created. The policy was designed to compel poor women, including mothers of very young children, to get off of welfare rolls and into paid employment.

supported by tax subsidies: *Occupational welfare* (employment-based "private" benefits) and *fiscal welfare* (redistribution through the tax code) programs (Titmuss, 1958). Analysis of how taxation works to sustain occupational and fiscal welfare is of more recent vintage (early examples include Hacker, 2002; Howard, 1997; Myles & Street, 1995; Sinfield, 1993; Street, 1996; Street & Ginn, 2001) and research is significantly less extensive (see Hacker, 2005) than for the direct spending programs that are the apparent centerpieces of modern welfare states. Sustained attention to the costs and outcomes associated with tax expenditures is virtually absent from the popular media, creating an information vacuum about the intricacies involved in the complex interaction of the U.S. tax system and taxpayer behavior. Yet, tax subsidies are enacted, expanded, funded, and sustained by policy decisions as deliberate as those of direct expenditure programs, although tax expenditures are much more difficult for citizens and policymakers to understand. For example, a decision to raise the cap on savings eligible for tax subsidies in individual retirement accounts (set at $10,500 in 2008) requires legislative action, just as surely as gradually raising the normal retirement age from 65 to 67 for Social Security for individuals born after 1937.

Burgeoning tax breaks in many countries provide public financial support for employer-provided defined benefit (DB) pensions and defined contribution (DC) retirement plans, important sources of income for current and future retirees (see Béland & Gran, 2008; Ginn, Street, & Arber, 2001). Compared to progressive redistribution under universal social insurance and social assistance, redistribution for occupational and fiscal welfare does not conform to common sense understanding of social justice or norms of fairness. That is because, under current arrangements, fiscal and occupational welfare programs most often flow from low-waged, benefit-poor, insecurely-employed individuals—the *pension vulnerable*—to high-waged, benefit-rich, securely-employed individuals—the *pension elite*.

In the United States, taxes subsidize occupational welfare through employment-based DB and DC plans, and fiscal welfare boosts savings capacity in individual retirement accounts (IRAs)[2] and Keough plans

---

[2] This chapter covers traditional retirement savings plans (individual, Keogh, 401(k) and 403(b)-type plans) that permit individuals to make pretax contributions up to particular dollar limits (which differ by type of plan, and sometimes by age of the individual) without having to pay income tax on the value of the contributions, thus "sheltering" that income from taxation. In such plans, the value of contributions and the interest or gains they earn are not taxed until money is withdrawn at retirement. Roth IRAs are not covered in this chapter. Contributions to Roth IRAs are also capped

(for the self-employed). Indirect spending helps many working-aged people prepare for retirement, yet consistent with neoliberal ideology and the individualist moral economy of the American welfare state, such benefits are valorized as privately earned and individually acquired. One hallmark, then, of U.S. occupational and fiscal welfare programs are their rather ironic "private" cachet despite the need for public investment to sustain them. Tax-subsidized plans are hybrid welfare state programs, not entirely public, but not exclusively private either. They depend on public resources, like Social Security and SSI to fund benefits, alongside contributions from employers on behalf of workers, or individuals for themselves. Unlike the universal coverage or pooled risk-sharing provided by Social Security and SSI, the value of tax subsidies go to discretionary[3] firm-level DB pensions (available only to certain workers in certain firms, with only small risk-sharing pools) or DC plans provided to (some) workers by (some) employers, or for individual IRAs and Keough plans.

Rhetorical attacks on social insurance by its neoliberal opponents have undermined confidence among younger Americans and have been coupled with attempts to retrench and/or privatize public direct expenditure programs (Ginn, Street, & Arber, 2001). One tactic has been to promote public subsidies to bolster "private" benefits, enticing beneficiaries out of public programs[4] and undermining the collective solidarity of social insurance (see Gilbert, 2002; Ginn, Street, & Arber, 2001; Hacker, 2002). However, tax expenditures can also be used in progressive ways (Schlesinger & Hacker, 2007). For example, judicious design of refundable tax credits for popular programs like the Earned Income Tax Credit (EITC) for working aged families in the United States (Porter & Dupree, 2001) and the Guaranteed Income Supplement (GIS) for elderly Canadians (Myles & Street, 1995; Street & Connidis, 2001) have provided carefully targeted, nonstigmatizing, relatively low-cost means of alleviating poverty and raising unacceptably low incomes for millions of citizens in both countries—key goals of welfare state policies.

Tax expenditures, thus, have a dual character: (1) potential as a useful public policy tool that can accomplish important social welfare goals and

---

but they are not tax deductible. Unlike traditional IRAs, withdrawals from Roth IRAs that have been held for 5 years and made after the age of 59.5 are not taxed.

[3] In some unionized workplaces, the employer is contractually obligated to provide a pension plan; in many others, DB or DC plans are at the discretion of the firm.

[4] One example is using public funds to entice beneficiaries out of traditional Medicare into Medicare +Choice; others include proposals to divert part of Social Security contributions to support private, individually held retirement accounts.

(2) utility as effective weapons in the arsenals of social insurance opponents, compensating some citizens to abandon their support and participation in social insurance. Whether tax expenditures are interpreted—and experienced—as tools for social justice or weapons used to dismantle solidarity depends on the specific details, quality of outcomes, and goals associated with particular tax expenditures: Who pays, who benefits, and which interests are served. Table 19.1 shows many details associated not only with tax expenditure programs, but also within the broader context of all types of public investment in retirement income.

Social insurance (Social Security) and social assistance (SSI) benefits are guaranteed by the capacity of the public to finance and share risk (paying taxes) and the government to honor claims. All taxpayers share the cost of providing for impoverished elderly beneficiaries under SSI, and all citizens could benefit if they needed to; all workers contribute to and receive benefits from Social Security (along with their dependents and survivors).

In contrast, indirect public expenditure funding comes from all income taxpayers, but not all taxpayers can share the benefits. Fiscal and occupational welfare generate public costs but insecure outcomes; in fact, there is often no retirement income guarantee at all. Future benefits depend on many factors. Receiving occupational benefits and their eventual value depend on tenure of employment, amount of employee/employer contributions to DC plans, and the fiscal capacity of large (mostly unionized) corporations and public sector employers (the last bastions of traditional DB pensions) to keep pension promises, during a period when many employers are abandoning traditional plans. The payoff for fiscal welfare depends on skill and luck: The investment acumen of the millions of individual DC retirement plan participants (in employment-based programs, or IRAs/Keoughs for individuals), many who are novice or unskilled investors; and (currently diminishing) returns, or even losses, in increasingly volatile equity markets.

Occupational welfare supported by tax expenditures is available when firms offer occupational pensions or retirement savings plans that qualify for tax subsidies. This criterion alone excludes a sizeable fraction of the working age population (and their dependents) from access to publicly subsidized occupational welfare because few small employers offer such programs. Even when firms offer eligible programs, some workers never benefit either by program design or by individual choice. For example, although occupational DB pensions have many advantages for workers lucky enough to be covered, restrictive eligibility, and vesting rules limits

Table 19.1

DIRECT AND INDIRECT PUBLIC EXPENDITURE PROGRAMS RELATED TO RETIREMENT INCOME IN THE UNITED STATES

	TYPE OF PUBLIC BENEFIT	PUBLIC FUNDING SOURCE	POPULATION SERVED	BENEFICIARIES	SOCIAL WELFARE OUTCOME	ANNUAL PUBLIC COSTS	MONTHLY BENEFITS, VARIOUS RECIPIENTS 65+	SOCIAL WELFARE OUTCOME
Social Assistance							***All individuals 65+***	
Supplemental Security Income (SSI)	Selective, means-tested cash income	General revenue	All citizens	Aged, blind, and disabled poor	Progressive selective benefits	$41.0 billion[a]	$623 (max indiv)[b] $924 (max couple)[b]	progressive
Social Insurance								
Social Security	Universal cash pensions	Payroll taxes	All workers and their families	Retirees (62 and older) plus dependents and survivors	Progressive universal benefits	$552.8 billion[a]	$2,116 (max indiv)[b] $1,044 (avg. retiree)[b] $1,178 (avg. man)[b] $ 905 (avg. woman)[b]	progressive
Occupational/fiscal Welfare							***Only eligible individuals***	
DB pensions and DC savings plans like 401(k) and 403(b) plans and annuities	Selective tax break for employees	General revenue	Workers in firms offering DB pensions and DC plans	Retirees from firms offering pensions and savings plans	Regressive selective benefits	$95.1 billion[a]	$15,000 (public annual median)[d] $6,840 (private annual median)[d]	regressive

(Continued)

Table 19.1

DIRECT AND INDIRECT PUBLIC EXPENDITURE PROGRAMS RELATED TO RETIREMENT INCOME IN THE UNITED STATES *(Continued)*

	TYPE OF PUBLIC BENEFIT	PUBLIC FUNDING SOURCE	POPULATION SERVED	BENEFICIARIES	SOCIAL WELFARE OUTCOME	ANNUAL PUBLIC COSTS	MONTHLY BENEFITS, VARIOUS RECIPIENTS 65+	SOCIAL WELFARE OUTCOME
Income from assets such as Individual DC retirement savings plans like IRAs and Keough plans	Selective tax break for individuals	General revenue	Individuals with surpluses to save in DC plans	Individuals who accrue savings in DC plans	Regressive selective benefits	$25.3 billion[a]	Only 24% receive more than $2,000 income from assets annually[c] $1,087 (median annual)[d]	regressive

[a] From *2008 Annual Report of the Board of Trustees of the Federal Old-Age and Survivors Insurance and Disability Insurance Trust Funds*, by Social Security Administration, 2008, released: April 10, 2008. Retrieved on November 20, 2008 from http://www.socialsecurity.gov/OACT/TR/TR08/tr08.pdf

[b] From *Fast Facts and Figures about Social Security: 2007*, by Social Security Administration, 2007, Washington DC: Social Security Administration, Office of Policy, Office of Research, Statistics, and Evaluation, SSA Publication No.13-11785, released: September, 2006. Retrieved November 20, 2008 from http://www.ssa.gov/policy/docs/chartbooks/fast_facts/2007/fast_facts07.pdf

[c] From *Social Security and retirement income adequacy* (Social Security Brief 25), by National Academy of Social Insurance, 2007, Washington: NASI Retrieved October 26, 2008, from http://www.nasi.org/usr_doc/SS_Brief_025.pdf

[d] From *Topics in aging: Income and poverty among older Americans in 2005*, by Congressional Research Service, 2006, Washington, DC: CRS, The Library of Congress. Retrieved November 24, 2008, from http://assets.opencrs.com/rpts/RL32697_20060921.pdf

eventual benefits even in those firms. Lack of portability of DB pensions across workplaces further restricts DB benefits and the value of the public subsidy mainly to long-term single-firm workers. Although with employment-based DC plans' portability increases their appeal among a mobile workforce, investment risk is entirely individualized and enrollment is seldom automatic, again limiting the value of the public investment to fewer individuals. Some workers choose current consumption of income over tax-deferred savings—sometimes because they do not fully understand the plans, others because they are unable to afford to make contributions to participate at all (Bell, Carasso, & Steuerle, 2005). Finally, many individuals work where occupational welfare is unavailable.

Fiscal welfare is still available for saving in approved IRAs or Keough plans (for the self-employed) to shelter individual income from taxes (up to a maximum contribution limit), similar to DC plans now in vogue with large employers. Contributions to DC plans are made with pretax dollars that enable individuals to reduce the cost of saving for retirement; of course, participation in DC plans of all types depends on having a surplus to save in the first place. Table 19.2 shows the percentage of all income from various sources for individuals 65 and older, alongside the percentage of 65 and older who receive income from various sources. Data in the table underscore how critically important Social Security benefits are to all Americans and demonstrate the unequal access to asset income (fiscal welfare) and pension income (occupational welfare), especially for minority Americans.

In just one example of the inequities embedded in current tax arrangements, as Table 19.2 shows, the distribution of different types of retirement income available across subgroups of retirees varies dramatically across race/ethnic groups. Similarly, unequal distributions occur across occupational groups, employment sector, full-time and part-time or seasonal workers, gender, and income level (Department of Labor, 2000). For all disadvantaged workers, direct public expenditure programs like Social Security and SSI represent the dominant source of income, often the only source of retirement income (Harrington Meyer & Herd, 2007; Street & Wilmoth, 2001).

Still, the unequal distribution of the capacity for individuals to benefit from occupational and fiscal welfare might not be interpreted by some as an equity problem, but for the public subsidy involved. After all, labor markets "value" jobs and occupations differently; high wages and employment-based benefits represent one part of wage packages. However, the public cost to taxpayers for indirect expenditures creates a

Table 19.2

PERCENTAGE OF INCOME FROM ALL SOURCES FOR INDIVIDUALS 65+ AND PERCENTAGE OF INDIVIDUALS 65+ RECEIVING ANY INCOME FROM SOURCE, BY RACE/ETHNICITY

	Percent of Total Annual Income Received from Source	Percent of Individuals Receiving Income from Source			
	ALL INDIVIDUALS 65+	*ALL 65+*	*WHITE*	*BLACK*	*HISPANIC*
Social Security	37	89	91	83	76
Asset income (fiscal welfare)	13	55	59	26	23
Pension income (occupational welfare)	19	43	43	28	20
Earnings	28	24	24	21	21
SSI	n/a	4	3	10	13
Other	3		n/a	n/a	n/a

Note: From Social Security Administration [SSA]. *Income of the Population 55 or Older: 2004*, by Social Security Administration, 2006, Washington DC: Social Security Administration, Office of Policy, Office of Research, Statistics, and Evaluation, SSA Publication No.13-11871, released: May 2006. Retrieved November 20, 2008, from http://www.ssa.gov/policy/docs/statcomps/income_pop55/2004/incpop04.pdf

perverse policy outcome when viewed through the lens of principled rationale for public investment in social welfare, creating a case of "upside down" targeting (Sinfield, 1993).

Where retirement income is concerned, social welfare outcomes of fiscal and occupational welfare are neither progressive (as advocates of redistribution and public insurance prefer), nor are they neutral and market driven (a core public policy tenet from a conservative perspective), and they certainly are not exclusively private or market-derived (as neoliberal ideology, if consistently applied, would demand). More than merely reproducing market-driven stratification within the American labor market, tax breaks for retirement income intensify stratification, creating regressive social welfare outcomes that improve the social welfare of higher-income individuals. Obviously, individuals with the highest income have the most "benefit rich" jobs in the first place. Not only are more high-income individuals more likely to have pension coverage through their employment, but their higher incomes also give them a greater capacity

Table 19.3

PERCENTAGE OF FAMILIES WITH PENSION COVERAGE, BY INCOME CATEGORY (2003)

INCOME RANGE	PERCENTAGE OF FAMILIES WITH PENSION COVERAGE
<$16,200	4.6
$10,200–30,999	21.4
$31,000–50,219	45.3
$50,220–81,513	64.4
≥$81,514	74.3

Note: From *Tax expenditures: Trends and Critiques*, by Congressional Research Service, 2006, Washington, DC: CRS, The Library of Congress. Retrieved November 24, 2008, from http://taxprof.typepad.com/taxprof_blog/files/RL33641.pdf

for surplus income to save for retirement and take advantage of tax benefits (see Table 19.3). Because marginal rates of taxation are modestly higher for high-income earners (the rate of income tax is slightly higher for high-income earners), even when middle- and high-income earners save the same amount in retirement plans, the value of the tax subsidy is greater for the higher-income individual.

Table 19.4 shows the marginal tax rate (the rate at which each additional dollar of income is taxed) for the different tax brackets for U.S. federal income taxes. Note that for the lowest-income individuals and families who would certainly struggle to find $2,000 to save out of meager

Table 19.4

VALUE OF INCOME TAX DEDUCTION FOR SAVINGS, BY TAX RATE (2008)

MARGINAL TAX RATE	SINGLE	MARRIED FILING JOINTLY OR QUALIFIED WIDOW(ER)	VALUE OF INCOME TAX REDUCTION ON $2000 OF RETIREMENT SAVINGS
10%	$0–$8,025	$0–$16,050	$200
15%	$8,026–$32,550	$16,051–$65,100	$300
25%	$32,551–$78,850	$65,101–$131,450	$500
28%	$78,851–$164,550	$131,451–$200,300	$560
33%	$164,551–$357,700	$200,301–$357,700	$660
35%	$357,701+	$357,701+	$700

incomes, that they would receive a $200 tax break (tax expenditure to support retirement savings in a Keough, 40l[k] or IRA). To make exactly the same $2,000 contribution into a retirement plan for individuals in the highest tax bracket, high-income tax payers receive a $700 tax break—$500 more than a low-income person or family who struggled to set money aside.

All individuals who cannot or do not participate in tax subsidized DB or DC retirement plans pay higher taxes than would otherwise be required because they work for the "wrong" employers or because their incomes are too low to generate surpluses to save (Ginn, Street, & Arber, 2001). Individuals who are responsible for unpaid care work, (dominantly women), minority Americans, workers in small firms, and the low-waged are disproportionately likely to be left out of indirect public expenditure for retirement income. As Table 19.1 demonstrated, the distribution of risk and reward differs considerably across the three main public expenditure components Americans depend on for retirement income, with clearly perverse outcomes related to fiscal and occupational welfare. For tax-subsidized programs, it is mainly the "unlucky"—the *pension vulnerable*—who disproportionately shoulder the burden of public spending that supports "private" retirement income.

DISCUSSION

There is no intrinsic property of tax expenditures that make them an inevitable choice for the provision of income adequacy in old age. Rather, deliberate political choices and the dominant neoliberal ideology drive a preference for pretense: Pretense that tax-subsidized retirement income is a private, individual accomplishment. Additionally, the pretense is predicated on a belief that this accomplishment was achieved through more desirable or appropriate vehicles than public Social Security benefits. But a dollar is a dollar, taxes are taxes, and dollars not collected for taxes because they instead fund retirement planning (for those who can afford it) are public resources with real value (that negatively impact those who cannot!).

Citizens finance the use of tax subsidies, in some cases for programs they can never use, just as surely as they pay for direct expenditure programs like Social Security, which they always stand to benefit from. Tax subsidies for "private" retirement benefits reproduce employment inequalities and reinforce rather than reduce income inequality in old age

(Ginn, Street, & Arber, 2001; Harrington Meyer & Herd, 2007). Under direct expenditure programs, who pays and who benefits is relatively easy to discern, but that is not the case for indirect public expenditures.

Having access to tax subsidized retirement savings and occupational pension benefits makes a big difference in the amount of later life income millions of currently retired Americans receive. Despite such obvious benefits to many individuals, tax-subsidized retirement programs exact hidden costs with only limited political oversight to assess whether the outcomes are worth the investment. Tax expenditures are expensive, channeling public resources away from other important tasks; they undermine the social solidarity of shared interests in social welfare, redistributing resources from lower-income taxpayers to more affluent ones; they attract little political or media attention, making current Social Security debates about the future of retirement income partial and inadequate (Estes, 2004; Ginn, Street, & Arber, 2001; Hacker, 2002; Street, 1996).

Despite these obvious flaws, reformed tax mechanisms could progressively redistribute resources in a more comprehensive retirement income system, by creating targeted benefits to improve the security and adequacy of benefits for low- and moderate-income earners. Such a program could operate similarly to EITC, offering refundable tax credits to low- and modest-income elders, who would be disproportionately unmarried, women, and minority individuals (see Myles & Street, 1995 and Street & Connidis, 2001 regarding the Canadian experience with guaranteed retirement income provided through the tax system). Social Security and SSI budgets are constantly monitored to ensure that the programs are efficiently administered, that benefits match the value of public investment, and that outcomes achieved with direct spending warrant high levels of public investment, reformers could choose to monitor tax expenditures more regularly, as is the case for EITC in current annual legislative oversight. Tax mechanisms can be designed in ways that explicitly serve the needs of low-income individuals while preserving the value of universal Social Security benefits for beneficiaries at all income levels—making social welfare outcomes of public expenditures more progressive overall. Alongside stabilization of Social Security benefits, implementing reforms that provide better incomes to future low- to moderate-income retirees could use the tax system as a way to create the political will—political buy-in because benefits are carefully targeted but nonstigmatizing, with a degree of middle class incorporation—to improve late life income.

Why have tax expenditures only recently attracted sustained attention among researchers, and still so little among the public? Partly, it is the sheer proliferation of fiscal welfare expenditures,[5] their increasingly noticeable impacts on public accounts,[6] and the increasing insecurity of the benefits they subsidize (Hacker, 2006). The valorization of individual self-sufficiency and the hidden role that fiscal welfare plays in the U.S. welfare state keeps the glare of public attention on Social Security reform, rather than on its shadowy cousin of indirect spending (Street & Ginn, 2001). Fiscal and occupational welfare had a profound impact on the contours of the mature 20th century American welfare state (Hacker, 2002; Quadagno & Street, 2005) and will no doubt shape its future. Yet, public concern expressed about the sustainability and affordability of expensive public programs like Social Security and Medicare has not been matched by attention to the unraveling, but increasingly expensive, shadow system of tax-subsidized benefits. The trick, then, may be to educate the public and policy makers to the social injustice and insecurity created by current tax expenditure arrangements. The benefits they subsidize are coming at greater public cost but with less secure benefits. Perhaps unveiling their perverse social welfare effects, cost, and growing insecurity can underscore the need for a more socially just outcome for the public investment, fostering a more creative and progressive use of redesigned tax expenditures to better support income security in old age.

DISCUSSION QUESTIONS

1. What are the two programs of tax expenditures discussed by Street? How does each program work?
2. Who are the pension vulnerable? Who are the pension elite? According to Street, how do tax expenditures connect these two groups of people?
3. How do social insurance and tax expenditures differ in their underlying values or principles and how they approach the distribution of resources? Why does Street believe the redistribution of resources through occupational and fiscal welfare "do not conform to common sense understanding of social justice?"

---

[5] According to the Joint Committee on Taxation (2008) tax expenditures have increased from around 60 in the JCT's first description of tax expenditures in 1972 to approximately 170 in 2007.

[6] The GAO (2005) estimated the revenue lost due to tax expenditures at $730 billion in 2004.

4 Street argues that tax expenditures in the United States have recently been used in ways that undermine social solidarity. Identify and explain one example of this outcome. Additionally, Street explains that tax expenditure policy can be used as a vehicle to achieve social justice. Identify and explain one example of using tax expenditures to achieve this outcome.

5 Street lists multiple characteristics of welfare state policy decisions. Select one of these characteristics and explain what it means. Select an example of a U.S. policy that illustrates this characteristic of policy making. Select an example of an international policy that illustrates this characteristic of policy making. What are some key differences in the character of the welfare state of the United States and that of the country in which the comparison policy is located?

REFERENCES

Béland, D., & Gran, B. (Eds.). (2008). *Public and private social policy: Health and pension policies in a new era.* Houndmills, England: Palgrave Macmillan.

Bell, E., Carasso, A., & Steuerle, C. E. (2005). *Strengthening private sources of retirement savings for low income families* (No. 5, The Ownership Project). Retrieved October 26, 2008, from http://www.urban.org/UploadedPDF/311229_private_sources.pdf

Congressional Budget and Impoundment Control Act of 1974, Pub. L. No. 93-344, § 3(3), (1974).

Congressional Research Service [CRS]. (2006a). *Topics in aging: Income and poverty among older Americans in 2005.* Washington, DC: CRS, The Library of Congress. Retrieved November 24, 2008, from http://assets.opencrs.com/rpts/RL32697_20060921.pdf

Congressional Research Service [CRS]. (2006b). *Tax expenditures: Trends and critiques.* Washington, DC: CRS, The Library of Congress. Retrieved November 24, 2008, from http://taxprof.typepad.com/taxprof_blog/files/RL33641.pdf

Department of Labor. (2000). Coverage status of workers under employer provided pension plans. Washington, DC: Office of Pension Research. Retrieved October 26, 2008, from http://www.dol.gov/ebsa/programs/opr/CWS-Survey/contents.htm

Esping-Andersen, G. (1990). *The three worlds of welfare capitalism.* Princeton, NJ: Princeton University Press.

Estes, C. L. (2004). Social Security privatization and older women: A feminist political economy perspective. *Journal of Aging Studies, 18*, 9–26.

GAO. (2005, September). *Tax expenditures represent a substantial federal commitment and need to be reexamined* (GAO-05-690). Washington, DC: GAO. Retrieved October 26, 2008, from http://www.gao.gov/new.items/d05690.pdf

Gilbert, N. (2002). *Transformation of the welfare state: The silent surrender of public responsibility*. Oxford: Oxford University Press.

Ginn, J., Street, D., & Arber, S. (Eds.). (2001). *Women, work and pensions: International issues and prospects*. Buckingham, England: Open University Press (OUP).

Hacker, J. S. (2002). *The divided welfare state: The battle over public and private social benefits in the United States.* New York: Cambridge University Press.

Hacker, J. S. (2005). Bringing the welfare state back in: The promise (and perils) of the new social history. *Journal of Policy History, 17*(1), 125–154.

Hacker, J. S. (2006). *The great risk shift: The new economic insecurity—And what can be done about it.* Oxford: Oxford University Press.

Harrington Meyer, M., & Herd, P. (2007). *Market friendly or family friendly? The state and gender inequality in old age.* New York: Russell Sage Foundation.

Hendricks, J. (2005). Moral economy and aging. In M. L. Johnson, V. L. Bengtson, P. G. Coleman, & T. B. L. Kirkwood (Eds.), *The Cambridge handbook of age and ageing* (pp. 510–517). Cambridge, UK: Cambridge University Press.

Howard, C. (1997). *The hidden welfare state: Tax expenditures and social policy in the United States*. Princeton, NJ: Princeton University Press.

Joint Committee on Taxation [JCT]. (2008, May 12). *A reconsideration of tax expenditure analysis* (JCX-37-08). Retrieved October 26, 2008, from http://www.house.gov/jct/x-37-08.pdf

Minkler, M., & Cole, T. (1999). Political and moral economy: Getting to know one another. In M. Minkler & C. L. Estes (Eds.), *Critical gerontology: Perspectives from political and moral economy* (pp. 37—49). Amityville, NY: Baywood Publishing Company.

Myles, J., & Street, D. (1995). Should the economic life course be redesigned? Old age security in a time of transition. *Canadian Journal of Aging, 14*(2), 335–359.

National Academy of Social Insurance [NASI]. (2007). *Social Security and retirement income adequacy* (Social Security Brief 25). Washington: NASI Retrieved October 26, 2008, from http://www.nasi.org/usr_doc/SS_Brief_025.pdf

Porter, K. H., & Dupree, A. (2001). *Poverty trends for families headed by working single mothers, 1993-1999*. Washington, DC: Center on Budget and Policy Priorities. Retrieved October 26, 2008, from http://www.cbpp.org/8-16-01wel.pdf

Quadagno, J., & Street, D. (2005). Antistatism in American welfare state development. *Journal of Policy History, 17*(1), 52–71.

Schlesinger, M., & Hacker, J. S. (2007). Secret weapon: The 'new' Medicare as a route to health security. *Journal of Health Politics, Policy and Law, 32*(2), 247–291.

Sinfield, A. (1993). Reverse targeting and upside down benefits: How perverse policies perpetuate poverty. In A. Sinfield (Ed.), *Poverty, Inequality and Justice* (pp. 29–48). Edinburgh: Edinburgh University Press.

Social Security Administration [SSA]. (2006). *Income of the Population 55 or Older: 2004*. Washington DC: Social Security Administration, Office of Policy, Office of Research, Statistics, and Evaluation, SSA Publication No.13-11871, released: May 2006. Retrieved November 20, 2008, from http://www.ssa.gov/policy/docs/statcomps/income_pop55/2004/incpop04.pdf

Social Security Administration [SSA]. (2007). Fast Facts and Figures about Social Security: 2007. Washington DC: Social Security Administration, Office of Policy, Office of Research, Statistics, and Evaluation, SSA Publication No. 13-11785, released: September, 2006. Retrieved November 20, 2008 from http://www.ssa.gov/policy/docs/chartbooks/fast_facts/2007/fast_facts07.pdf

Social Security Administration [SSA]. (2008). *2008 Annual Report of the Board of Trustees of the Federal Old-Age and Survivors Insurance and Disability Insurance Trust Funds,* released: April 10, 2008. Retrieved on November 20, 2008 from http://www.socialsecurity.gov/OACT/TR/TR08/tr08.pdf

Street, D. (1996). The politics of pensions in Canada, Great Britain, and the United States: 1975-1995. Unpublished PhD dissertation, Tallahassee: Florida State University.

Street, D., & Cossman, J. S. (2006). Greatest generation or greedy geezers? Social spending preferences and the elderly. *Social Problems, 53*(1), 75–96.

Street, D., & Connidis, I. (2001). Creeping selectivity in Canadian women's pensions. In J. Ginn, D. Street, & S. Arber (Eds.), *Women, work and pensions: International issues and prospects* (pp. 158–178). Buckingham, England: OUP.

Street, D., & Ginn, J. (2001). The demographic debate: A gendered political economy of pensions. In J. Ginn, D. Street, & S. Arber (Eds.)*Women, work and pensions: International issues and prospects* (pp. 31–43). Buckingham, England: OUP.

Street, D., & Wilmoth, J. (2001). Social insecurity: Women and pensions in the US. In J. Ginn, D. Street, & S. Arber (Eds.)*Women, work and pensions: International issues and prospects* (pp. 120–141). Buckingham, England: OUP.

Surrey, S. S. (1973). *Pathways to tax reform: The concept of tax expenditures.* Cambridge, MA: Harvard University Press.

Surrey, S. S., & McDaniel, P. R. (1985). *Tax expenditures.* Cambridge, MA: Harvard University Press.

Titmuss, R. M. (1958). *Essays on "the welfare state."* London: Allen and Unwin.

PART V

Teaching Social Insurance: Critical Pedagogy and Social Justice

Part V: Teaching Social Insurance: Critical Pedagogy and Social Justice

Introduction

LEAH ROGNE

Scholars in this volume have been guided by a framework of critical gerontology, which seeks to provide alternative theoretical frameworks, a scientific epistemology, concrete information, and emancipatory knowledge to address concerns of social inequality and social justice. Within critical gerontology, the political economy perspective, now considered part of mainstream gerontological theory, examines old age and aging as social constructions that may be understood only in the context of the larger social forces of politics, class, and social status and in the context of cultural identities such as race, ethnicity, gender, and able bodiedness.

It follows, therefore, that the approach to pedagogy on social insurance should be a critical one, focusing on participatory approaches to learning, emancipatory knowledge, and the application of that knowledge in the public arena to create social change. In addition, because a critical understanding of the educational institution that "recognizes the political nature of all educational interventions" (Mayo, 1999, p. 24), education on social insurance must be undertaken with an awareness of the power of the frames that have come to dominate the debate and have shaped the consciousness of students and the public in general and their ideas about the future of social insurance programs.

In research on teaching social insurance in higher education (Estes, Grossman, Rogne, Hollister, & Solway, 2008), the editors of this book found educators facing a number of barriers, including their own limited knowledge about social insurance and their limited knowledge about existing curricula and resources on the subject. Institutional ageism was also found to be a significant challenge as a persistent elder-as-other attitude distances young people from older adults and their concerns. In addition, as a result of dominance in the media of the "twin ideologies" of neoliberalism and neoconservativism (Estes, Biggs, & Phillipson, 2003, p. 57), educators are often confronted with their students' deeply held, negative assumptions about entitlements and the role of the government. One professor reported, "I always have a moment when I say: 'How many of you say Social Security won't be there when you get old?' Nearly everyone raises their hand" (Estes et al., 2008, p. 27). As current efforts to establish some kind of universal health care system in the United States gain momentum at the same time as assaults on Social Security and Medicare continue, effective education on social insurance will became even more important.

The chapters presented thus far in this volume provide valuable information about various aspects of the history and development of social insurance, the contours of the debate, and some recommendations for the future. In the last section, scholars who are knowledgeable about social insurance as well as experienced classroom teachers share their ideas on how to engage students and empower them to be active participants in the decisions that will determine its future. In the spirit of critical pedagogy, these teaching strategies are designed to help foster the development of what Aronowitz and Giroux (1986) called "transformative intellectuals" who not only recognize the power relations and political struggles embodied in the debates on social insurance, but who also see their legitimate roles as actors in efforts to advance the cause of social progress and the common good.

In chapter 20, historian Andrew Achenbaum suggests ways to teach the history of social welfare, identifying sources of historical data that give voice to those who reside in the margins of American society and elaborating on the need to address the complex and varied set of power relations operating at different historical moments. He provides his own experience teaching the history of social welfare, from the Babylonians to the George W. Bush, in an effort to illustrate the complexity of this work and the successes one can have as an educator. Teaching social insurance in the college classroom is as much a struggle for inclusion as any in history and one that is likely to be met with derision and/or disinterest on the part of students. However, Achenbaum argues that through both explicit and implicit means the history of social insurance can be offered as a relevant force that has shaped the nation and continues to impact contemporary policy debates.

In chapter 21, social work professor Patricia Cianciolo argues that because of the nature the debate about social insurance in this country, "teaching without any semblance of values or conviction is unimpassioned, unrealistic, and sells both students and their professors short" (p. 402, this volume). Beginning with a compelling personal story, Cianciolo makes the case that a wide public, including college students, should know about the basics of Social Security and Medicare and what is at stake in the various reform proposals. Cianciolo outlines resources on teaching on social insurance from a political economy perspective, including sources on financing and solvency issues, ways to evaluate reform proposals, criteria for appropriate policy analysis, and ways to apply concepts from moral philosophy to the social insurance debate. She identifies a wide variety of sources of information from a variety of perspectives, including foundations, think tanks, interest groups, university centers, and the media.

Finally, in chapter 22, gerontologist Joanne Grabinski advocates for learning experiences that are relevant to and meaningful in the personal world of the learner. She suggests a number of strategies and environments that help learners transition from teacher-centered pedagogical methods to andragogical or learner-centered models of learning. Drawing on Bloom's Cognitive and Affective Domains of Bloom's Taxonomy of Educational Objectives, Grabinski shares learner-centered strategies for use in facilitating education about social insurance for students in gerontology-specific or aging-related courses at institutions of higher education (community colleges, colleges, universities, and professional schools), along with some advice for facilitators new to andragogy and the study of social insurance.

Both Cianciolo and Grabinski provide a wide variety of resources, many of them online, for educators and students to find out information on Social Security and Medicare and examine various aspects of the social insurance debate. All three authors provide inspiration to educators as well as useful information for professors who want to inform their students about social insurance and empower students to be actively engaged in the decisions that will determine the future of social insurance in this country.

REFERENCES

Aronwitz, A., & Giroux, H. A. (1986). *Education under siege: The conservation, liberal and radical debate over schooling*. New York: Routledge.

Estes, C. E., Biggs, S., & Phillipson, C. (2003). *Social theory, social policy and ageing: A critical introduction*. Berkshire, UK: Open University Press.

Estes, C. L., Grossman, B. R., Rogne, L., Hollister, B. A., & Solway, E. (2008). *Teaching social insurance in higher education*. Washington, DC: AARP.

Mayo, P. (1999). *Gramsci, Freire and adult education: Possibilities for transformative action*. London: Zed Books.

20

Make History Ground-Breaking by Teaching Essential History: Putting Social Security in U.S. History Syllabi

W. ANDREW ACHENBAUM

A certain paradox pervades the teaching of U.S. history. The fewer number of key players an instructor introduces into the narrative, the smoother the story line. This lecturing tactic has the advantage of raising the likelihood that an acceptable percentage of the listening audience will grasp some (ideally most) of the central pedagogical lessons of the presentation. Conversely, the historian's didactic message becomes muddled and disjointed as she or he mixes diverse faces and disparate roles into the tale being told. Students checking their e-mail have difficulty listening to a chorus of speakers conveyed by a single human voice. Diluting lecture content nonetheless carries its own risks: It strips away the multiple perspectives and activities integral to a given historical event that might, if apprehended, convey that rich sense of irony and contingency to human actions.

Nor is it simply the polarity of the two approaches—one homogenized, the other contested—that make it hard to find common ground in teaching U.S. history. Historians invariably disagree over content. One of my favorite teachers managed to teach the entire survey course without once invoking the Civil War; he considered the event peripheral to the motifs he wanted to invoke. Especially in survey courses, as more and more historical actors compete for space in a discourse that begins and ends by the clock, the issue of packaging can become acute. To add a lecture on the Conservationist Movement may require an instructor to shave time off a lecture on Gilded Age politics.

Current cohorts of undergraduates and graduate students rarely encounter professors who dwell primarily on the lives and accomplishments of dead white men and, as a consequence, assign minor parts to all other historical actors. My generation 4 decades ago would not have characterized the Great Man pedagogy of recounting the American saga in such derisive terms, though it must be quickly added that few of us knew any other way of probing the past. Winners wrote chronicles (or had amateurs or professional writers write them) that celebrated their virtues and muted their foibles. Losers rarely were acknowledged. And the rest—mostly women, members of minority groups, people with disabilities, and ordinary families in rural and urban settings barely getting by—got scant attention (if their lives and communal experiences were recognized at all).

The central themes of the textbooks and teachers of my undergraduate days in retrospect seem chauvinistic and bombastic. They heralded an American exceptionalism that defied all aphorisms about the rise and fall of great powers in world history. Americans were a people of plenty, whose borders were safely insulated by large oceans and weaker nations. Americans were bound to achieve their Manifest Destiny. The historical record, thus unfolding, revealed the steady progress of U.S. triumphalism in a world in which Good countries (will) inexorably vanquish Evil ones. "The American Century" that Henry Luce extolled in 1942 now seems illusory, more than a little embarrassing in its pretense. Within 25 years of its promulgation, Americans had witnessed too many disappointments, broken promises, violent acts, as well as tragedies at home and abroad to sustain the myth that God somehow is the Great White Father of our own Yankee Doodle Dandy.

For nearly 4 decades, a contrapuntal theme has swept graduate seminars and undergraduate lecture halls. It took shape with the rise of the so-called new social history, itself forged in the dramatic upheavals of the 1960s. Blacks in the South and northern ghettos, contrary to stereotypes and conventional wisdom, proved that they were not pawns. Reexamining the historical record underscored that blacks played a significant role in changing their place in the United States. Just as 19th-century historians discarded images of "Sambo" in recounting the dynamics of work and family in antebellum slave quarters, so too have 20th-century Americanists underscored that leaders in black communities were at the forefront of the struggle to end segregation and other racial disparities.

Similarly, instructors recognized that women were not merely handmaidens in the historical processes unfolding in the First New Republic. Women of all ranks mobilized their peers to demand educational and social reforms. Women were at the vanguard of the abolitionist movement and the temperance movement. Immigrant women defied deeply instilled ethnic norms as they worked outside the home to keep their family networks intact. Transcending barriers of class, race, religion, and ethnicity, more and more women joined forces to claim their identities and distinctive voices.

The demography of teaching history changed along with the message after 1970. White, middle-class men no longer dominated the professorial ranks. Classrooms in elite centers of learning as well as in community colleges in remote parts of the country themselves became more heterogeneous. Race theory, feminist theory, and queer theory permeated a discipline not known for its theoretical moorings because fresh ways of thinking raised new questions and illuminated hitherto obscure facets of the American experiences. History instructors have been assiduously reworking texts and discourses in books, lectures, and discussions so as to privilege the visions and struggles of women since 1619, when the first boatload of European women arrived at Jamestown. No longer content to silence or trivialize the roles that anonymous Americans played in making U.S. history, most lecturers seized the opportunity to recount the travails of a widening sphere of minorities (racial, ethnic, class, sexual, and religious), whose diversity sustains the nation's energy.

All these changes undercut the "big message" that long had dominated the unfolding of U.S. history. Few instructors these days talk about Pax Americana, or celebrate claims of hegemony. U.S. history teachers are more likely to characterize the American melting pot—long vaunted for its tolerance—as a cauldron of hatred, distrust, and misgivings. Based on the latest scholarship, it becomes harder to privilege the legacy of winners from the prophecies of losers. History professors generally portray efforts to bind wounds caused by culture wars as episodic so that they can move on to the next clash along racial, gender, ethnic, religious, or regional lines. This approach to teaching U.S. history certainly affords a richer version of the past than I was taught. Yet, lost in the transformative mayhem has been much sense of the connective tissues that have knit together, however fragilely, a nation of people with little sense of how their democratic legacy persists from generation to generation.

There is a middle way to teaching U.S. history that melds themes of consensus and conflict, of disparities and comities, of continuities and changes. This middle way gives significant emphasis to social welfare issues as well as to the needs and demands of the aged and the aging. Such facets of the American experiences have commanded remarkably little attention during the last half century in undergraduate syllabi or graduate students' reading lists. Social welfare history lies at the margins of social and political history. Few study the history of age and aging. The historical omission is unsettling, because silence contributes to ignorance. Social welfare themes, to judge from their current valance in seminar rooms and lecture halls, seem as pertinent in the grand scheme of things as the relevance of historic preservation efforts after Sherman's army marched by. In an aging society, instructors rarely prepare future generations to appreciate how a concatenation of demographic, economic, political, and social vectors converging over the past 6 decades will affect their careers and social relationships.

Social welfare history deserves a fuller recounting by U.S. historians. Not only is caring for the sick, the poor, the orphan, and the old an important responsibility of any political order to fulfill, but it also helps us conjoin disparate facets of the historical puzzle. Defining and prescribing care for "worthy" dependents has since the colonial era been an important (if not foremost) concern at various levels of government and within local philanthropic bodies. Here, to state the obvious, the preferences and prejudices of dead white men and their "ladies bountiful" have been apparent in policy orientations and programmatic shifts. The documents and artifacts of the rich are not the only pieces of historical social welfare evidence at our disposal, however. We also have historical data by age, gender, race, ethnicity, occupation, and place of origins collected in almshouses and census records. In court hearings and admissions files, we can "hear" the now still voices of the poor and their kin.

After instructors have identified the historical actors, they can turn their lectures to identifying who "controlled" the poor and how "they" did it. Here, effective pedagogy requires a fresh, revisionist approach. Typically, instructors, presuming (incorrectly) that "control" is an effective deterrent to civic disorder, pitted rich and poor in one-sided power struggles. In a fresh retelling, emerge diverse stories of compassion for and by some groups and fear by rich and poor alike of other segments of the vulnerable. Students grasp history when the narrative gets beneath the overriding desire to remove physically or institutionally unsavory groups, and the narrator probes altruism tarnished and mitigating circumstances behind poverty.

There is no straightforward, neat teleological thread that takes professors and students alike from the Elizabethan Poor Laws to the origins of the 1935 Social Security Act. The ideological underpinnings and policy dimensions of the most important measure of the New Deal are not without precedent, to be sure. Still, the unpacking of the legislative details truly depends on a "thick" understanding of the political economy of the times and the pragmatic policy making conducted in Washington. Surely, late 19th-century corporate pension plans and old-age dependency provisions passed by several states before the Great Depression served as prototypes for aspects of various titles of the 1935 Act. These hardly exhaust the treasure trove. How, for instance, do we tease out the relative importance to be ascribed to Constitutional precedents, to a series of failed federal and state-level initiatives, to efforts by unions and Townsendites, as well as to international experiences in giving philosophical and bureaucratic mooring to one of the most important pieces of omnibus legislation in U.S. history? Having been on both sides of the podium, I know that it takes more than a sentence or two in a rushed lecture, spent summarizing alphabet agencies created by Franklin D. Roosevelt in his first 100 days and his first term, to do justice to the creation of Social Security.

That said, few lecturers assert that the Social Security Act of 1935 laid the foundation for the American welfare state. Nor do they go on to note that the 1939 amendments, with its emphases on familial versus employee needs and on providing a minimal level of support rather than a benefit based on contributions, altered the thrust of the original legislation. (For more on the 1935 Act and 1939 amendments, see p. 391.) The absence is not for want of materials: The original documents are readily available on line; there are several dozen highly competent historical monographs from which to take talking points.

One problem, I think, is that instructors are afraid that the origins of Social Security are boring. They do not believe that exposing their audiences to the unknowns in the policy matrix, or the clash of individual and institutional interests, actually can make for lively theatre. Furthermore, most historians, preferring to reconstruct history on its own terms, are loath to apply lessons of the past to present-day challenges. So amidst periodic pleas by presidents and pundits to "privatize" Social Security, few instructors revisit the past to explain why FDR thought that imposing taxes on wages would prevent any Congress from "scrapping" his Social Security system. In their silence, a teachable moment is lost. Explaining the strengths and flaws in the original Social Security legislation might influence students to (re)consider why some of their fears about the program's future solvency are unfounded.

Ironically, from a lecturer's perspective, the most interesting part of Social Security history has taken place since the Great Society. As its architects anticipated, the program grew to be the largest U.S. domestic program, affecting the well-being of more individuals than any other federal measure. Social Security is probably our most successful antipoverty initiative. Disparities—especially by race and gender—present at the outset have been reduced over time, though anomalies persist. Despite its successes, the system has been on the defensive for 25 years. History untold, unspoken, allows Social Security's detractors a platform larger than the historical facts warrant.

This is why the omission from undergraduate and graduate syllabi of this landmark legislation, and subsequent attempts to discredit or diminish Social Security clout, is so astounding. Ignoring the ways that Social Security has transformed the fabric of U.S. social relationships diminishes efforts to reconstruct the American experiences. The history of Social Security is not just about demographic projections and fiscal outlays. The system, which lies at the heart of the compact between the government and the governed, affects ordinary people of all races and creeds, from all walks of life. Once the third rail of American politics, the future Social Security requires now constant vigilance, lest rising cohorts of citizens forget its importance in the lives of their (grand)parents as well as their own future well-being. Social Security's triumphs and travails make for gripping history, if only teachers were to tell its story with passion.

What follows is one historian's effort to insinuate social welfare history, and especially Social Security, into a graduate level course on the history of U.S. policy making. And then, more poignantly, I recount the ways in which I have tried (with mixed success) to convince teaching assistants and undergraduates that learning something about Social Security's history would make them better citizens.

PUTTING SOCIAL SECURITY IN A GRADUATE-LEVEL U.S. SOCIAL WELFARE HISTORY COURSE

For 6 years, I have offered a Historical Research Seminar on U.S. Social Welfare in the Graduate College of Social Work at the University of Houston. Every second-year student must take one of two research seminars, both of which happen to meet at the same time.

I begin the first class saying that the best seminar of the term will be the discussion of the 1935 Social Security Act and its 1939 amendments. I tell them that by the time we get done with that session, they will have a better handle on current politics. Some students nod approvingly—I know that type, I was a brownnoser once too. Some look blankly—they are the audience I want to reach—skeptical but teachable. Some are typing furiously on their laptop; for some reason, I doubt that they are recording my comments.

We begin with the Babylonians, move to the ancient Hebrews and Jesus movements, turn to the Greeks and Romans, and then end up with Islam and the pre-Reformation Roman Catholic Church. The purpose is twofold. On the one hand, I want to emphasize the importance of the need to attend to the "stranger" in any civic society, dating back as far into recorded history as we can probe. On the other hand, I want to suggest the permeability of the lines of responsibility between the public and private sectors in caring for strangers in need. (I readily acknowledge the historical possibility of ignoring pleas for help or escorting undesirables to the frontiers.)

To reinforce these two themes, I pay considerable attention to the Elizabethan Poor Laws. I stress that these measures set the precedent for all subsequent initiatives in the New World. When New York became a British colony, for instance, its measures took precedence over Dutch codes. Certain motifs were central in the Poor Laws: The individual bore responsibility for his or her well-being in the face of the vicissitudes of life; the family (broadly defined) was the primary backup; the private sector formed the next line of defense; and by default, grudgingly because its intervention involved raising taxes, the State (in this class, the local county or community) stepped in. Though "welfare" in the sense of caring for the needy was mentioned neither in the Declaration of Independence nor in the Constitution, the 1787 Ordinances governing the Northwest Territories nonetheless replicated the spirit of these Elizabethan poor laws.

I pay little attention to the antebellum period except to lay out the horrors of the almshouse, which people at the time thought was an improvement over existing ways of helping the poor. I force debates in the class over who was considered "worthy" of support and who was undeserving. I ask students to consider the merits of age-integrated provisions, especially if such places housed criminals, orphans, the insane, and the desperately ill. I indicate that private individuals, often with first-hand experience with almshouse residents, began to create distinctive institutions for special segments of the population. Lest the historical pattern I am weaving in lectures and discussions becomes too predictable, I try to shock students short by talking about Franklin Pierce's 1854 veto of Dorothea Dix's appeal for federal funding for homes for the deaf and insane. My support of Pierce's decision confuses them: I insist that there was, at the time, no provision for federal intervention, however noble the cause. Hence, the president acted wisely. All along, I portray a fear of federal intervention at all levels of society that is eerily familiar.

I spend a week on the Civil War. I want to show how the public health movement arose from the filth of battleground hospitals, from university-based instructors, and from forward looking state-level agencies. This partnership, borne in a national crisis, suggests (to me) how radical change from the bottom up emerges in an emergency situation. I insinuate that Social Security would be forged in a time of crisis with grassroots support for federal intervention. To illustrate a top-down approach, I analyze the Freedman's Bureau, a Radical Republican effort to afford newly freed slaves and their families land, education, and the right to vote.

I use the emerging urban-industrial order to demonstrate the ways that immigrants, especially through their religious organizations, cared for the needy in their own community. Americans historically preferred to rely on "voluntary associations" in the private sector in dealing with dependency. Hence, social welfare history resembles a patchwork quilt. I indicate that the continuing withdrawal of segments of the almshouse population made most poorhouses de facto old-age homes. In addition, I stress the growing dependence of ordinary Americans and officials during the last decades of the 19th century on the expertise of professional bodies, which needed "scientific" credibility to advance social issues.

By the early years of the 20th century, I portray (with mordant irony) the federal government as the chief supporter of older people: Washington gave pensions to Yankee Civil War veterans and their dependents who happened to be old, but it steadfastly resisted any proposals to assist veterans of the industrial revolution. Indeed, I indicate that Progressive reformers paid less attention to the plight of old-age dependency than to the needs of children, their mothers, and to disabled or unemployed workers. I note, with sadness, the rise and fall of the Shepphard-Towner Act (1920–1929), which aided children and poor mothers. An early victim of the Great Depression, the measure would find a second life in titles of the 1935 Social Security Act. However, its fate challenges our assumption that federal measures, once enacted, become sacrosanct.

Until now, students were expected to do the assigned reading, but I rarely worried about how carefully they had wrestled with primary and secondary sources. On the week in which we discussed Social Security, the class was told to mark up the report of the Committee of Economic Security, the 1935 Act, and the 1939 Amendments. I read out loud the concluding paragraphs of the first document as if I were rehearsing the preamble to the Constitution. I understood the theme of the Act's architects to be a balance between liberal/conservative, like Europe/distinctively American, traditional/innovative. I underlined the plainness of the words—as value-free as is the Preamble—to embellish the architects' desire to strike a middle ground.

Then, guiding my students along, I marveled at the uncertainties written into the law. Did you notice? No firm estimate of what percentage of the elderly population would be dependent in Title I, no clear distinction between "employer" and "employee" in Title II, yet an assiduous attempt to avoid a Constitutional showdown by disentangling social insurance function (Title II and Title III) from finance (Title VII and Title VIII). By the time we are done with the exercise, students generally feel as if they got their tuition's worth; they understand the original Act.

Then, the bombshell. We turn to the 1939 amendments, first stressing the difference between "equity" and "adequacy." (This distinction is not apparent.) Analogies to private insurance do not work, I point out, because we are talking about "social insurance." I quietly indicate that, thanks to the passage of the 1939 amendments, Social Security went bankrupt before the first paycheck was issued. Why? The government decided to cover a greater percentage of the citizenry than were contributing to the system. In Texas, such pronouncements cause hearts to flutter.

Then, I offer a twofold conclusion, which sets the stage for the rest of course. If you are a conservative, then bemoan the fact that the 1935 Act never got implemented, but do not claim that modern-day politicians have violated its principles. Historical honesty requires you to acknowledge instead that original provisions were superseded before they ever took effect. In addition, if you are a liberal, then rejoice that a recession caused an expert panel of advisors to rework the 1935 measure to make it more generous and more inclusive. But recognize that World War II precluded the further liberalizations promised in the 1939 amendments. By 1944, Roosevelt had become Dr. Win the War.

I then spend time talking about the "politics of incrementalism," which aptly defined Social Security policy making for the next 3 decades. In addition, I try to disassociate images of "welfare" from notions of "poor people," by suggesting the social security outlays have largely been benefits for middle-class wage earners and their families. To demonstrate this, I devote considerable time to showing that the bureaucratic language establishing eligibility criteria under Social Security adversely affected the status of women and minorities from 1940 to 1960 without being blatantly sexist or racist. In addition, I use the G.I. Bill as a model "welfare" measure, which boosted the earnings and educational capacities of "worthy" recipients.

My treatment of social insurance in the Great Society is more circumspect than I expressed myself 25 years ago: Dramatizing the importance of Medicare, Medicaid, and the Older Americans Act. I, nonetheless, point out that these measures were enacted at the end of Lyndon B. Johnson's legislative initiatives. That they survived when other measures were rescinded gives them a relative significance they might otherwise not have had at their inception.

I spend as much time on Nixon as on Johnson for two reasons. First, Nixon's role in boosting Social Security benefits and imposing a cost-of-living adjustment deserves praise, as does his consolidation of various state-based welfare programs under Supplemental Security Income. The 1972 Social Security amendments were a significant development in the history of social insurance. Election-year politics made him Machiavellian, but to a greater benefit to older Americans than I would be tempted to portray him. Second, it is worth remembering that Nixon coined the term the "New Federalism." This concept devolved the actual allocation of resources to states as they determined to place their priorities. In addition, this set the stage for the neoconservative revolution under which we still live. States traditionally, even in the contemporary era, have been the primary site for the ebb and flow of social welfare history.

Aware that most of my students are more conservative and polite than I, I try to be as circumspect in my vitriol as I can be in recounting the last 35 years of social welfare history. It is hard to be dispassionate, after all, in describing how Ronald Reagan and David Stockman viewed cutting Social Security benefits as part of their larger war on entitlements. When Congress rebuffed the president's measure as draconian, Reagan gamely had to sign a bipartisan measure, the 1983 amendments to the Social Security Act, which (in my opinion) remains the basis for any meaningful reform of Title II. Once again, I make students read the legislative particulars so that they can sense the delicate balancing of Democratic/Republican, liberal/conservative concerns. I let students deduce for themselves the inherent flaw in President George H. W. Bush's Catastrophic Coverage Act. And I paint the Clinton years as ones of missed opportunities, especially in terms of developing and implementing a national health care plan. I cannot pretend to temper my contempt for the second Bush's ill-fated attempt to privatize Social Security, but I do dispassionately attest to importance the coalition forged by old-age interest groups like AARP and concerned academics in enacting Medicare, Part D.

Then, I try to put these recent presidential actions into broader context. We talk about ageism. We talk about Americans for Generational Equity. We talk about the power of statistics as if they were divinations. We talk about fear, especially our collective vulnerability in the wake of Hurricane Ike, and about bad things that might occur during future tropical storms. We move, living so close to New Orleans, to the stigma of race and class, from Jamestown to the post-Katrina world. We talk about continuing gender inequities, despite advances in professional education and family laws. And this brings us back to the beginning of the course, to a discussion of the "stranger," to reflections on civic responsibility. The trend line is deliberately messy, which is intentional, if my students are to have a keener appreciation for the complexities and contrarieties of the past. They leave the course recognizing that Social Security rests at the cornerstone of social welfare history.

SUBVERSIVE WORK: MAKING ROOM FOR SOCIAL SECURITY IN THE U.S. SURVEY

Survey courses of U.S. history differ from graduate seminars on U.S. social welfare history in at least three ways. First, most surveys last more than one term, extending over the academic year. In northern schools, the end of the Civil War (1865) serves as the cut-off, thus allowing for a measure of regional legerdemain. In the South, teachers begin the second half of the survey with the end of Reconstruction (1877), when the Yankees went home, and conditions resumed for the planter class as normally as they could, amidst the ruins.

Second, deans and department chairs have a greater stake in how the survey course is taught than they invest in a graduate seminar. To the extent that enrollments in the introductory history courses help to determine a department's future faculty lines, there is an incentive to have the best lecturers in the trenches. (At one institution where I taught, however, a contrary logic prevailed. Graduate students ran the survey courses so that research-driven faculty would not have to bother with pandering to novices.)

Third, by design and happenstance, determining the "time" to be allocated to competing interests and issues counts more in structuring the survey course far more than in an upper-level class. If race matters to an instructor, for example, then she or he may actually foreshadow the second half of the course with a lecture or two on slavery and the collapse of political discourse in Washington, DC, and across regions during the 1850s. Race would loom large as a topic in the 24 remaining lectures of the term. Recounting the accomplishments and shortcomings of the Reconstruction might take a week. An entire lecture would be given to the educational and political differences between Booker T. Washington and W. E. B. DuBois. A lecturer probably would allocate another class to the 20th-century migration of African Americans up north, surely one to the importance of jazz (in the cultural history of the 1920s), and a third to the experiences, at home and abroad, of blacks during World War II. Most historians would require two to three lectures to do the Civil Rights movement justice, followed with a lecture on the underclass and possibly one on the significance of race and class in the wake of Katrina.

That would leave such an instructor 13 lectures to cover 26 presidents, Populism, Progressivism, the New Deal, the New Frontier, and the neoconservatives. Economically, attention must be paid to the Great Depression, four panics, and post-World War II affluence. Undergraduates love to hear about wars. And into the mix must be made space for women, Native Americans, new professionals, immigrants, fundamentalists, Hispanics, gays and lesbians, and people with disabilities. Given the attention accorded global warming and water shortages, surely a case can be made for a lecture respectively on the rise and fall of conservationism and on riparian rights on the Great Plains. (I am assuming there no longer is the need to enunciate Great Themes or to end the survey course's series of lectures on a hortatory note—though Obama's presidency may cause fresh interpretations of the civic order. I leave no room for in-class examinations.)

The possibilities are endless. The choices, like it or not, are ideological. To decide to devote 20 minutes to Pine Ridge might entail shaving minutes off the discussion of Stonewall. It is a zero-sum game, even with take-home finals, and discussion sections that compensate for materials given short shrift by the instructor.

Missing, of course, from this menu is any discussion of social insurance. While preparing to teach the survey course of U.S. history since 1865 at the University of Michigan a decade ago, I offered my eight teaching assistants a preview of my course syllabus. Within minutes, virtually all of them objected to my spending a week on the New Deal, especially my recommendation for a full lecture on the 1935 Social Security Act and the 1939 amendments. Why?, they asked. Because it is the single most important piece of social legislation thus far in U.S. history, I responded. Social Security's details are tedious, they claimed. How can the plight of destitute women, disenfranchised blacks, and galvanized older people not make for a great lecture, I retorted. Then they mentioned omissions in my lecture topics—where was the rise of modern medicine, the 1893 Chicago World's Fair? Ford's assembly line deserved attention if I were truly interested in mass consumption. The debate, nasty at times, continued for 20 minutes. It ended when I reminded my assistants that I was the primary instructor. Glaring at eight snarling faces is not the best way to begin a term.

The lecture on Social Security went well, though I admit that attendance was noticeably lighter. The follow-up discussion in sections (except mine, naturally) were desultory. Teaching assistants can make or break a survey. Although the lecture has remained a mainstay when I teach the course, I have never succeeded in convincing a colleague to follow my example, and to do likewise.

Why is this the case? On one level, I think it reflects market-driven exigencies. Undergraduates expect to hear somewhere in the course about the sinking of the Maine. They cringe when reminded about the horrors of the Holocaust and Hiroshima. They fantasize about whether their lecturer was at Woodstock—or at least takes comfort that she or he knows what it is. They do not expect to join 300 other students in taking notes on the differences between Old-Age Assistance (Title I) and Old-Age Insurance (Title II) in the Social Security Act of 1935.

On a deeper level, I think the lack of interest in social insurance is ageist. Social Security is for senior citizens, and undergraduates think that they congregate in temples of youth. This dichotomy fuels their own fears of growing older, with the visceral horror of lacking the means to make a miserable existence tolerable. At the same time, they manage to deny the value of learning enough about the historical record to ask questions about their future selves. Indeed, most find it difficult to gaze imaginatively ahead while keeping an eye on the past.

If my diagnosis is correct, and I believe it is, then the remedy is straightforward. Insisting on one lecture in a survey course on the original Social Security Act and the 1939 amendments is probably as radical a move that I can make pedagogically. The rest must be subversive, insinuating "age" into familiar accounts of race, gender, and class in the sweep of U.S. history. So, in the face of tawdry urban politics in the Gilded Age, I duly mention Populist reforms, but I also emphasize what the federal government was willing to do for aging Civil War veterans. I introduce students to the G.A.R., to prepare them for Townsendites. In the same lecture, I take them to the military home in Dayton, Ohio, where 6,000 Union men receive start-of-the-art social services and medical care. A bit later, I end the lecture on Progressivism, pointing out that the largest single outlay in the federal budget in 1917 went to grants for veterans and their aging dependents. I do not hesitate to point out that Congress rejected analogies to underwriting old-age industrial pensions. Congress was not blind to factory conditions or to the incidence of disabilities caused by accidents, I remind students. Lawmakers consciously chose not to make the latter condition a priority, partly out of fiscal conservatism, partly out of ethnic prejudice, partly out of lack of immediate contact with the vicissitudes of lower-class immigrant life.

The lecture I give on Social Security in the survey course differs from the graduate seminar. For openers, it is more melodramatic. Despite Roosevelt's generosity to older paupers when governor of New York, as president he was not moved to address old-age dependency until he had dealt with the crises in major sectors of the economy, such as banking, the work force, the stock market, and agriculture. By the time he was willing to act, more than 2 years into his administration, the safety net for elders was torn asunder. Unemployment rates among those over age 65 exceeded all other age groups. Savings were lost as banks collapsed. Leaders could not honor pension promises made by corporations and unions, because their institutions lacked resources. Philanthropic agencies, surprised by the length and depth of the Great Depression, had exhausted funds. Families tried to help, but they were having difficulty feeding their own children. Most state governments were on the verge of bankruptcy. So, Washington was the last hope, the only hope.

However, federal officials were not the only pivotal actors. I give more credence at the lectern to the impact of the Townsend movement than I do in my writing. On the one hand, this tact sets the stage for the emergence of the gray lobby, a critical component of a lecture I give on "social movements," which sweeps the terrain from *now* to evangelicals. On the other hand, it sets up my argument for the genesis of the second civil-rights movement, in which I claim that the steady use of the judicial system by African Americans sufficed to cause fissures in the Jim Crow system, before Brown v. the Board of Education (1954) or the nonviolent methods advanced by Dr. Martin Luther King. Like older people in the 1930s, those hitherto un(der)spoken in the United States were in fact prime movers of their own emancipation.

Older people make cameo appearances in recent American history, beyond the discussion of AARP in the social movements lecture. I dwell on the elder lobby's role in attaining Medicare and Medicaid. I stress the role of older people worldwide networking for environmental causes. In my last lecture, I introduce the notion of societal aging, insisting that social insurance is the best contract existing across generational lines.

The life of an academic is, for better and for worse, solitary. I write at home. I teach behind closed doors. I have written this essay in the hopes that it will give others ideas for introducing social insurance and (old) age into history curricula at the undergraduate and professional levels. It is an uphill struggle. There is much to be done. Perhaps this essay will empower others to follow my example or, better yet, devise more compelling ways to teach a rising generation why these topics matter so much.

DISCUSSION QUESTIONS

1. Why is an understanding of the debates over Social Security important to students?
2. Achenbaum argues that Social Security has "transformed the fabric of U.S. social relationships." Give examples of how this has occurred.
3. With all the competing topics that one might cover in a U.S. history course, what argument does Achenbaum make for the inclusion of the story of Social Security?
4. Achenbaum describes significant changes in the teaching of American history over the last 4 decades. What are some

of these changes? What impact have these changes had on how history is taught?

5 Achenbaum references a "middle way to teaching U.S. history." What does he mean by this? What are the other forms of teaching to which he refers?

21 Teaching Collaborative Learning and Continuing Education Strategies about Social Security and Medicare

PATRICIA K. CIANCIOLO

INTRODUCTION

My first personal experience with Social Security benefits occurred when I was 19 years old, soon after my mother had died. I vividly remember receiving the first check for $50—it was both a blessing and a curse. The benefits attempted to replace a portion of my mother's lost earnings for our family; however, no amount of money could bring her back again. There were eight children and, like many families, both my parents had to work to make ends meet. My father even had to work two jobs for a number of years. One of my brothers was born with profound developmental disabilities and was not expected to live very long. He is now 52 years old, living in a medium-sized residential facility with other children and adults whose mental and physical disabilities prevent them from living fully independent lives. He receives Social Security adult dependent child survivor benefits on my father's account, which helps to pay a portion of his care while Medicaid pays the rest. None of my siblings could afford the near $70,000 annually it would take to do this.

These examples illustrate some of the basic goals of social insurance programs. The death of a spouse at a young age or the birth of a child who is profoundly disabled is hardly expected. For the majority of older adults in the United States, Social Security and Medicare benefits provide a basic "floor of protection" for income and health security (Kaiser Family Foundation, 2007; Social Security Administration (SSA), 2007) that differs considerably from private insurance. Social Security provides cash benefits to more than 49 million men, women, and children in the United States (SSA, 2007), while Medicare provides health care coverage to 43 million aged and disabled individuals (Congressional Budget Office, 2007; Kaiser Family Foundation, 2007). Social Security represents the largest share of aggregate income for older adults, making its importance to income security in old age unmistakable (SSA, 2007, p. 6). Social insurance programs entail the redistribution of resources from one group to another (Benavie, 2006; Century Foundation, 2005; Marmor & Butler, 2000; Marmor & Mashaw, 2006), lift the majority of older adults out of or keep them from falling into poverty, and are especially critical to women and people of color (Boivie & Weller, 2007; Gonyea, 2005; Kaiser Family Foundation, 2007; SSA, 2007).

Although data illustrate the relevance of these programs to the well-being of older adults and their families, politicians debate a number of reform efforts that are likely to result in unintended consequences. Conservatives and liberals alike have initiated such proposals, with the Medicare Modernization Act of 2003 being the most recent and major change to take effect. Due to the scope and complexity of the Social Security and Medicare programs, and the magnitude of the impact that any alterations have and will have on the collective citizenry of the United States, it is essential that the public be well informed. Collaborative teaching and learning strategies in college classes and the use of continuing education programs offered by institutions of higher learning represent effective ways to accomplish this goal. This chapter discusses these educational strategies and provides resources to teach about Social Security and Medicare and current reform efforts.

THE SOCIAL INSURANCE DEBATE AND THE ROLE OF HIGHER EDUCATION

There are a number of factors that have led to a "crisis mentality" related to Social Security and Medicare. Some of those factors are the march of the baby boomers toward retirement, increased longevity, spiraling health care costs, lowered fertility rates, and a decline in the dependency ratio (Rettenmaier & Saving, 2007). To be sure, these variables are and will continue to exert a strong influence on both programs and need to be addressed. Should these so-called crises lead to radical alterations such as dismantling or partial privatization? Or is it in the best interest of U.S. citizens for the government to maintain the social insurance principles and features of these programs, making needed incremental changes? These are economic, political, and value-oriented issues and are difficult for the average person, much less the seasoned scholar, to decipher. The purpose of Social Security (1935) and Medicare (1965) have not changed since their inception, but the rhetoric has. The rhetoric is ushering in numerous proposed changes to "fix" Social Security and Medicare, and is skewed toward a conservative agenda (Altman, 2005; Binstock, 2006; Diamond & Orszag, 2004; 2005; Estes & Svihula, 2007; Herd, 2005; Kingson, 2007; Marmor & Mashaw, 2006; Williamson, 2007).

Higher education in the United States has been the venue for providing the environment to introduce, critically analyze, and debate ideas. It is also where the acquisition of knowledge and skills can be obtained to meet the needs of a changing and dynamic economic and social landscape (Cianciolo & Henderson, 2003; U.S. Department of Labor, 2000). Higher education, however, is not immune from societal influences and pressures. Mitchell (2007, p. 48) discusses a culture war taking place in higher education between the "traditionalists" and the "modernizers," the latter of which have adopted a corporate versus collective model. Traditionalists hold dear the notions of academic freedom, shared governance, and the pursuit of truth through education and intellectual inquiry. The modernizers would prefer to administer higher education as a streamlined, efficient, and rapidly adaptable organization with the primary purpose of job training, minimizing the value of a liberal arts foundation that promotes intellectual inquiry and informed debate. Mitchell (2007) articulates the need for the two opposing groups to embrace what he calls a "commitment to deliberative democracy on campus" (p. 49), and reminds us of the dual nature of the educational environment, which is "aimed at providing students with the education necessary to make them not only good workers, but also good citizens" (p. 50). His notion of the university embraces the value of the "common good" that promotes an environment where the collective university becomes "both teachers and learners in cooperative inquiry" (p. 51). In another article "Impassioned Teaching," Caughie (2007), a feminist scholar, argues, "classrooms today seem to be more like talk shows with the professor as host, than forums for intellectual inquiry . . . too many teachers feel their job is to acknowledge any and all opinions offered on the topic being studied. Not to do so is to risk being exposed as someone intent on indoctrinating rather than teaching them" (p. 56).

Most academics are committed to a particular perspective or subject area, and have spent years cultivating that knowledge. A balanced approach to teaching is essential to be sure; however, teaching without any semblance of values or conviction is unimpassioned, unrealistic, and sells both students and their professors short. The very nature of the debate about Social Security and Medicare reform is value-laden, and politically and economically charged. Exposure to information that educates citizens about the complexities in these debates is essential.

COLLABORATIVE LEARNING AND CONTINUING EDUCATION AS TEACHING STRATEGIES

Collaborative Learning

A significant number of students and citizens, in general, do not make the connection between social policy decisions and real life circumstances. Public policy, professional practice, and everyday lives of individuals are indeed connected and educating students about this connection is fundamental (Cianciolo, Henderson, Kretzer, & Mendes, 2002; Cianciolo & Henderson, 2003; Popple & Leighninger, 2008). Collaborative learning strategies have been documented to have three important outcomes: (1) the creation of a classroom environment where students are actively engaged in their own education (Steiner, Stromwell, Bruzzy, & Gerdes, 1999); (2) student accountability for their own learning (Johnson & Johnson, 1994); and (3) the reduction of competition by rewarding group performance and cooperation (Johnson & Johnson, 1981). The role of teachers who use collaborative learning changes from the traditional position of imparting knowledge to one of facilitator of learning (Deering, 1989) and focuses on providing students with the types of resources needed to accomplish their educational goals. This is often accomplished through the use of structured groups that have specific tasks (Cianciolo & Henderson, 2003; Kluge, 1990).

Collaborative learning is an effective strategy to use when teaching about Social Security and Medicare reform because it involves students in the subject matter, promotes mastery of new policy content, and ultimately educates them about the connection between policy change and the lives of real people, including themselves. As an alternative to giving a student a project and expecting them to find relevant materials, the teacher provides students with resources that offer multiple perspectives, and it is the students' responsibility to utilize the resources to facilitate their own education and that of their peers. Group projects create an environment in which students and their colleagues become immersed in the topic, while at the same time fostering discussion, debate, and critical assessment about materials presented. When group efforts about topics such as Medicare and Social Security reform are presented to the class as a whole, a much more in-depth dialogue takes place.

Continuing Education

Most professionals are required to obtain continuing education to maintain licensure and practice competencies, which largely serves as a safeguard for the public whom they serve. What about the average person who wants to continue life-long learning or other audiences not wanting to spend time in a semester-long course, but are interested in the subject? As mentioned earlier in this chapter, institutions of higher education have the dual purpose of educating a competent workforce and producing good citizens (Mitchell, 2007). Continuing education programs represent an avenue to accomplish this goal and can be used as a mechanism to teach about Social Security and Medicare reform. According to Bash (2003), continuing education programs have had to be innovative and flexible in serving adult learners for the past 50 years, and in the 21st century, the proportion of adult learners is expected to increase. The need for faculty to incorporate technology and less traditional pedagogy into continuing education programming will persist, and as Bash (2003) states "strategies—like collaboration and harnessing the learner's own experience—if they hope to achieve transformative learning" (p. 36).

An example of one type of continuing education programming that has been used at the university where the author teaches is the use of "hot topics" courses. These courses are designed to be intensive educational sessions built around a topic considered to have high interest to community, student, and nonstudent populations. The courses can be physically located on campus, in the community such as a public library, or use an electronic format. The general structure for the "hot topics" course is a 3 to 4 week session for one credit, either on consecutive Saturdays, or one evening a week. Students are graded on a satisfactory/unsatisfactory system if taken for college credit. Most participants taking such courses are nondegree participants. Courses can be offered by a faculty member of the university without going through the normal academic curriculum review process, whereas a nonfaculty members' proposal must be reviewed by the College of Graduate Studies. Sponsorship of "hot topics" courses is through the College of Graduate Studies, and coordinated through the university's Continuing Education department. There is a cost, which varies depending on graduate/undergraduate degree status, although individuals older than 62 years of age benefit from a credit waiver program. One of the greatest benefits of the "hot topics courses is that it provides an alternative venue for faculty and experts to provide important educational opportunities (M. J. Falcon & C. B. Hadley, personal communication, September 18, 2007).

An example of a "hot topics" course developed at the author's institution was one on Living Wills, offered in the fall of 2005. It was taught by a philosophy faculty member who used his expertise in applied ethics (Cooper, 2004) as a way to teach about and evaluate current issues and reform efforts surrounding living wills and their use in the United States (D. E. Cooper, personal communication, September 18, 2007). The "hot topics" format offers potential for teaching about Social Security and Medicare reform in a nontraditional university format, with the opportunity to attract a diverse audience and provide a venue in which accurate information about reforms can be discussed, debated, and critically analyzed.

CONTENT AND RESOURCES FOR TEACHING ABOUT SOCIAL SECURITY AND MEDICARE REFORM

Political Economic Perspectives and Social Insurance

A number of academics representing multiple disciplines have studied Social Security and Medicare and their proposed reforms. This section will discuss some works that are useful teaching resources. The discussion is by no means exhaustive as the literature is vast, constantly evolving, and can be overwhelming. The majority of works discussed, argue that radical changes are uncalled for, that the Social Security and Medicare programs have and continue to protect the health and income security of older adults as they were intended to do, and that incremental change is the best policy option to "fix" them.

Since the author completed her dissertation on older women and income security in old age (Cianciolo, 1991), she has used the work of Myles (1984) in teaching about the origins of old-age policies in the United States. Myles identifies the "retirement principle" and the "liberal-democratic state" as ideological perspectives, which legitimized the removal of older workers from the labor force, and underpinned the political-economic framework for the development of income maintenance policies for the aged. The works of Olson (1982) and Quadagno (1983; 2005) are additional sources that use a political-economic framework to discuss how old-age policies have developed and continue to be molded in the present. Although increased longevity has exacerbated challenges to the retirement principle, and the baby boomers promise to strain the budgets of Social Security and Medicare in the United States, democratic principles mandate the state with responsibility for the protection of citizen rights (Marmor & Butler, 2000; Marmor & Mashaw, 2006; Myles, 1984;). Estes and associates (2001), in their political economy of aging, critically examine social structural factors that create and perpetuate health and income disparities in old age. The political economy of aging perspective emphasizes the confluence of race, class, and gender in maintaining these disparities.

Enter "the great risk shift" that Hacker (2006; 2007) identifies in terms of aging public policies. This risk shifting includes both private market and governmental efforts to place more responsibility on the shoulders of average citizens to secure their own health and retirement security. Income instability, coupled by catastrophic medical expenses, personal bankruptcy filings, and debt for working Americans is moving them precariously off the path of attaining health and income security in old age, and Hacker (2007, pp. 5, 6) argues this predicament will necessitate more, not less, governmental supports.

The works of Ghilarducci (2007) and Munnell (2007) provide further elucidation on the economic inability of average- and low-income earners in particular to secure their futures in old age. The movement away from defined benefit to defined contribution retirement plans has decreased not increased retirement security for most Americans, and has actually subtracted from their savings rate (Ghilarducci, 2007, p. 9). Today's retirees are living in the "best of times," and many factors have and will contribute to a more risky financial outlook in the future (Munnell, 2007). The National Retirement Risk Index (NRRI), developed by the Center for Retirement Research at Boston College, has determined that 43% of baby boomers and Generation Xers will have a difficult time maintaining their preretirement income levels (Munnell, 2007, p. 16). The factors most likely to be contributing to this situation are: "1). A decline in Social Security replacement rates due to the rise in two-earner couples and the increase in Social Security's Normal Retirement Age (NRA); 2) lower pension replacement rates as a result of the shift from defined benefit to defined contribution plans; and 3) lower annuity payments due to the dramatic decline in real interest rates" (Munnell, 2007, p. 17).

Most of the previous discussion focuses on retirement security, where Moon (2007) identifies similar obstacles in terms of health security and Medicare changes. The risk shifting taking place within the Medicare program is evidenced by reform proposals that could lead to the development of vouchers, usurping its basic benefit package with a fixed amount the government would pay per beneficiary per year. In essence, the voucher proposal carries the privatization scheme already occurring within Medicare one step further—the first step was the passage of the Medicare Prescription Drug, Improvement, and Modernization Act (MMA) of 2003 (Butler, 2007; Marmor, 2007; Oliver, Lee, & Lipton, 2004). Another political force sculpting a "fix" for Medicare comes from the centrists, both Democrats and Republicans, who view Medicare as unaffordable (White, 2007, p. 221).

The tension between the goals of a market-based economic system and a democratic polity has led to the "commodification" of social programs addressing health and income security for older adults, placing market-based goals ahead of social needs (Estes, 1979; 2001a). The role of the media in forwarding this agenda and promoting a "climate of fear" related to Social Security and Medicare solvency has additionally had a marked influence on current reform efforts (Binstock, 2006; Estes, 2001b; Estes & Svihula, 2007).

Evaluating Reform Proposals

Reform proposals largely fall into three categories: maintenance of benefits, reducing benefits, and/or changing the mix of private/public provisions (Cianciolo & Henderson, 2003, p. 213). Evaluation of proposed reform efforts for the Social Security and Medicare programs is a complex, but necessary undertaking. But how should one evaluate the proposals, based on what criteria, and using what fundamental premise regarding the nature and intent of social insurance programs? The following provides some suggestions to accomplish a framework for accomplishing this goal.

Policy Analysis

Social welfare policy is proposed, passed, evaluated, and modified in a constantly changing and fluid environment. The individuals who make policy are not a homogenous group nor are those who are affected by social policies. Thus, policy analysis needs to take into consideration a myriad of factors. Bardach (1996) has developed an eight-step path for conducting a policy analysis. In a nutshell, it includes the following: defining the problem, assembling evidence about it, developing alternative solutions to the problem, selecting criteria to evaluate the alternatives, projecting what the outcomes will be of a given alternative, confronting tradeoffs, adopting a policy option, and discussing the entire process (Bardach, 1996, p. 2).

In terms of Social Security and Medicare reforms, some basic policy analysis questions would be: Who is defining the problems involving Social Security and Medicare? Is this definition representative of all views? What evidentiary material is available about both intended and unintended consequences of suggested reform proposals? Policy analysis is an attempt to take the multiple factors involving a particular policy and applying scientific methods to critically analyze which alternative(s) will hopefully produce the greatest good for the most people. Additional questions that are central to evaluating reform efforts from a policy analysis perspective are related to ensuring program solvency, providing adequate benefits, and whether the policy alternative will increase or decrease public confidence in the programs.

Applied Ethics

The application of moral agency or ideal theory in applied ethics, which find its origins in the discipline of philosophy, can provide some useful guidelines for evaluating reform proposals related to Social Security and Medicare. At the foundation of these social insurance programs is the value of providing a "basic floor of protection" for income and health security in old age by virtue of citizenship. In essence, profit should not theoretically outweigh the ability to obtain adequate health care or prevent some degree of financial security in old age for any group (Myles, 1984). The use of a "model decision procedure" (Cooper, 2004, pp. 43–45), incorporating moral agency or ideal theory allows for establishing what basic principles should guide policy makers in their deliberations about how to "fix" these programs.

Another concept used in moral philosophy is beneficence, often formalized in professional code of ethics, which articulates the moral imperative that professionals have in terms of promoting the well-being of those they serve (Jansson, 1999). Because of the inequalities, which capitalist economies produce, protection of the most vulnerable and attempts to eradicate structural inequality are important. Social Security and Medicare, as mentioned earlier in this chapter, attempt to redistribute scarce resources from one group to another. Some reasonable questions deriving from this orientation would be: What are the constraints and facilitating factors that any given reform proposal represents, in terms of the basic value premise of these programs? What consequences would a reform alternative have on vulnerable groups? Who are the winners and losers? Is this morally justifiable?

Social Security and Medicare Finances and Solvency

Each year, the Boards of Trustees for Social Security and Medicare make reports to Congress related to the financial solvency and projected solvency of these programs. Most people mistakenly rely on the media to provide them with accurate information about the financial status of Social Security and Medicare. The public at-large is unaware of the significance of estimating low-, high-, and intermediate-cost projections of the Social Security and Medicare trust funds. Although cumbersome to wade through, these reports are very important in understanding reform proposals and correcting misinformation about the all but certain bankruptcy of these programs. The 2007 Annual Report for the Boards of Trustees for Social Security and Medicare is available electronically at www.ssa.gov/OACT, and a summary of the 2007 Annual Reports at www.ssa.gov/OACT/TRSUM/trsummary.html.

The National Academy of Social Insurance and the American Academy of Actuaries (2007) provide further interpretation of the Trustees Reports, in a more succinct, comprehensible fashion. The AARP Public Policy Institute, AARP's "Divided We Fail" campaign, and the AARP Office of Academic Affairs alert interested individuals to the publication of useful, educational materials. Reno and Gray (2007) authored a Social Security brief, *Social Security Finances: Findings of the 2007 Trustees Report,* published by the National Academy of Social Insurance, which is available electronically at http://news.aarp.org/UM/T.asp?A910.52851.3896.4.904209. An additional Issue Brief published in April 2007, by the American Academy of Actuaries, *Medicare's Financial Condition: Beyond Actuarial Balance,* is available electronically at the same address.

The Social Security Administration's Web site (www.ssa.gov), and the Centers for Medicare and Medicare Services Web site (www.cms.gov), provide access to basic information on program structure, eligibility requirements, coverage, a benefit calculator, and a plethora of statistical information on program costs, beneficiary characteristics, and so forth. The *Social Security Bulletin*, a major publication of the Social Security Administration, contains informative articles about reform issues such as current challenges in securing adequate retirement income (Engen, Gale, & Uccello, 2005), how Social Security will deal with increased life expectancies and declining fertility rates (Reznik, Shoffner, & Weaver, 2005/2006), how individual retirement accounts are working in other countries (Kritzer, 2005), and providing a program and policy history of Social Security (Martin & Weaver, 2005).

The Government Accountability Office (GAO) (www.gao.gov), a prominent audit, evaluation, and investigative arm of Congress established in 1921, provides timely in-depth analyses on Social Security and Medicare issues. Three GAO publications useful for teaching about current reform efforts are *Social Security Reform: Preliminary Lessons from Other Countries' Experiences*, released in June 2005; *Retirement Security: Women Face Challenges in Ensuring Financial Security in Retirement*, released in October 2007; and *Health Care 20 Years from Now: Taking Steps to Meet Tomorrow's Challenges*, released in September 2007.

The Congressional Budget Office (CBO) (www.cbo.gov) began operation in 1975 and is another source of information related to health care spending in the United States. It produced a study titled *The Long-Term Outlook for Health Care Spending* in November 2007, which provides the CBO's estimates of federal spending on Medicare and Medicaid and all other national health care (CBO, 2007, p. 1).

Additional governmental units that are resources and should be well known to aging experts that deal with social policy issues impacting the aged in general are the Administration on Aging (www.aoa.gov), the National Institute on Aging (http://www.nia.nih.gov/) and the U.S. Senate Select Committee on Aging (http://aging.senate.gov/).

Foundations, Think Tanks, Interest Groups, and University Centers

Foundations. A number of foundations provide nonpartisan, in-depth analysis of health and income security issues. Two that are especially useful to teaching about Social Security and Medicare reforms are The Century Foundation (TCF) founded in 1919, and the Henry J. Kaiser Family Foundation (KFF) established in 1948. These foundations produce publications that are well written and researched that multiple audiences will find germane and accessible. TCF produces a series called *The Basics*, which includes Social Security and Medicare Reform and is available at www.tcf.org. The KFF, with its emphasis on health care issues recently published *Medicare: A Primer* in March 2007, which is accessible at www.kff.org. These resources are helpful in gaining an understanding of basic program structure and reform efforts.

Think Tanks. The Brookings Institution (www.brookings.edu) and the Urban Institute (www.urban.org) established in 1918 and 1968, respectively, have more liberal leanings. The Employee Benefit Research Institute (www.ebri.org) was established in 1978 as a result of the passage of the Employment Retirement Income Security Act of 1974, and it has the express purpose of focusing on research and education on economic security and employee benefits issues. All three organizations conduct research on health and income security issues, commissioning scholars from differing political and theoretical perspectives to foster critical debate about social insurance reform proposals.

The American Enterprise Institute (www.aei.org) was established in 1943 and was the first of the conservative think tanks. The CATO Institute (www.cato.org) was founded in 1977, and the Heritage Foundation (www.heritage.org) began in 1973. During the 1970s and 1980s, there was a national political shift to a conservative agenda. This agenda also began to target older Americans for taking disproportionate resources away from younger generations (Binstock, 2007). In teaching about Social Security and Medicare reforms, it is important to provide students with resources that offer an array of perspectives related to reforms. That said, it is equally important to articulate the basic political-economic perspectives of the organization disseminating the information.

Interest Groups. A host of interest groups are vested in the same direction Social Security and Medicare reforms take. The largest and probably most well known is AARP (www.aarp.org), which was established in 1958 as the American Association of Retired Persons. The *AARP Bulletin* is one of the most widely read of the organizations' publications, reaches a significant audience, and routinely carries stories about Social Security and Medicare. Two such examples are Bethell's (2007, pp. 11–13) article "Keeping It Afloat" about why we need to maintain Social Security, and Barry's (2007, pp. 20–21) article "The Going Gets Tougher," related to the precipitous drop in drug plans covering brand name drugs under

MMA's Prescription Drug coverage. Since the launching of the "Divided We Fail" campaign in 2005, AARP has made concerted efforts to form crucial alliances with other groups to educate the public about reforms that could undermine the social insurance functions of Social Security and Medicare. The Public Policy Institute and Office of Academic Affairs of AARP, mentioned earlier in this chapter, provide invaluable resources pertinent to the Social Security and Medicare debate and can be accessed through the AARP Web site (www.aarp.org).

The National Committee to Preserve Social Security and Medicare (www.ncpssm.org), which formed in 1982, sends out regular updates to members and interested individuals. Other organizations worth exploring for content relevant to Social Security and Medicare reform are the Center for American Progress (www.americanprogress.org), the National Women's Law Center (NWLC) (www.nwlc.org), and the Older Women's League (OWL) (www.owl-national.org), the last two focus on how reform proposals will impact women in particular.

University Centers. There are many universities that have centers dedicated to studying aging issues. Two that are especially noteworthy in terms of health and retirement security policy research are the Center for Policy Research, housed in the Maxwell School of Citizenship and Public Affairs at Syracuse University, and the Center for Retirement Research at Boston College (CRR). Aside from the research undertaken by the Center for Policy Research faculty at Syracuse University, it has served as a training and resource site for academics from around the country to learn how to get aging public policy content into their courses (Cianciolo, Henderson, Kretzer, & Mendes, 2002; Cianciolo & Henderson, 2003). Policy briefs and other publications are available through the center's Web site (http://www-cpr.maxwell.syr.edu/).

The CRR at Boston College was established in 1998 through a grant from the Social Security Administration and has goals related to conducting research, disseminating information, and promoting scholarly interest in retirement issues. A recent publication released by CRR, authored by Brown, Hassett, and Smetters (2005), "Top Ten Myths of Social Security Reform," takes a critical look at current reform proposals offered by both proponents and opponents of these plans. CRR's Web site and publications can be accessed at www.bc.edu/crr.

Media. Reputable magazines, newspapers, and television programs are important tools for teaching about Social Security and Medicare reforms.

The mass media exerts an enormous influence on the public, promulgating sound bits that often do not accurately inform. Unfortunately, it is often the case that what people hear or read through these resources becomes absolute truth. The media, however, can be a terrific springboard for debate and critical analysis of Social Security and Medicare reform efforts. The author routinely uses articles from a variety of newspapers and magazines such as *The New York Times*, *The Christian Science Monitor*, and *Newsweek*.

The Public Broadcasting System (PBS) has a program called *Frontline*, which produces documentaries on a number of topics. One recent example of a *Frontline* production useful in terms of teaching about Social Security is "Can I Afford to Retire" (2006), produced by Rick Young, which addresses recent societal changes that will make it difficult for baby boomers to have a secure retirement. Using different sources of information and various mediums in teaching about Social Security and Medicare reforms can effectively enhance learning and support the in-depth discussion and critical analysis these issues need and deserve.

CONCLUSION

This chapter has suggested that the use of collaborative learning and continuing education in higher education can represent important vehicles to teach about Social Security and Medicare reforms. Because of the importance Social Security and Medicare hold in terms of the income and health security of older adults and their families, it is crucial to educate students and the broader community about reform proposals. For those teaching about these programs and their reforms, a significant number of resources have been provided in this chapter to foster knowledge about what is available. Both seasoned and unseasoned teachers can use these resources to stay current and/or develop competency in negotiating the often confusing and contradictory world of reform of social insurance programs in the United States.

DISCUSSION QUESTIONS

1. How can you find out more information about current proposed changes to social insurance programs?

2 How should one go about doing policy analysis and applying ethical principles to evaluate proposals for reform of Social Security and Medicare?
3 Why is it important to include information from a variety of points of view in teaching about social insurance?
4 Based on the readings in this volume, what compelling scenarios or stories such as Cianciolo's could you construct about vulnerable groups who depend on Social Security and/or Medicare?

REFERENCES

Altman, N. J. (2005). *The battle for Social Security: From FDR's vision to Bush's gamble*. Hoboken, NJ: John Wiley & Sons, Inc.

American Academy of Actuaries. (2007, April). *Medicare's financial condition: Beyond actuarial balance (Issue Brief, 1-7)*. Washington, DC: Author.

Bardach, E. (1996). *The eight-step path of policy analysis: A handbook for practice*. Berkeley, CA: Academic Press.

Barry, P. (2007, December). The going gets tougher. *AARP Bulletin*, *48*(11), 20–21.

Bash, L. (2003, January/February). What serving adult learners can teach us. *Change*, *35*(1), 32–37.

Benavie, A. (2006). *Social Security under the gun: What every citizen needs to know*. New York: Palgrave/MacMillan.

Bethell, T. N. (2007, May). Keeping it afloat. *AARP Bulletin*, *48*(5), 11–13.

Binstock, R. H. (2006, Winter). Social Security and Medicare: President Bush and the delegates reject each other. *Public Policy & Aging Report*, *15*(1), 9–12.

Binstock, R. H. (2007). Is responsibility across generations politically feasible? In R. A. Pruchno & M. A. Symer (Eds.), *Challenges of an aging society: Ethical dilemmas, political issues* (pp. 285–308). Baltimore: The Johns Hopkins University Press

Boivie, I., & Weller, C. E. (2007, August). *An oldie but a goodie: The importance of Social Security as a source of retirement income*. Washington, DC: Center for American Progress. Retrieved October 27, 2008, from www.americanprogress.org/issues/2007/08/social_security.html

Brown, J., Hassett, K., & Smetters, K. (2005). Top ten myths of Social Security reform. (CRR WP 2005-11). Chester Hill, MA: Center for Retirement Research at Boston College. Retrieved October 27, 2008, from http://crr.bc.edu/images/stories/Working_Papers/wp_2005-11.pdf?phpMyAdmin=43ac483c4de9t51d9eb41

Butler, S. (2007). Assessing the returns from the new Medicare drug benefit. In R. A. Pruchno & M. A. Symer (Eds.), *Challenges of an aging society: Ethical dilemmas, political issues* (pp. 397–419). Baltimore: The John Hopkins University Press.

Caughie, P. L. (2007, July-August). Impassioned teaching. *Academe*, 54–56.

Century Foundation (2005). The basics (Rev.ed.). New York: Author. Retrieved November 8, 2008, from http://www.tcf.org/Publications/RetirementSecurity/SocialSecurityBasicsRev2005.pdf

Cianciolo, P. K. (1991). Economic insecurity: The experience of women 62 and over under Social Security's Title I and II programs, 1935-1977. *Dissertation Abstracts International* (UMI No. 9107775).

Cianciolo, P. K., Henderson, T.L., Kretzer, S., & Mendes, A. (2002). Promoting collaborative learning strategies in aging and public policy courses. *Gerontology & Geriatric Education, 22*(2), 47–61.

Cianciolo, P. K., & Henderson, T. L. (2003). Infusing aging and public policy content into gerontology courses: Collaborative learning methods to teach about Social Security and Medicare. *Educational Gerontology, 29*(3), 217–233.

Cooper, D. E. (2004). *Ethics for professionals in a multicultural world.* Upper Saddle River, New Jersey: Pearson Education, Inc.

Congressional Budget Office. (2007, November). *The long-term outlook for health care spending* (Publication No. 3085). Washington, DC: Author. Retrieved October 27, 2008, from http://www.cbo.gov/ftpdocs/87xx/doc8758/11-13-LT-Health.pdf

Deering, P. D. (1989, October). *An ethnographic approach for examining participants' construction of a cooperative learning class culture.* Paper presented at the annual meeting of the American Anthropological Association, Washington, DC (ERIC Document Reproduction Service No. ED 319 083).

Diamond, P. A., & Orszag, P. R. (2004). *Saving Social Security: A balanced approach.* Washington, DC: Brookings Institution Press.

Diamond, P. A., & Orszag, P. R. (2005). Saving Social Security: The Diamond-Orszag plan. *The Economists' Voice, 2*(1), article 8, 1–8. Retrieved November 8, 2008, from http://www.bepress.com/ev/vol2/iss1/art8

Engen, E. M., Gale, W. G., & Uccello, C. E. (2005). Lifetime earnings, Social Security benefits, and the adequacy of retirement wealth accumulation. *Social Security Bulletin, 66*(1), 38–57.

Estes, C. L. (1979). *The aging enterprise.* San Francisco: Jossey-Bass.

Estes, C. L. (2001a). Political economy of aging: A theoretical framework. In C. L. Estes & Associates (Eds.), *Social policy & aging: A critical perspective* (pp. 1–22). Thousand Oaks, CA: Sage.

Estes, C. L. (2001b). Crisis, the welfare state, and aging. In C. L. Estes & Associates (Eds.), *Social policy & aging: A critical perspective* (pp. 95–117). Thousand Oaks, CA: Sage.

Estes, C. L., & Associates (Eds.). (2001). *Social policy & aging: A critical perspective.* Thousand Oaks, CA: Sage.

Estes, C. L., & Svihula, J. (2007, March). Social Security politics: Ideology and reform. *Journal of Gerontology: Social Sciences, 62B*(2), S79–S89.

Ghilarducci, T. (2007, Spring). Pressures on retirement income security. *Public Policy & Aging Report, 17*(2), 8–12.

Gonyea, J. G. (2005, Summer). The economic well-being of older Americans and the persistent divide. *Public Policy & Aging Report, 15*(3), 1, 3–11.

Government Accountability Office (2005, June). Social security reform: Preliminary lessons from other countries' experiences (Publication No. GAO-05-810T). Washington, DC: Author. Retrieved November 8, 2008, from http://www.gao.gov/new.items/d05810t.pdf

Government Accountability Office (2007, September). *Health care 20 years from now: Taking steps today to meet tomorrow's challenges* (Publication No. GAO-07-1155SP

Health Care Forum). Washington, DC: Author. Retrieved November 8, 2008, from http://purl.access.gpo.gov/GPO/LPS87664

Government Accountability Office (2007, October). *Retirement security: Women face challenges in ensuring financial security in retirement* (Publication No. GAO-08-105 Retirement Security). Washington, DC: Author. Retrieved November 8, 2008, from http://www.gao.gov/new.items/d08105.pdf

Hacker, J. S. (2006). *The great risk shift: The assault on American jobs, families, health care, and retirement – And how you can fight back*. New York: Oxford University Press.

Hacker, J. S. (2007, Spring). The great risk shift: Issues for aging and public policy. *Public Policy & Aging Report, 17*(2), 1, 3–7.

Herd, P. (2005). Universalism without the targeting: Privatizing the old-age welfare state. *The Gerontologist, 45*(3), 292–298.

Jansson, B. S. (1999). *Becoming an effective policy advocate: From policy practice to social justice*. Pacific Grove, CA: Brooks/Cole.

Johnson, D. W., & Johnson, R. T. (1981). Effects of cooperative and individualistic learning experiences on interethnic interaction. *Journal of Educational Psychology, 73*, 454–459.

Johnson, D. W., & Johnson, R. T. (1994). *Learning together and alone: Cooperative, competitive, and individualist learning* (4th ed.). Englewood Cliffs, NJ: Prentice Hall.

Kaiser Family Foundation (2007, March). *Medicare: A primer*. Menlo Park, CA: Author. Retrieved November 4, 2008, from http://www.kff.org/medicare/upload/7615.pdf

Kingson, E. R. (2007). Setting the agenda for Social Security reform. In R. A. Pruchno & M. A. Symer (Eds.), *Challenges of an aging society: Ethical dilemmas, political issues* (pp. 332–345). Baltimore: The John Hopkins University Press.

Kluge, L. (1990). *Cooperative learning*. Arlington, VA: Educational Research Service.

Kritzer, B. E. (2005). Individual accounts in other countries. *Social Security Bulletin, 66*(1), 31–37.

Marmor, T., & Butler, S. (2000). Individual choice versus shared responsibility: Debate on social insurance reform. In S. Burke, E. Kingson, & U. Reinhardt (Eds.), *Social Security and Medicare: Individual risk vs. collective risk and responsibility* (pp. 71–86). Washington, DC: National Academy on Social Insurance.

Marmor, T. R. (2007, February). Medicare's politics. *Journal of Health Politics, Policy and Law, 32*(1), 307–315.

Marmor, T. R., & Mashaw, J. L. (2006, March). Understanding social insurance: Fairness, affordability, and the "modernization" of Social Security and Medicare. *Health Affairs, 25*(3), w114–w134. [Web Exclusive]. Retreived November 20, 2008, from http://globalag.igc.org/pension/us/socialsec/2006/fair.pdf

Martin, P. P., & Weaver, D. A. (2005). Social Security: A program and policy history. *Social Security Bulletin, 66*(1), 1–14.

Mitchell, J. (2007, November–December). A communitarian alternative to the corporate model. *Academe*, 48–51.

Moon, M. (2007, Spring). Risky Medicare: Vouchers, private plans and defined contributions. *Public Policy & Aging Report, 17*(2), 13–15.

Munnell, A. H. (2007, Spring). Risk in motion: The National Retirement Risk Index. *Public Policy & Aging Report, 17*(2), 16–19.

Myles, J. (1984). *Old age and the welfare state: The political economy of public pensions*. Boston: Little, Brown and Company.

Oliver, T. R., Lee, P. R., & Lipton, H. L. (2004). A political history of Medicare and prescription drug coverage. *The Milbank Quarterly, 82*(2), 283–354.

Olson, L. K. (1982). *The political economy of aging: The state, private power and social welfare*. New York: Columbia University press.

Popple, P. R., & Leighninger, L. (2008). *The policy-based profession: An introduction to social welfare policy analysis for social workers* (4th ed.). Boston: Pearson Education, Inc.

Quadagno, J. (1983). *The transformation of old age security: Class and politics in the American welfare state*. Chicago: University of Chicago Press.

Quadagno, J. (2005). *One nation uninsured: Why the U.S. has no national health insurance*. New York: Oxford University Press.

Reno, V. P., & Gray, J. (2007, April). *Social Security finances: Findings of the 2007 Trustees Report* (Brief #24). Washington, DC: National Academy of Social Insurance. Retrieved October 27, 2008, from http://news.aarp.org/UM/T.asp?A910.52851.3896.4.904209

Rettenmaier, A. J., & Saving, T. R. (2007). *The diagnosis and treatment of Medicare*. Washington, DC: American Enterprise Institute.

Reznik, G. L., Shoffner, D., & Weaver, D. A. (2005/2006). Coping with the demographic challenge: Fewer children and living longer. *Social Security Bulletin, 66*(4), 37–45.

Social Security Administration. (2007, September). Fast facts & figures about Social Security, 2007 (SSA Publication No. 13-11785). Washington, DC: Author. Retrieved October 27, 2008, from http://www.ssa.gov/policy/docs/chartbooks/fast_facts/2007/fast_facts07.pdf

Steiner, S., Stromwall, K. L., Brzuzy, S., & Gerdes, K. (1999). Using cooperative learning strategies in social work education. *Journal of Social Work Education, 35*, 253–264.

U.S. Department of Labor. (2000). What work requires of schools: A scan report for America 2000. Retrieved November 8, 2008, from http://wdr.doleta.gov/SCANS/whatwork/whatwork.pdf

White, J. (2007, April). Protecting Medicare: The best defense is a good offense. *Journal of Health Politics, Policy and Law, 32*(2), 221–246.

Williamson, J. B. (2007). Social Security reform and responsibility across generations: Framing the debate. In R. A. Pruchno & M. A. Symer (Eds.), *Challenges of an aging society: Ethical dilemmas, political issues* (pp. 311–331). Baltimore: The John Hopkins University Press.

Young, R. (Producer). (2006). *Can I afford to retire*? [Frontline Series]. Washington, DC: PBS Home Video.

22

Beyond Lectures and Tests: Facilitating Applied and Interactive Social Insurance Learning Experiences in Gerontology Courses

C. JOANNE GRABINSKI

Assignment 1: Illustrate the history of Social Security on a chronological timeline. Start with the enactment of the Social Security Act and note changes to the Act up to the present time.

Assignment 2: Your mother asks you for assistance in determining if she is eligible to collect Social Security, and if so, (1) when she will be eligible to collect Social Security and (2) how she goes about applying for it.

Each of these assignments is an appropriate beginning level assignment about Social Security, one of several *social insurance* programs in the United States. Both assignments ask the learner to provide factual information. What differentiates the two assignments is that one is teacher-centered and the other is learner-centered. Assignment 1 asks the learner to identify information that the teacher considers to be important for the learner to know, whereas Assignment 2 asks the learner to identify information that is of some personal relevance.

Learning experiences that are relevant to and meaningful in the personal world of the learner are more likely to have a greater impact on the learner. They require the learner to move beyond rote memorization, hypothetical cases, and generic applications. They move both the teacher and the learner from teacher-centered pedagogical methodologies to learner-centered models, such as *andragogy* (Knowles, 1984), *heutagogy* (Kenyon & Hase, n.d.; Hase & Kenyon, 2000), and *transformative learning* (Cranston, 2006; Mezirow & Associates, 2000; Mezirow, 1991).

The purpose of this chapter is to encourage those who teach about *social insurance* to adopt a learner-centered orientation and to do so specifically through the approach of *andragogy*. Using andragogical learning strategies and creating learner-centered classroom environments, teachers and other learning facilitators help their students transition from pedagogical to andragogical styles of learning. To work toward accomplishment of this purpose, the author:

- Presents a working definition of *social insurance*,
- Provides a rationale for use of learner-centered strategies and learning environments for courses and other learning experiences related to *social insurance*,
- Differentiates between teacher-centered *pedagogy* and learner-centered *andragogy*,
- Illustrates the use of two domains—Cognitive Domain and Affective Domain—from Bloom's Taxonomy of Educational Objectives as a tool to use in the development of learner-centered experiences specific to *social insurance*,
- Suggests an array of applied, interactive, and learner-centered strategies that can be adapted for use in gerontology-specific or gerontology-related courses and other learning experiences in which *social insurance* is a focus or topic,
- Offers some advice for learning facilitators who are new to andragogy, and
- Recommends some excellent sources of information on *social insurance* and related issues.

TEACHING ABOUT SOCIAL INSURANCE

Rosenblatt (2007), a senior fellow of the National Academy of Social Insurance, describes *social insurance* as follows:

> Life is filled with risks. Uncertainty is the rule because nobody can predict with confidence his or her future state of wealth or health. Families once

> bore the primary responsibility for caring for their individual members in bad times, but modern industrial society has scattered family members to different jobs in different locations. Certain risks we have agreed to confront as a society, rather than as individuals. Citizens have decided, through the political system, that we need financial protection against some of life's difficulties that are hard to face as individuals. These include old age, ill health, unemployment, disability that makes it impossible to work, injury on the job, and death of a family breadwinner. For all of these conditions, we rely on help from social insurance programs, which are financed by workers and employers. Social insurance programs include Social Security, which pays benefits to retired and disabled workers and their families and to families of deceased workers; Medicare, which pays for health care for those over 65 and disabled adults under age 65; Workers' Compensation, which pays for wage replacement and medical care for those injured or killed on the job; and Unemployment Insurance, which provides partial wage replacement for those who have lost their jobs.

As defined, *social insurance* is a complex topic. Although connections exist between at least two (Social Security and Medicare) of the four programs identified in defining *social insurance*, each of the four programs has unique aspects that add to the complexity of understanding required by learning facilitators and learners alike. In addition, Social Security and Medicare have age-specific entry points for program recipients, whereas Worker's Compensation and Unemployment Insurance are based on employment status or work-related situations for program-eligible workers of all ages. For those who continue to work after they begin to draw on Social Security and Medicare, situations that create the need for Worker's Compensation and/or Unemployment Insurance may present more dire complications and consequences.

In many gerontology-specific courses, the scope of what is considered to be *aging policy* includes the Older Americans Act, Social Security, Medicare, and, perhaps, the Age Discrimination in Employment Act, but excludes the other two *social insurance* programs (Worker's Compensation and Unemployment Insurance). In gerontology-related courses (e.g., Elders and Their Families/Family Development in Later Life and Sexuality and Aging taught by the author), discussion about policy infrequently touches on *social insurance* programs and issues except as it relates directly to a specific topic or situation. For example, Social Security, Medicare, and Medicaid are considered in regard to income and insurance limitations for custodial grandparents whose sole or primary income source is Social Security. In other required or elective courses, the inclusion of *social insurance* might be determined by how aging is defined. Is aging viewed as being normal, successful, and productive or as a stage of decline, disability, and disease?

Because of factors such as those noted above, it becomes even more vital for *social insurance* to become more visible in the gerontology curriculum at institutions of higher education (i.e., community colleges, colleges/universities, and professional schools). For learners to recognize and understand the complexity of older persons' lives, *social insurance* learning experiences need to be designed so as to engage and involve the learners in realistic ways via assignments and activities that are personally and/or professionally connected to their own lives. This requires learning facilitators to move away from (or at least lessen) the use of teacher-centered approaches toward the implementation of more learner-centered approaches and learning environments.

FROM TEACHER-CENTERED TO LEARNER-CENTERED APPROACHES

Pedagogy refers to teaching children. In this model, the teacher is the authority who makes decisions about what is to be learned, how it is to be learned, and when it is to be learned. The student is a passive learner or, at best, is reactive to the teacher's instructions. *Andragogy* refers to the art and science of facilitating adult learning (Knowles, 1984). It is a learner-centered approach in which the teacher and the learner collaborate in the design of the learning experience. Instead of being the "fountain of all relevant knowledge," the teacher becomes a "learning facilitator, mentor, and guide." As an active collaborator, the learner takes on equal (or at least more) responsibility for diagnosing his or her learning needs, setting learning goals and objectives, identifying necessary human and material resources, and evaluating learning outcomes. In andragogy, these facets of learning are usually approached in linear fashion.

Based on the writings of Smith (1999, 1996) and Knowles (1984), Table 22.1 presents assumptions that can be made about learners in a comparison of pedagogy and andragogy. A major goal of this chapter is to assist gerontology and geriatrics educators and professionals working in the field of aging to move from the use of teacher-centered pedagogical approaches to adopt a learner-centered andragogical orientation to the learning experiences they directly or indirectly facilitate.

Table 22.1

ANDRAGOGY VS. PEDAGOGY: ASSUMPTIONS ABOUT LEARNERS*

PEDAGOGY	ANDRAGOGY
Learner's Self-Concept: *As a person matures, his self-concept moves from one of being a dependent personality toward one of being a self-directed human being.*	
Learner is a dependent personality; learner submissively carries out teacher's directions	Learner is self-directing (or becomes self-directing through transitional assistance from the teacher, who transists from teacher to facilitator/guide of adult learning)
Learner's Level of Experience: *As a person matures, he accumulates a growing reservoir of experience that becomes an increasing resource for learning.*	
Learner enters an educational activity with little or no useful life experience upon which to build new learning	Learner enters an educational activity with greater volume and quality of life experience upon which to base new learning
Learner's Readiness to Learn: *As a person matures, his readiness to learn becomes oriented increasingly to the developmental tasks of his social roles.*	
Learner is ready to learn when told to learn; readiness to learn is primarily a function of learner's age or grade in school	Learner readiness is based on need to know or do something so as to perform successfully a personal developmental task or a work-related task
Learner's Orientation to Learning: *As a person matures, his time perspective changes from one of postponed application of knowledge to immediacy of applications, and accordingly, his orientation toward learning shifts from one of subject-centeredness to one of problem-centeredness.*	
Subject-centered orientation to learning; learning is seen as an a process to acquire prescribed subject-matter content	Life-centered, task-centered, or problem-centered orientation to learning
Learner's Motivation to Learn: *As a person matures, the motivation to learn is internal.*	
Learner is motivated primarily by external expectations or mandates of teachers and parents, competition for grades, consequences of failure, desire to advance to next grade in school, or peer pressure to succeed	Learner is motivated more by internal motivators (e.g., self-esteem, recognition, higher quality of life, greater self-confidence, self-actualization) than by external motivators (e.g., a better job, or a salary increase) or learning for the sake of learning

*Italicized statements are direct quotes from Smith (1996); nonitalicized assumptions are adapted from Knowles (1984).

Learning facilitators need to keep in mind that many more learners are entering into learning experiences as adults in their middle or later years. It cannot be assumed, though, that these adults are already functioning as adult learners. Some will need nurturing to blossom as adult learners and others will need support, encouragement, and transitional learning experiences designed to facilitate their transition from pedagogical to andragogical learners.

Such nurturance might be even more essential for learning related to the complex knowledge base and operational processes of *social insurance* policy and programs. One way to assist learners in this transition from one learning style to another is to shape course content and processes in ways that allow the learners to progress from recognition or memorization of basic content knowledge toward using that information to identify and resolve personal or client social insurance problems, analyze related policy, and recommend changes in program rules and regulations, so as to better meet the needs of older persons. Employing a framework of learning objectives, such as Bloom's Taxonomy of Educational Objectives, is an effective way to stay on track in shaping learning experiences that allow learners to progress from simple to complex levels of learning about social insurance.

BLOOM'S TAXONOMY OF EDUCATIONAL OBJECTIVES

Bloom and associates posited that there are three domains of learning: cognitive, affective, and psychomotor. The Cognitive Domain is designated as rational learning, with an emphasis on thinking and knowing (Bloom & Krathwohl, 1956), and the Affective Domain is designated as emotional learning, with an emphasis on caring and feelings (Krathwohl, Bloom & Masia, 1956). The Psychomotor Domain, emphasizing physical learning, will not be considered in this chapter. For each domain, five or six levels of learning were identified (see Table 22.2).

The levels of learning in each domain are hierarchical in nature. This means that a higher level of learning, such as Cognitive Domain, Level 4: Reasoning, requires prior relevant learning at Levels 1, 2, and 3 so that the learner has an adequate foundation on which to base Level 4 learning experiences. The lower levels of each domain of learning tend to be less complex, and might be seen as more teacher-centered in orientation, especially for courses and other learning experiences intended to introduce learners to a topic. As indicated in Table 22.2, the complexity

Table 22.2

BLOOM'S TAXONOMY OF EDUCATIONAL OBJECTIVES FOR TWO DOMAINS (COGNITIVE AND AFFECTIVE), WITH LEVEL OF COMPLEXITY AND CONTINUUM FROM TEACHER-CENTEREDNESS TO LEARNER-CENTEREDNESS

LEVEL	COGNITIVE DOMAIN			AFFECTIVE DOMAIN
		Most Complex	Learner-Centered	
		↑	↑	
6	**Evaluation**	↑	↑	
5	**Synthesis**	↑	↑	**Characterization**
4	**Analysis**	↑	↑	**Organization**
3	**Application**	↑	↑	**Valuing**
2	**Comprehension**	↑	↑	**Responding**
1	**Knowledge**	↑	↑	**Receiving**
		↑	↑	
		Least Complex	Teacher-Centered	

Note. Adapted from "*Back to the future: From pedagogy to andragogy... and beyond,*" *by Grabinski, C. J., November 2006, In J. Wood (Chair), Gerontology and geriatric education: Moving from teacher-centered to learner-centered strategies and environments.* Preconference workshop conducted at the annual meeting of the Gerontological Society of America, Dallas, TX.

increases as one moves up the hierarchy of levels and this provides an excellent opportunity to move from teacher-centeredness at lower levels to learner-centeredness at higher levels. This does not exclude, however, the potential to use learner-centered approaches at lower levels (as shown in the earlier Assignment 2).

Using these domains to shape learning experiences begins with writing both the course syllabus and the assignments using behavioral objectives written in the proper domain and at levels that match the level of learning expected of students in the course. Lists of relevant verbs have been formulated by various educators for use in writing behavioral objectives (see Table 22.3).

For example, the two assignments at the beginning of this chapter are written at Level 2 of the Cognitive Domain. The first assignment asks the learner to *illustrate* the history of Social Security on a chronological timeline, and the second assignment implies that the learner should *describe*, *explain*, *interpret,* or *summarize* information about her or his mother's eligibility for Social Security and how to go about applying for it if she is eligible. The Cognitive Domain examples in Table 22.4 demonstrate how assignments on the same topic should vary at each of the domain's

Table 22.3

BLOOM'S COGNITIVE AND AFFECTIVE DOMAINS: DEFINITIONS AND VERB EXAMPLES

COGNITIVE DOMAIN	AFFECTIVE DOMAIN
Rational Learning: Emphasis on thinking and knowing	Emotional Learning: Emphasis on caring and feelings
Level 6: Evaluation: Making a Judgment	
Ability to judge the value of ideas, methods, materials, procedures, and solutions by developing and/or using appropriate criteria.	
Verbs for stating learning objectives:	
appraise, ascertain, assess, choose, compare, conclude, contrast, critique, decide, defend, discriminate, evaluate, interpret, judge, justify, resolve, select, support, validate, weigh	
Level 5: Synthesis: Creating	**Level 5: Characterization: Internalizing a Set of Values**
Ability to put parts and elements together into new forms; emphasizes creativity and originality.	Ability to integrate beliefs, ideas, and attitudes into a total philosophy of life or world view.
Verbs for stating learning objectives:	
categorize, combine, compile, compose, conceive, create, design, develop, devise, establish, formulate, generate, integrate, invent, make, manage, modify, organize, originate, plan, propose, rearrange, reconstruct, reorganize, revise, rewrite, set up, write	act upon, advocate, behave, characterize, conform, continue, defend, devote, display, disclose, encourage, exemplify, exhibit, expose, function, incorporate, influence, maintain, pattern, perform, practice, preserve, question, serve, support, uphold
Level 4: Analysis: Reasoning	**Level 4: Organization: Arranging Values Systematically**
Ability to break material into its constituent parts and to determine the relationship of these parts to each other and to the whole.	Ability to organize values, determine interrelationships among them, and establish a hierarchy of the dominant values.
Verbs for stating learning objectives:	
analyze, associate, breakdown, classify, compare, contrast, determine, differentiate, discriminate, distinguish, divide, illustrate, infer, outline, point out, relate, separate, subdivide	adapt, adhere, adjust, alter, arrange, classify, combine, compare, complete, conceptualize, disclose, establish, group, order, organize, rank, rate, reveal, synthesize, systematize

COGNITIVE DOMAIN	AFFECTIVE DOMAIN
Level 3: Application: Using Ideas	**Level 3: Valuing: Developing Attitudes**
Ability to use what is remembered and comprehended	Ability to accept the worth of an object, idea, belief, or behavior and also show a preference for it
Verbs for stating learning objectives:	
apply, change, compute, construct, demonstrate, develop, discover, dramatize, employ, estimate, illustrate, interpret, manipulate, modify, operate, organize, predict, produce, prepare, relate, show, solve, transfer, use	adopt, approve, assume responsibility for, behave according to, choose, commit, desire, endorse, exhibit loyalty for, express, form, initiate, invite, join, prefer, recognize, sanction, seek, share, show concern for, show continuing desire to, use resources to
Level 2: Comprehension: Understanding and Explaining	**Level 2: Responding: Doing Something about the Phenomenon**
Ability to grasp the meaning and intent of the material	Ability to perceive a particular situation, idea, or process and, in responding, to do something with or about it
Verbs for stating learning objectives:	
convert, decode, describe, explain, give examples, generalize, illustrate, interpret, paraphrase, restate, tell in one's own words, summarize	accept responsibility to, agree to, answer freely, ask, assist, care for, communicate, comply, conform, consent, contribute, cooperate, discuss, follow, follow-up, greet, help, indicate, inquire, obey, participate, pursue, question, react, read, reply, report, request, respond, seek, select, visit, volunteer
Level 1: Knowledge: Recalling, Remembering, and Recognizing	**Level 1: Receiving: Attending and Becoming Aware**
Ability to identify and remember material in a form very close to that in which it was originally encountered	Ability to merely become aware of a situation, idea, or process
Verbs for stating learning objectives:	
cite, define, describe, identify, label, list, match, name, recall, recite, recollect, reproduce, state	accept, acknowledge, attend, be alert, be aware, show awareness of, note, notice, pay attention to, listen, perceive, view, watch

Note. Adapted from "*Back to the future: From pedagogy to andragogy . . . and beyond,*" by Grabinski, C. J., November 2006, In J. Wood (Chair), *Gerontology and geriatric education: Moving from teacher-centered to learner-centered strategies and environments.* Preconference workshop conducted at the annual meeting of the Gerontological Society of America, Dallas, TX.

Table 22.4

LEARNER-CENTERED ACTIVITIES: COGNITIVE DOMAIN

Topic: Older Women's Eligibility for Social Security Benefits

Level 6: Evaluation: Making a Judgment

Activity: Your mother is having second thoughts about her decision to not wait until her full Social Security retirement age to begin receiving benefits. Validate her decision.

Level 5: Synthesis: Creating

Activity: Your mother decides to begin receiving Social Security benefits now rather than waiting until her full Social Security retirement age. Develop a strategy that will allow her do this without being penalized for earning too much in each year between now and her full Social Security retirement age.

Level 4: Analysis: Reasoning

Activity: Using your mother's Social Security contribution history and her current level of contribution, determine if it would be better for your mother to wait until full retirement age to begin receiving Social Security benefits.

Level 3: Application: Using Ideas

Activity: Using your mother's Social Security history and current contribution level, compute what her benefits will be if she retires at full retirement age.

Level 2: Comprehension: Understanding and Explaining

Activity: Your mother asks you for assistance in determining if she is eligible to collect Social Security and, if so, (1) when she will be eligible to collect benefits and (2) how she goes about applying for them. Summarize this information for your mother.

Level 1: Knowledge: Recalling, Remembering, and Recognizing

Activity: Identify (1) the specific age (in years and months) at which your mother will be eligible to receive Social Security benefits and (2) the month and year in which this will occur.

six learning levels. One major outcome of framing course syllabi and assignments according to Bloom's hierarchical taxonomy of educational objectives is that the learning outcomes and the evaluation criteria are clearly implied in the behavioral objectives.

MORE LEARNER-CENTERED STRATEGIES

Here are examples of some of the applied, interactive, and learner-centered strategies that have been used successfully in courses that are gerontology-specific (e.g., Policy & Aging) or related (Family Development in Later Life):

- Debate: When learners self-select and self-direct debate of social insurance issues of specific interest to them, they appear to be more open to listening to, learning about, and debating issues that are less central to their own lives. To effectively use debate as a learning tool, however, the learners need to first receive good instruction about the debate process and must agree to follow formal debate processes and rules. Rather than the course instructor serving as the debate trainer, this would be a wonderful opportunity to enlist high school and college debate teams to do the training. When high school debaters become the trainers for college/university-level learners, education about social insurance programs and issues is accomplished with both age cohorts of learners.
- Fact or fiction?: During a recent television news commentary show, the commentator stressed the importance of fact checking rather than just accepting the spoken/written "facts" presented by political candidates, reporters, and other media personnel. Turning learners into fact checkers creates a dynamic learner-centered process when the student self-directs the assignment by choosing the source (e.g., television news show, newspaper article or column, internet blog) and the specific "facts" to check.
- Comparative profiles of older adults: Gender is an important variable in social insurance policy and programs. Within the current elderly population of the United States, there are gender gaps in social insurance eligibility and benefits for older men and older women, with women often being severely disadvantaged. One way to explore these gender differences is to have learners develop case studies, based on their parents or grandparents (or both), in which they compare the eligibility status and subsequent benefits for their fathers and grandfathers with those of their mothers and grandmothers. A caveat in using this as a required learning experience is that some learners may find that one or more older relatives is unwilling to disclose the necessary personal information.
- Primer or program on social insurance program(s): Working in teams or as a whole class group, learners develop a primer about a social insurance program for a specific group of older adults (e.g., elderly relatives, a discussion group at the local senior center, attendees of congregate meal site educational program, residents of a continuing care residential center). Using an interactive process

in which they first visit with the older adults to determine the type of information wanted or needed by these elders makes this a real life learning experience. The answers to the questions can be delivered in one or more formats (e.g., printed primer, interactive presentation-discussion session). To extend the intergenerational nature of this learning experience, have the elders and students work in integrated teams to prepare and deliver the primer information.

- Hearing testimony: State and federal legislators frequently hold informal drop-in sessions and formal hearings to gather constituent input on reauthorization or changes in existing policy/programs and on proposed policy (e.g., reauthorization of the Older Americans Act, changes in Social Security or Medicare policy). Have learners identify an issue of personal interest and then prepare to testify at a related hearing. A variation on this learning experience would be to have the learners prepare letters or e-mail messages related to a social program policy issue of personal concern.
- Inbox: The mailboxes of faculty members in higher education are fertile ground for learner-centered learning experiences related to policy. Several years ago, a letter from a state official requested input on the renewal of the state's Temporary Assistance for Needy Families (TANF) regulations. The timing of this request was perfect as students in a course on aging families were considering the needs of older adults who were custodial grandparents of grandchildren younger than age 18. Assignments related to this topic were revised as the professor asked the students to help prepare the requested input. The conjointly formulated input focused on the needs of grandparents older than age 65. Through a series of individual and team assignments, along with whole group open dialogue, the final input document was a product of all course participants (not just the professor), and students were cited as first authors of the document. Although this activity was not specific to a social insurance program or policy, this strategy can be adapted easily to requests for input about such programs.
- Selection of course reading materials: Course instructors are constantly faced with the task of selecting required and recommended readings for their courses. After too many complaints about instructor-selected materials, it seemed worthwhile to invite students to become involved in the selection process. Students in a current course were invited to work with the instructor to select

reading materials to be used the next time the course was offered. Several students accepted the invitation. This allowed not only a wider array of materials to be considered, but also turned into a semester-long process through which planned course topics were addressed. As a result, some reading materials got an actual test-run during the current semester, and additional students joined the review team as the semester progressed. Students in the course the next time around benefited from the more diverse readings and reading sources. Another outcome was that not only did they actually read the required materials, but they also enriched the in-class discussions with supplemental readings they brought to class.

ADVICE FOR LEARNING FACILITATORS NEW TO ANDRAGOGY

Learning facilitators who are new to andragogy may experience resistance from learners who are used to teacher-centered lectures, term papers, and exams; although they often complain about such processes, students may prefer to have the teacher carry full responsibility for the total learning experience. For teachers, changing one's teaching routine and processes can be discomforting and difficult, especially if one already has spent considerable time and effort in preparing assignments, lecture notes, quiz/test/exam questions, course handouts, and other course materials and resources that fit a pedagogical style of teaching. Change can be threatening for both the students and teachers. The following advice is offered to help smooth your transition from pedagogy only to using at least some andragogical approaches.

- Explain to your students, at the beginning of the course and at specific points in the course, where such a change has been made, what you are changing, and why you are making such changes. This may be of greater importance for students who already have taken a course from you than for students who are new to the subject and/or to you as a professor.
- Start slowly. Although you might be really excited about your new understanding of andragogy and are ready to jump into it full force, both you and your students need time to make the transition from pedagogical to andragogical approaches. Start by incorporating only one or two learner-centered assignments and processes into

the course plan; expand use of this approach as both you and the students gain confidence in and comfort with this learning orientation.

- Create a safe and supportive classroom environment that pays attention to all three aspects—physical, emotional, and social—of the learning environment. Rearrange seating so that learners face each other rather than sitting with their backs to each other and their faces only toward the professor. Rather than standing at the lectern in the front of the room, sit among the learners and move around as the semester progresses so that you sit beside and face different learners in each class session. Design at least the first few attempts at learner-centered assignments without grades attached to them, and assess learner outcomes for these assignments through learner-feedback instruments that allow each learner to be a co-evaluator of the learning experience.
- When the assignment requires learners to present to an external audience, allow for in-class rehearsals prior to the formal presentation.
- Stay alert for learning opportunities that present themselves in the midst of the semester and then be flexible enough to use an opportunity when it occurs (see the Inbox strategy discussed earlier). Students may be more open to this if you give them some advance notice that you may use such an experience with them if the opportunity arises and provide them with an example of something you have done in the past.
- Adopt a teaching colleague who uses adult learning styles as a mentor and guide to help you through your early attempts at using learner-centered strategies and assignments.

RECOMMENDED RESOURCES

The following are some of the many excellent resources where learning facilitators can find information about social insurance programs and related issues:

- National Academy of Social Insurance (NASI) at http://www.nasi.org: This is the most thorough source of information on social insurance programs. NASI publications include a *Reporters Sourcebook on Social Insurance*, which is a primer for journalists;

information about current NASI projects; and other types of publications (e.g., briefs, fact sheets, conference proceedings, books, and *Social Insurance Update*, a bimonthly newsletter). Student Opportunities include listings of and links to current internship opportunities and, at times, information about social insurance-related student awards and funding opportunities. A very valuable component of the NASI Web site is the links they provide, especially in regard to links to Social Insurance-Related Federal Agencies.

- Social Security Administration (SSA) at http://www.ssa/gov: SSA is another key source of updated and accurate information about Social Security and Medicare.
- National Committee to Preserve Social Security and Medicare (NCPSSM) at www.ncpssm.org: NCPSSM is a membership organization, dedicated to protecting, preserving, promoting, and ensuring financial security, health, and well-being for current and future aging Americans through advocacy, education, and provision of services at the grassroots level.
- Current Awareness in Aging Research E-Clippings (CAAR): This is an e-mail subscription service (free of charge) provided through the Data and Information Services Center, Social Sciences Research Services, at the University of Wisconsin-Madison. Subscribers receive current information on aging-specific or aging-related policy, including Social Security and other social insurance programs, retirement and pension issues, and research. Categories of information include U.S. National News, U.S. State News, International News, and Medical/Science News. Informational messages are sent once or twice daily most weekdays. To subscribe, send a request to caar1@ssc.wisc.edu.
- AARP at www.aarp.org: Considerable information on Social Security and, at times, other social insurance programs, is available on AARP's Web site. Also, *Teaching Gerontology* is a subscription (free of charge) e-newsletter edited by Harry R. Moody, AARP Office of Academic Affairs. To subscribe, send a request to hrmoody@aarp.org.
- Women's Institute for a Secure Retirement (WISER) at www.wiserwomen.org: WISER's mission is to offer women information about their long-term financial security and issues that affect that security. For example, WISER and the Heinz Family Philanthropies recently published an e-book, *What Women Need*

to Know About Retirement, that is available free of charge as a .PDF download.

- Institute for Women's Policy Research (IWPR) at www.iwpr.org: IWPR is an independent, nonprofit research organization that addresses women's needs that are related to economic and social policy through five program areas: poverty, welfare and income security; work and family; employment, education, and economic change; health and safety; democracy and society.

DISCUSSION QUESTIONS

1. Describe the benefits of a learner-centered approach to teaching about social insurance.
2. Describe the role of the teacher in the learner-centered approach to teaching about social insurance.
3. Propose a level 5 teaching strategy that meets the requirements of the level in both the cognitive and affective domain and that illustrates some basic principle of social insurance.

REFERENCES

Bloom, B. S., & Krathwohl, D. R. (1956). *A taxonomy of educational objectives: The classification of educational objectives. Handbook I: Cognitive domain.* New York: Longman.

Cranston, P. (2006). *Understanding and promoting transformative learning: A guide for educators of adults* (2nd ed.). San Francisco: Jossey-Bass.

Grabinski, C. J. (2006, November). *Back to the future: From pedagogy to andragogy . . . and beyond.* In J. Wood (Chair), *Gerontology and geriatric education: Moving from teacher-centered to learner-centered strategies and environments.* Preconference workshop conducted at the annual meeting of the Gerontological Society of America, Dallas, TX.

Hase, S., & Kenyon, C. (2000). From andragogy to pedagogy. *UltiBASE Articles.* Retrieved November 9, 2008, from http://ultibase.remit.edu.au/Articles/dec00/hase2.htm

Kenyon, C., & Hase, S. (n.d.). Moving from andragogy to heutagogy in vocational education. Retrieved November 9, 2008, from http://www.tafe.swinburne.edu.au/profdev/learnbydesign/pdfs/andragogy_paper.pdf

Knowles, M. S. (Ed.). (1984). *Andragogy in action: Applying modern principles of adult learning.* San Francisco: Jossey-Bass.

Krathwohl, D. R., Bloom, B. S., & Masia, B. B. (1956). *Taxonomy of educational objectives: The classification of educational objectives. Handbook II: Affective domain.* New York: David McKay Co.

Mezirow, J. (1991). *Transformative dimensions of adult learning*. San Francisco: Jossey-Bass.

Mezirow, J., & Associates. (2000). *Learning as transformation: Critical perspectives on a theory in progress*. San Francisco: Jossey-Bass.

Rosenblatt, R. (Compiler). (2007). What is Social Insurance? *Sourcebook*. Retrieved January 21, 2008, from http://www.nasi.org/publications3901/publications.htm

Smith, M. K. (1996). *Andragogy. The encyclopedia of informal education.* Retrieved November 9, 2008, from http://www.infed.org/lifelonglearning/b-andra.htm

Epilogue: From the Audacity of Hope to the Audacity of Action

CARROLL L. ESTES, LEAH ROGNE, BRIAN R. GROSSMAN, BROOKE A. HOLLISTER, AND ERICA SOLWAY

As this book goes to press and we reflect on where we were at the time of the inception and writing of the book, it is clear that the political and economic circumstances surrounding the debates about social insurance and social justice have markedly changed. And these circumstances have made it unquestionably clear that social insurance as a foundation of our economic and health security is more important now than ever.

The presidential election of Barack Obama occurred as the United States began to be rocked by a series of "meltdowns" including the subprime mortgage crisis, the collapse of the investment banking industry, and the massive decline in stock values on Wall Street. We now know the crisis is much deeper, more complex, and lasting, embracing the credit card and automobile industries, the unemployment of more than 10 million people, two Middle East wars, a severe recession, gaping social inequality, a dysfunctional health care system with high and increasing numbers of uninsured and skyrocketing unaffordable costs, and the wipe-out of more than $3 trillion (and up) in American retirement savings held in private pensions.

Mirroring the United States destabilization, the globalization of market capitalism has reproduced destabilization and financial meltdown for many other nations. Unfortunately, these global trends follow the International Monetary Fund's (IMF) and the World Bank's (WB) arduous promotion of private pension capitalism and health care privatization as conditions of foreign loans. These and other structural adjustment policies imposed by the IMF, WB, and World Trade Organization have diminished the social and economic health of developing nations and stripped them of their safety net programs. In some cases, these lending agencies have even forbidden nations from providing agricultural subsidies, thus robbing their peoples of capacity for sustainable agriculture within their borders. Likewise developed nations (e.g., the United Kingdom) have been encouraged to "reform" and compromise their state-supported safety nets of retirement and health security.

Our analysis is that the situation is a clear case of *the excesses of capitalism and a deficit of democracy*. The consequences are millions of distressed and dispossessed homeowners, unemployed and underemployed persons, children without opportunity and health care, and virtually all working families spiraling downward.

The United States of America is immersed in what experts and ordinary people are experiencing as crises on all sides of our lives. There is fear bordering on panic (in the United States and globally) with lurching, plummeting stock markets and the seemingly endless bad economic numbers including galloping joblessness climbing to double digits and accelerating individual and corporate bankruptcies, further wiping out retirement savings and health insurance coverage for millions.

Nevertheless, there is a mixed sense of hope and high expectation for the new president. Mr. Obama, the nation's first African American president, now in the early days of his new administration, confronts a mountain of problems with an economy that is cratering and a crisis of confidence in our system that is profound and deepening. As we know, crises—however they come about (socially constructed and objectively rendered)—provide the nation's power elite the opportunity for bold and radical action. This crisis also provides an opportunity for the grass roots to mobilize. A giant window of potential social change has opened. And with it will be the "mother" of all class struggles, gender struggles, and race and ethnic struggles, among others. The issues at the heart of this nation starkly underscore the crucial importance of social insurance and the peril of the choices that will be made concerning the nation's economic and health security.

No one in the United States is unaffected, particularly the 44 million elders, the 77 million baby boomers, the children, and the generations to follow. Perhaps not surprisingly, the assistance that is needed for the people from the state is far outweighed by the trillions of dollars already spent by the state to backstop the engines of capitalism, beginning with its financial institutions.

Attending to the "demand" part of the classical economic paradigm (getting the working people of this nation back to work and making good on the intent of the nation's social insurance programs) is very out of balance with the trillions of dollars already allocated by the state in an attempt to jump-start the supply and liquidity of capital. How can anyone but the rich buy anything without a major jump-start on the social needs of the people?

The distress, chaos, and extreme uncertainty in this historical period are a culmination of the New Gilded Age, for which Reagan's 1980 election laid the ideological foundation. The current period, which has been called the Era of Empire, has been produced through political, economic, and ideological struggles won largely by conservatives that have affirmed and reaffirmed the legitimacy and sanctity of the market above all (Estes, 1991). Corporate welfare from the state in the form of tax-breaks and state subsidies to private capital have mushroomed—to great reward of the military industrial complex, the medical industrial complex, and U.S. and global financial capitalism.

For nearly 3 decades, the nation's social insurance programs (such as Social Security and Medicare) and the elderly have been under relentless attack. With regard to social insurance, the virulent ageism targeted against the old is manifested in the portrayal of the old as greedy geezers and in the contention of privatization advocates that demographic aging is, itself, a global and societal crisis that makes social insurance for retirement, disability, and medical care unsustainable in the United States and elsewhere. This fallacious argument has been pivotal to the advancement of U.S. state policies to privatize Social Security and Medicare. There has been an intentional risk shift (Hacker, 2006) from the state to the individual, orchestrated by the Republican Congress between 1994 and 2006 and dramatically accelerated by the White House during the last 8 years.

Also during this period, the treatment and rights of citizens have atrophied and been directly assaulted at the hand of harsh identity politics and the religious right, blurring the lines between church and state. The recent denial of the right to same-sex marriage in California is an example in point. The new American nativism through the war on immigrants is another.

With these forces gripping the United States, foreboding and disturbing forms of cleavage, disadvantage, and distrust have been stoked along the lines of race, class, gender, sexual orientation, generation, disability, and immigration status. With millions unemployed and joblessness growing, issues of "the end of work" and "the end of retirement" have taken center stage. The tensions between capital and labor are implicit if not explicit. Even the right to work itself is threatened and, with it, the loss of security, human dignity, and the American dream for all generations. Such conditions clearly imperil the lives of the old and young alike. The vital role of the state is unveiled, as it has always been in the failure of the market. Regrettably, we find ourselves woefully unprepared because the dominant market rhetoric has so desensitized us to notions of the common good, the collective, the communal, and our inevitable interdependence.

As a consequence, we now are ill-prepared, culturally, politically, and structurally in terms of state policy to address the multiple and intertwined crisis tendencies facing the American people. The market paradigm has dominated the corridors of power, the airwaves, and cyberspace for so long that the alternative paradigm of collective good, the commons, and shared risk and responsibility has been seriously repressed. The national debate is now expanding to encompass conversations concerning the rationale and need for a safety net in the nation. As the failures of the market and the greed that has consumed the promise of our way of life are revealed, the case for social insurance becomes more apparent in the urgency of this political and economic moment.

Presently, the working people of the nation are poised for the battle of this century for the soul of democracy.

The question is how the Obama presidency and the new Congress will structure and implement the state's response to the three major arenas of crisis that test us now: the legitimation crisis of capital, the legitimation crisis of the state, and the legitimation crisis of democracy (Estes, 2008). The future of social insurance is, at base, an issue of social justice.

In another time of crisis, Franklin D. Roosevelt accepted the 1932 Democratic Party nomination for president with a bold call: "Let us all here assembled constitute ourselves prophets of a new order of competence and of courage. This is more than a political campaign; it is a call to arms. Give me your help, not to win votes alone, but to win in this crusade to restore America to its own people" (Roosevelt, 1938, p. 647). Likewise, it is imperative now that the President, Congress, and the American people move boldly and courageously from the audacity of hope to the audacity of action.

REFERENCES

Estes, C. L. (1991). The Reagan legacy: Privatization, the welfare state & aging. In J. Myles & J. Quadagno (Eds.), *States, labor markets, and the future of old age policy* (pp. 59–83). Philadelphia: Temple University Press.

Estes, C. L. (2008, October 25). *Old age in America: A study in crisis*. Paper presented at the Annual Meeting of the American Public Health Association, San Diego, CA.

Hacker, J. (2006). *The great risk shift*. New York: Oxford University Press.

Roosevelt, Franklin D. (1938). The public papers and addresses of Franklin D. Roosevelt 1928–1932 (vol. 1, p. 647). New York: Random House.

Index